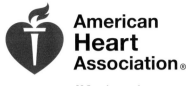

American Heart Association

life is why™

American Academy of Pediatrics

DEDICATED TO THE HEALTH OF ALL CHILDREN™

PEDIATRIC ADVANCED LIFE SUPPORT

PROVIDER MANUAL

© 2016 American Heart Association
ISBN 978-1-61669-559-0
Printed in the United States of America

First American Heart Association Printing October 2016
10 9 8 7 6 5

Acknowledgments

The American Heart Association thanks the following people for their contributions to the development of this manual: Ricardo A. Samson, MD; Stephen M. Schexnayder, MD; Mary Fran Hazinski, RN, MSN; Reylon Meeks, RN, BSN, MS, MSN, EMT, PhD; Lynda J. Knight, MSN, RN, CPN; Allan de Caen, MD; Jonathan Duff, MD, MEd; Mary Ann McNeil, MA, NRP; Mary E. McBride, MD, MEd; Cindy Brownlee, BSN, RN; Jeffrey M. Berman, MD; Farhan Bhanji, MD, MSc(Ed); Kelly D. Kadlec, MD; Mark A. Terry, MPA, NREMT-P; Adam Cheng, MD; Aaron Donoghue, MD, MSCE; Claire R. Wells, AC-PNP; Sallie Johnson, PharmD, BCPS; Holly Capasso-Harris, PhD; and the AHA PALS Project Team.

To find out about any updates or corrections to this text, visit **www.heart.org/cpr**, navigate to the page for this course, and click on "Updates."

To access the Student Website for this course, go to **www.heart.org/eccstudent** and enter this code: pals15

Contents

Contents

Part 2
Review of BLS and AED for Infants and Children — **15**

Part 3
Systematic Approach to the Seriously Ill or Injured Child — **29**

Part 4
Recognition and Management of Cardiac Arrest   69

Contents

Part 5
Effective Resuscitation Team Dynamics   105

Part 6
Recognition of Respiratory
Distress and Failure   113

Part 7
Management of Respiratory
Distress and Failure **129**

Resources for Management of
Respiratory Emergencies **147**

Contents

Part 9
Management of Shock   197

Contents

Part 12
Post–Cardiac Arrest Care

Contents

life is why.™

At the American Heart Association, we want people to experience more of life's precious moments. That's why we've made better heart and brain health our mission. It's also why we remain committed to exceptional training—the act of bringing resuscitation science to life—through genuine partnership with you. Only through our continued collaboration and dedication can we truly make a difference and save lives.

Until there's a world free of heart disease and stroke, the American Heart Association will be there, working with you to make a healthier, longer life possible for everyone.

Why do we do what we do?
life is why.

Life Is Why is a celebration of life. A simple yet powerful answer to the question of why we should all be healthy in heart and mind. It also explains why we do what we do: Lifesaving work. Every day.

Throughout your student manual, you will find information that correlates what you are learning in this class to **Life Is Why** and the importance of cardiovascular care. Look for the **Life Is Why** icon (shown at right), and remember that what you are learning today has an impact on the mission of the American Heart Association.

We encourage you to discover your **Why** and share it with others. Ask yourself, what are the moments, people, and experiences I live for? What brings me joy, wonder, and happiness? Why am I partnering with the AHA to help save lives? Why is cardiovascular care important to me? The answer to these questions is your **Why.**

Instructions

Please find on the back of this page a chance for you to participate in the AHA's mission and **Life Is Why** campaign. Complete this activity by filling in the blank with the word that describes your **Why.**

Share your "_____ **Is Why**" with the people you love, and ask them to discover their **Why.**

Talk about it. Share it. Post it. Live it.   #lifeiswhy   #CPRSavesLives

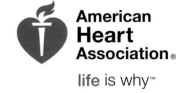

American **Heart** Association®
life is why™

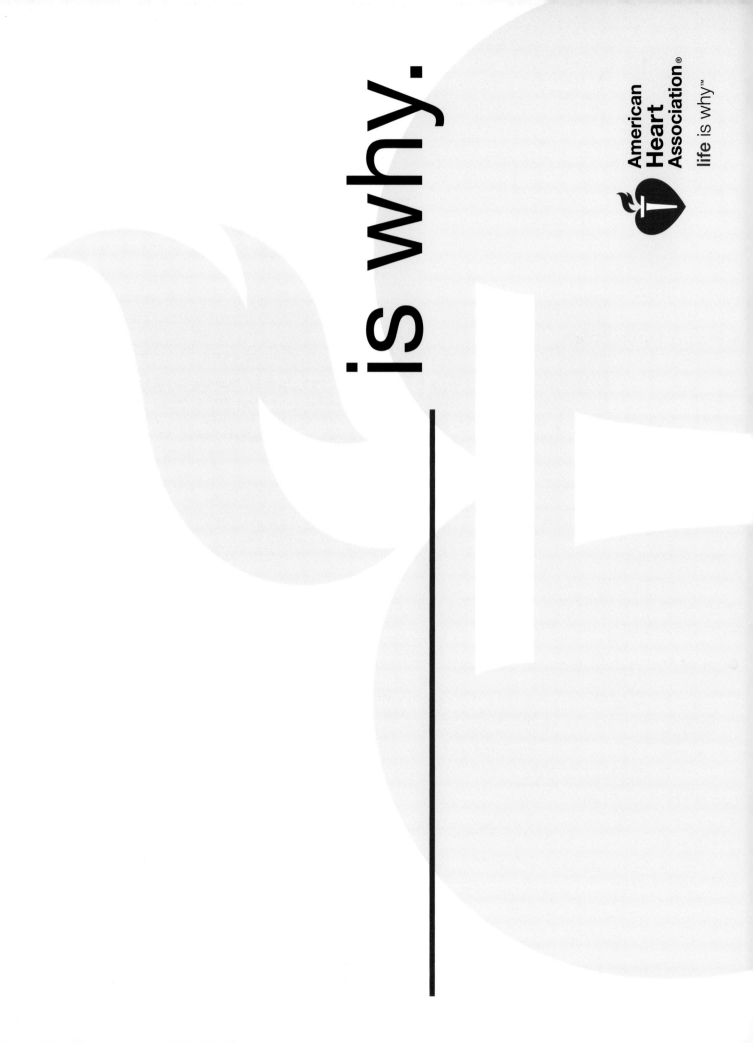

is why.

American Heart Association®

life is why™

Part **1**

Course Overview

Course Objectives

The Pediatric Advanced Life Support (PALS) Provider Course is designed for healthcare providers who either direct or participate in the management of respiratory and/or cardiovascular emergencies and cardiopulmonary arrest in pediatric patients. Precourse preparation, didactic instruction, and active participation in skill stations and simulated cases will be used to enhance the recognition of and intervention for respiratory emergencies, shock, and cardiopulmonary arrest.

During the course, you will actively participate in a series of case scenario practices with simulation. These simulations are designed to reinforce important concepts, including

- Identification and treatment of problems that place the child at risk for cardiac arrest
- Application of a systematic approach to pediatric assessment
- Use of the evaluate-identify-intervene sequence
- Use of PALS algorithms and flowcharts
- Demonstration of effective resuscitation team dynamics

Goal of the PALS Provider Course

The goal of the PALS Provider Course is to improve outcomes for pediatric patients by preparing healthcare providers to effectively recognize and intervene in patients with respiratory emergencies, shock, and cardiopulmonary arrest by using high-performance team dynamics and high-quality individual skills.

Learning Objectives

Upon successful completion of this course, you will be able to

- Perform high-quality cardiopulmonary resuscitation (CPR) per American Heart Association (AHA) basic life support (BLS) recommendations
- Differentiate between patients who do and do not require immediate intervention
- Recognize cardiopulmonary arrest early and begin CPR within 10 seconds
- Apply team dynamics
- Differentiate between respiratory distress and failure
- Perform early interventions for respiratory distress and failure
- Differentiate between compensated and decompensated (hypotensive) shock
- Perform early interventions for the treatment of shock

- Differentiate between unstable and stable patients with arrhythmias
- Describe clinical characteristics of instability in patients with arrhythmias
- Implement post–cardiac arrest management

Course Description

To help you achieve these objectives, the PALS Provider Course includes

- BLS competency testing
- Skills stations
- Case scenario discussions and simulations
- Case scenario testing stations
- An exam

BLS Competency Testing

What You Will Be Expected to Do

You must pass 2 BLS tests to receive an AHA PALS Provider course completion card.

BLS Skills Testing Requirements
• Child CPR and AED Skills Test • Infant CPR Skills Test

How to Prepare

The PALS Provider Course does not include detailed instructions on how to perform basic CPR or how to use an automated external defibrillator (AED). You must know this in advance. Consider taking a BLS course if necessary.

Before taking the PALS Provider Course, review the following resources in the *PALS Provider Manual* to prepare for taking the BLS tests:

Resource	See
BLS skills testing checklists	Appendix
Table 18. Summary of High-Quality CPR Components for BLS Providers	"Part 4: Recognition and Management of Cardiac Arrest"
Pediatric Cardiac Arrest Algorithm	"Part 4: Recognition and Management of Cardiac Arrest"

Skills Stations

What You Will Be Expected to Do

The course includes the following skills stations:

- Airway Management
- Rhythm Disturbances/Electrical Therapy
- Vascular Access

During the skills stations, you will have an opportunity to practice specific skills and then demonstrate competency. Below is a brief description of each station. During the course, you will use the skills station competency checklists while practicing the skills. Your instructor will evaluate your skills based on the criteria specified in these checklists.

How to Prepare

See the Appendix for the skills station competency checklists, which list detailed steps for performing each skill.

Airway Management Skills Station

What You Will Be Expected to Do

In the Airway Management Skills Station, you will need to demonstrate your understanding of oxygen (O_2) delivery systems and airway adjuncts. You will have an opportunity to practice and demonstrate competency in airway management skills, including

- Insertion of an oropharyngeal airway
- Effective bag-mask ventilation
- Oropharyngeal airway and endotracheal (ET) tube suctioning
- Confirmation of advanced airway device placement by physical examination and an exhaled CO_2 detector device
- Securing the ET tube

If it is within your scope of practice, you may be asked to demonstrate advanced airway skills, including correct insertion of an ET tube.

How to Prepare

Review the following topics in the *PALS Provider Manual* before the course to learn more about airway management skills:

Topic	See
Bag-Mask Ventilation	"Resources for Management of Respiratory Emergencies" at the end of Part 7
Endotracheal Intubation	

Rhythm Disturbances/Electrical Therapy Skills Station

What You Will Be Expected to Do

In the Rhythm Disturbances/Electrical Therapy Skills Station, you will have an opportunity to practice and demonstrate competency in rhythm identification and operation of a cardiac monitor and manual defibrillator. Skills include

- Correct placement of electrocardiographic (ECG) leads
- Correct paddle/electrode pad selection and placement/positioning
- Identification of rhythms that require defibrillation
- Identification of rhythms that require synchronized cardioversion
- Operation of a cardiac monitor
- Safe performance of manual defibrillation and synchronized cardioversion

How to Prepare

Consider taking a BLS course if necessary to learn about cardiac monitoring and manual defibrillation. Review the following resources in the *PALS Provider Manual* before the course to help you with rhythm identification, cardiac monitoring, and manual defibrillation:

Resource	See
Rhythm Recognition Review	Appendix
Management: Pediatric Bradycardia With a Pulse and Poor Perfusion Algorithm	"Part 11: Management of Arrhythmias"
Management of Tachyarrhythmias	"Part 11: Management of Arrhythmias"
Table 18. Summary of High-Quality CPR Components for BLS Providers	"Part 4: Recognition and Management of Cardiac Arrest"
Pediatric Cardiac Arrest Algorithm	"Part 4: Recognition and Management of Cardiac Arrest"

Vascular Access Skills Station

What You Will Be Expected to Do

In the Vascular Access Skills Station, you will have an opportunity to practice and demonstrate competency in intraosseous (IO) access and other related skills. In this skills station you will

- Insert an IO needle
- Summarize how to confirm that the needle has entered the marrow cavity
- Summarize/demonstrate the method of giving an intravenous (IV)/IO bolus
- Use a color-coded length-based resuscitation tape to calculate correct drug doses

How to Prepare

Review the following topics in the *PALS Provider Manual* before the course to learn more about vascular access skills:

Topic	See
Intraosseous Access	"Resources for Management of Circulatory Emergencies" at the end of Part 9
Color-Coded Length-Based Resuscitation Tape	

PALS Case Scenario Discussions and Case Scenario Practice With Simulations

What You Will Be Expected to Do

In the learning stations, you will actively participate in a variety of learning activities, including

- Case scenario discussions, using a systematic approach for evaluation and decision making
- Case scenario practice with simulations

In the learning stations, you will apply your knowledge and practice essential skills both individually and as part of a team. This course emphasizes effective team skills as a vital part of the resuscitative effort. You will receive training in effective team behavior and have the opportunity to practice as a team member and a team leader.

How to Prepare	The focus of the PALS Provider Course is to teach you to use a systematic approach when caring for a critically ill or injured child. You will need to read and study the entire *PALS Provider Manual* to understand all the necessary concepts.

PALS Case Scenario Testing Stations

What You Will Be Expected to Do	At the end of the course, you will participate as a team leader in 2 case scenario testing stations to validate your achievement of the course objectives. You will be permitted to use the PALS Pocket Reference Card and the *2015 Handbook of Emergency Cardiovascular Care for Healthcare Providers* (ECC Handbook). These simulated clinical scenarios will test the following:

- Ability to evaluate and identify specific clinical conditions covered in the course
- Recognition and management of respiratory and shock emergencies
- Interpretation of core arrhythmias and management by using appropriate medications and electrical therapy
- Performance as an effective team leader

A major emphasis of this evaluation will be your ability to direct the integration of BLS and PALS skills by your team members according to each member's scope of practice.

How to Prepare	Review the following topic in the *PALS Provider Manual* before the course to prepare yourself to participate as a team leader in the case scenario testing stations:

Topic	See
Roles of the Team Leader and Team Members	"Part 5: Effective Resuscitation Team Dynamics"

Exam

What You Will Be Expected to Do	The exam measures the mastery of cognitive skills. Each student must score at least 84% on the exam to meet course completion requirements. As part of the new education methodologies, the AHA has adopted an open-resource policy for exams administered online through an eLearning course and in a classroom-based course.

Open resource means that students may use resources as reference while completing the exam. Resources could include the Provider Manual, either in printed form or as an eBook on personal devices; any notes the student took during the provider course; the ECC Handbook; the *2015 AHA Guidelines Update for CPR and ECC*; posters; etc. *Open resource* does not mean open discussion with other providers or the instructor.

How to Prepare	Prepare *before the class* by completing the Precourse Self-Assessment to identify any deficiencies in your knowledge of these topics and by reading and studying the *PALS Provider Manual*. Locate your PALS Pocket Reference Card and become familiar with the resources available for your reference. See the "Precourse Preparation" and "Course Materials" sections below for more information.

Prepare *during the class* by actively participating in the instructor-led case scenario discussions and case scenario practice with simulations.

Precourse Preparation

To successfully pass the PALS Provider Course, *you must prepare before the course*. Do the following:

- Take the Precourse Self-Assessment
- Make sure you are proficient in BLS skills
- Practice identifying and interpreting core ECG rhythms
- Study basic pharmacology and know *when* to use *which* drug
- Practice applying your knowledge to clinical scenarios

Precourse Self-Assessment

 You should complete the Precourse Self-Assessment on the AHA PALS Student Website before the PALS Provider Course. See the section "PALS Student Website" for details about how to access this resource. Print your certificate of completion and bring it with you to the course. Because the PALS Provider Course does not teach algorithms, ECG recognition, pharmacology, or BLS skills, use the Precourse Self-Assessment to identify any deficiencies in your knowledge of these topics. The Precourse Self-Assessment will provide a summary of your strengths and weaknesses. Increase your knowledge by studying the applicable content in the *PALS Provider Manual* or other supplementary resources, including the PALS Student Website.

BLS Skills

Strong BLS skills are the foundation of advanced life support. Everyone involved in the care of pediatric patients must be able to perform high-quality CPR. Without high-quality CPR, PALS interventions will fail. For this reason, each student must pass the Child CPR and AED and Infant CPR Skills Tests in the PALS Provider Course. *Make sure that you are proficient in BLS skills before attending the course.*

See the section "BLS Competency Testing" in the Appendix for testing requirements and resources.

ECG Rhythm Identification

You must be able to identify and interpret the following core rhythms during case scenario practice with simulations and case scenario tests:

- Normal sinus rhythm
- Sinus bradycardia
- Sinus tachycardia
- Supraventricular tachycardia
- Ventricular tachycardia
- Ventricular fibrillation
- Asystole

The ECG rhythm identification section of the Precourse Self-Assessment will help you evaluate your ability to identify these core rhythms and other common pediatric arrhythmias. If you have difficulty with pediatric rhythm identification, improve your knowledge by studying the section "Rhythm Recognition Review" in the Appendix. The AHA also offers self-directed online courses on rhythm recognition. These courses can be found at **OnlineAHA.org**.

Basic Pharmacology

You must know basic information about drugs used in the PALS algorithms and flow-charts. Basic pharmacology information includes the indications, contraindications, and methods of administration. You will need to know *when* to use *which* drug based on the clinical situation.

The pharmacology section of the Precourse Self-Assessment will help you evaluate and enhance your knowledge of medications used in the course. If you have difficulty with this section of the Precourse Self-Assessment, improve your knowledge by studying the *PALS Provider Manual* and the ECC Handbook.

Practical Application of Knowledge to Clinical Scenarios

 The practical application section of the Precourse Self-Assessment will help you evaluate your ability to apply your knowledge when presented with a clinical scenario. You will need to make decisions based on

- The Systematic Approach Algorithm and the evaluate-identify-intervene sequence
- Identification of core rhythms
- Knowledge of core medications
- Knowledge of PALS flowcharts and algorithms

Be sure that you understand the Systematic Approach Algorithm and the evaluate-identify-intervene sequence. Review the core rhythms and medications. Be familiar with the PALS algorithms and flowcharts so that you can apply them to clinical scenarios. Note that the PALS Provider Course does not teach the details of each algorithm. Sources of information are the *PALS Provider Manual,* PALS Student Website, and ECC Handbook.

Course Materials

 The PALS Provider Course materials consist of the *PALS Provider Manual,* the PALS Pocket Reference Card, and supplementary material on the PALS Student Website.

PALS Provider Manual

The *PALS Provider Manual* contains material that you will use *before, during, and after the course.* It contains important information that you need to know to effectively participate in the course, so *please read and study the manual before the course.* This important material includes concepts of pediatric evaluation and the recognition and management of respiratory, shock, and cardiac emergencies. Some students may already know much of this information; others may need extensive study before the course.

The manual is organized into the following parts:

Part		Read to Learn More About...
1	**Course Overview**	What you need to know before the course, how to prepare for the course, and what to expect during the course
2	**Review of BLS and AED for Infants and Children**	Child and infant high-quality CPR, bag-mask ventilation, and 1- and 2-rescuer CPR
3	**Systematic Approach to the Seriously Ill or Injured Child**	The systematic approach; Pediatric Assessment Triangle, initial impression; and evaluate-identify-intervene sequence, including the primary assessment, secondary assessment, and diagnostic tests
4	**Recognition and Management of Cardiac Arrest**	Signs of cardiac arrest and terminal cardiac rhythms; resuscitation and medical and electrical therapy
5	**Effective Resuscitation Team Dynamics**	Roles of team leader and team members; how to effectively communicate as a team leader or team member
6	**Recognition of Respiratory Distress and Failure**	Basic concepts of respiratory distress and failure; how to identify respiratory problems according to type and severity
7	**Management of Respiratory Distress and Failure**	Intervention options for respiratory problems and emergencies
8	**Recognition of Shock**	Basic concepts of shock; shock identification according to type and severity
9	**Management of Shock**	Intervention options for shock according to etiology
10	**Recognition of Arrhythmias**	Clinical and ECG characteristics of bradyarrhythmias and tachyarrhythmias
11	**Management of Arrhythmias**	Medical and electrical therapies for bradyarrhythmias and tachyarrhythmias
12	**Post–Cardiac Arrest Care**	Post–cardiac arrest evaluation and management
	Appendix	Checklists for BLS competency testing, skills station competencies, and case scenario practice with simulations; a brief rhythm recognition review

Throughout the *PALS Provider Manual*, you will find specific information in the following types of boxes:

Type of Box	Contains
Foundational Facts	**Foundational Facts** boxes contain basic information that will help you understand the topics covered in the course.
Critical Concepts	Pay particular attention to the **Critical Concepts** boxes. These boxes contain the most important information that you must know.
Identify and Intervene	**Identify and Intervene** boxes contain information about an important evaluation or an immediate lifesaving intervention.
FYI	**FYI** boxes contain advanced information that you can use to increase your knowledge but that is not required for successful course participation.
Life Is Why	**Life Is Why**™ boxes describe why taking this course matters.

Remember to take this manual with you to the course.

PALS Pocket Reference Card

The PALS Pocket Reference Card is a valuable learning aid and contains the following resources:

- Vital Signs in Children
- Pediatric Septic Shock Algorithm
- Drugs Used in PALS
- Pediatric Color-Coded Length-Based Resuscitation Tape
- Pediatric Cardiac Arrest Algorithm—2015 Update
- PALS Systematic Approach Algorithm
- Pediatric Bradycardia With a Pulse and Poor Perfusion Algorithm
- Pediatric Tachycardia With a Pulse and Poor Perfusion Algorithm
- PALS Management of Shock After ROSC Algorithm

Be sure to take your PALS Pocket Reference Card with you to the course. You will use it as a reference during the case scenario discussions and the exam.

PALS Student Website

 Go to the PALS Student Website to access the Precourse Self-Assessment. Here you will also find additional information about basic PALS concepts.

PALS Student Website URL

 The URL for the PALS Student Website is

www.heart.org/eccstudent.

To enter the website, you will need the access code found at the bottom of page ii in the front of your *PALS Provider Manual.*

Complete the Precourse Self-Assessment Before the Course

The Precourse Self-Assessment is a vital part of your preparation for the course. Feedback from this assessment will help you identify gaps in your knowledge so that you can target specific material to study.

The Precourse Self-Assessment has 3 parts:

- ECG rhythm identification
- Pharmacology
- Practical application

Complete these assessments *before the course* to identify gaps in and improve your knowledge. Print out your certificate of completion and take it with you to the course.

Course Completion Requirements

To successfully complete the PALS Provider Course and obtain your course completion card, you must do the following:

- Actively participate in, practice, and complete all skills stations and learning stations
- Pass the Child CPR and AED and Infant CPR Skills Tests
- Pass an exam with a minimum score of 84%
- Pass 2 PALS case scenario tests as a team leader

Science Update

The PALS Provider Course has been updated to incorporate the recommendations of the *2015 AHA Guidelines Update for CPR and ECC*. Every few years, hundreds of international resuscitation scientists and experts evaluate, discuss, and debate thousands of scientific publications. They reach consensus on the best treatments based on the evidence that they have evaluated. These consensus recommendations form the basis for the development of the guidelines. The *2015 AHA Guidelines Update for CPR and ECC* is based on the largest review of resuscitation literature ever published. Some recommendations are new, whereas others modify previous recommendations. The following list highlights many of the key recommendations for pediatric basic and advanced life support.

Major Science Changes in 2015

Some of the major science changes in 2015 include

- In specific settings, when treating pediatric patients with febrile illnesses, the use of restrictive volumes of isotonic crystalloid leads to improved survival. This contrasts with traditional thinking that routine aggressive volume resuscitation is beneficial.
- Routine use of atropine as a premedication for emergency tracheal intubation in non-neonates, specifically to prevent arrhythmias, is controversial. Also, there are data to suggest that there is no minimum dose required for atropine for this indication.
- If invasive arterial blood pressure monitoring is already in place, it may be used to adjust CPR to achieve specific blood pressure targets for children in cardiac arrest.
- Amiodarone or lidocaine is an acceptable antiarrhythmic agent for shock-refractory pediatric ventricular fibrillation and pulseless ventricular tachycardia (pVT) in children.
- Epinephrine continues to be recommended as a vasopressor in pediatric cardiac arrest.
- For pediatric patients with cardiac diagnoses and in-hospital cardiac arrest in settings with existing extracorporeal membrane oxygenation protocols, extracorporeal CPR (ECPR) may be considered.
- Fever should be avoided when caring for comatose children with return of spontaneous circulation (ROSC) after out-of-hospital cardiac arrest. A large randomized trial of therapeutic hypothermia for children with out-of-hospital cardiac arrest showed no difference in outcomes whether a period of moderate therapeutic hypothermia (with temperature maintained at 32°C to 34°C) or the strict maintenance of normothermia (with temperature maintained 36°C to 37.5°C) was provided.
- Several intra-arrest and post–cardiac arrest clinical variables were examined for prognostic significance. No single variable was identified to be sufficiently reliable to predict outcomes. Therefore, caretakers should consider multiple factors in trying to predict outcomes during cardiac arrest and in the post-ROSC setting.
- After ROSC, fluids and vasoactive infusions should be used to maintain a systolic blood pressure above the fifth percentile for age.
- After ROSC, normoxemia should be targeted. When the necessary equipment is available, oxygen administration should be weaned to target an oxyhemoglobin saturation of 94% to 99%. Hypoxemia should be strictly avoided. Ideally, oxygen should be titrated to a value appropriate to the specific patient condition. Likewise, after ROSC, the child's $PaCO_2$ should be targeted to a concentration appropriate to each patient's condition. Exposure to severe hypercapnia or hypocapnia should be avoided.
- It is hoped that these changes will result in more lives saved.

Immediate Chest Compressions (C-A-B vs A-B-C)

The *2010 AHA Guidelines for CPR and ECC* recommended a change in the CPR sequence from A-B-C (Airway-Breathing-Circulation/Compressions) to C-A-B (Compressions-Airway-Breathing). After a review of the literature, the C-A-B sequence for BLS was reaffirmed. Consistency in the order of compressions, airway, and breathing for CPR in victims of all ages may be easiest for rescuers who treat people of all ages to remember and perform. Maintaining the same sequence for adults and children offers consistency in teaching.

Emphasis on High-Quality CPR

High-quality CPR is essential. Without the foundation of effective BLS, even the most advanced life support measures will fail.

High-quality CPR is critical during cardiac arrest to provide adequate blood flow to the brain and vital organs. Compressions generate blood flow. Every time compressions are interrupted, blood flow is drastically reduced. When chest compressions are resumed, it takes several compressions before blood flow reaches the level it was before the interruption.

Critical elements of high-quality CPR include the following:

Push fast	• Push at a rate of 100 to 120 compressions per minute for infants, children, and adolescents.
Push hard	• Push with enough force to depress the chest at least one third the depth of the chest. This is about 1½ inches (4 cm) in infants and 2 inches (5 cm) in children.
	• Once children have reached puberty, the recommended adult compression depth of at least 2 inches (5 cm), but no more than 2.4 inches (6 cm), is used for the adolescent of average adult size.
Allow complete chest recoil	• *Release completely*, allowing the chest to completely recoil after each compression. This allows the heart to refill with blood.
Minimize interruptions	• Try to limit interruptions in chest compressions to 10 seconds or less or as needed for interventions (eg, defibrillation). Ideally, compressions are interrupted only for ventilation (until an advanced airway is placed), rhythm check, and actual shock delivery.
	• Once an advanced airway is in place, provide continuous chest compressions without pausing for ventilation.
Avoid excessive ventilation	• Each rescue breath should be given over 1 second. Each breath should result in visible chest rise.
	• When there is no advanced airway in place, deliver compressions and ventilation in a 30:2 ratio for single rescuer and a 15:2 ratio for 2 or more rescuers.
	• After an advanced airway is in place, deliver 10 breaths per minute (1 breath every 6 seconds), while continuous chest compressions are given. Be careful to avoid excessive ventilation.

Life Is Why

High-Quality CPR Is Why

Early recognition and CPR are crucial for survival from cardiac arrest. By learning high-quality CPR, you'll have the ability to improve patient outcomes and save more lives.

Fluid Resuscitation

Rapid identification and intervention of shock is an essential component of pediatric resuscitation. Although the cornerstone of the treatment of shock has always been early, rapid administration of isotonic fluids, administration of bolus IV fluids in children with febrile illness in settings with limited access to critical care resources (ie, mechanical ventilation and inotropic support) should be given with extreme caution. Treatment should also include an individualized plan for each patient that is based on frequent clinical assessment before, during, and after fluid therapy is given. Research has shown that excessive fluid boluses given to febrile patients can lead to complications, especially in resource-limited settings where other critical care therapies are not readily available.

Atropine for Endotracheal Intubation

In previous guidelines, the use of atropine was recommended before endotracheal intubation. Recent studies are conflicting, however, as to whether atropine prevents bradycardia and other arrhythmias. There is no evidence to support the routine administration of the drug as a premedication in emergency situations.

Invasive Hemodynamic Monitoring During CPR

If the child arrests in a critical care environment, invasive hemodynamic monitoring catheters are often in place at the time of the arrest. When such devices are already in place, it is reasonable for an advanced provider to use the arterial (and central venous) pressure measurements from these devices to guide the performance of CPR.

Antiarrhythmic Medications for Shock–Refractory Ventricular Fibrillation or pVT

Previous guidelines suggested that amiodarone was preferred over lidocaine as drug therapy for the treatment of shock-refractory ventricular fibrillation or pVT in children. However, one recent multi-institutional registry retrospective study of pediatric in-hospital resuscitation found that neither amiodarone nor lidocaine was associated with improved survival to hospital discharge. The new guidelines allow providers to choose either amiodarone or lidocaine for shock-refractory rhythms.

Vasopressors for Resuscitation

Recent guidelines state that it is reasonable to give epinephrine during cardiac arrest. However, use of this drug has been downgraded slightly in Class of Recommendation. Although recent studies have shown that epinephrine was associated with improved ROSC and survival to hospital admission, it did not improve survival to hospital discharge.

ECPR Compared With Standard Resuscitations

For children with an underlying cardiac condition who experience an in-hospital cardiac arrest, ECPR may be considered if they are unresponsive to conventional CPR. However, ECPR should only be performed in a setting where appropriate protocols, expertise, and equipment are available.

Targeted Temperature Management

- For children who are comatose after cardiac arrest, either in-hospital or out-of-hospital, providers should monitor temperature continuously and also treat fever aggressively for the first several days.
- For comatose children resuscitated from out-of-hospital cardiac arrest, it is reasonable for caretakers to maintain either 5 days of normothermia (36°C to 37.5°C) or 2 days of initial continuous hypothermia (32°C to 34°C) followed by 3 days of normothermia. For children remaining comatose after in-hospital cardiac arrest, there are insufficient data to recommend hypothermia over normothermia.
- A prospective, multicenter study showed no difference in functional outcome at 1 year between those who received either therapeutic hypothermia or normothermia.
- There are insufficient data to recommend therapeutic hypothermia over normothermia for children who are comatose after in-hospital cardiac arrest.

Intra-Arrest and Post-Arrest Prognostic Factors

When trying to predict outcomes of a cardiac arrest, multiple factors should be considered. These factors will inform your decision to continue or terminate resuscitative efforts and will also inform your prognosis concerning recovery after cardiac arrest.

Post–Cardiac Arrest Fluids and Inotropes

Once ROSC has been achieved for a child, it is recommended that caregivers use inotropes and vasopressors to maintain a systolic blood pressure above the fifth percentile for age of the patient. To identify the fifth percentile for systolic blood pressure, use the formula 70 mm Hg + (age in years × 2) (see Table 11: Definition of Hypotension by Systolic Blood Pressure and Age in Part 3). To maintain this, advanced caregivers should use intra-arterial blood pressure monitoring to continuously assess blood pressure and identify and treat hypotension. This vigilance is important because recent studies have shown that children who experience post-ROSC hypotension have worse survival and neurologic outcome.

Post–Cardiac Arrest PaO_2 and $PaCO_2$

After ROSC, it may be reasonable for rescuers to titrate oxygen administration to achieve normoxemia, which is an oxygen saturation of 94% or above. When possible, oxygen should be weaned to target an oxyhemoglobin saturation within the range of 94% to 99%. The goal should be to strictly avoid hypoxemia. A large study demonstrated that achieving and maintaining normoxemia was associated with improved survival to pediatric intensive care unit discharge, compared with hyperoxemia. Similarly, ventilation strategies for post-ROSC patients should target a $PaCO_2$ that is appropriate for each patient while avoiding extremes of hypercapnia or hypocapnia. Adult studies demonstrate worse patient outcomes associated with hypocapnia after ROSC.

Part 2

Review of BLS and AED for Infants and Children

Overview

This Part describes BLS for infants and children and discusses use of an AED in infants and children younger than 8 years.

The following age definitions are used in BLS:

- *Infants* are less than 1 year of age (excluding the newly born).
- *Children* are from 1 year of age to puberty. Signs of puberty include chest or under-arm hair on boys and any breast development in girls.

Learning Objectives

At the end of this Part, you will be able to

- Perform high-quality CPR for a child
- Perform high-quality CPR for an infant
- Describe the importance of early use of an AED for infants and children younger than 8 years of age
- Demonstrate the appropriate use of an AED for infants and children younger than 8 years of age

Life Is Why

Life Is Why

At the American Heart Association, we want people to experience more of life's precious moments. What you learn in this course can help build healthier, longer lives for everyone.

BLS for Infants and Children

BLS Healthcare Provider Pediatric Cardiac Arrest Algorithm for the Single Rescuer

The BLS Healthcare Provider Pediatric Cardiac Arrest Algorithm for the Single Rescuer outlines steps for a single rescuer of an unresponsive infant or child (Figure 1). Refer to this algorithm as you read the steps below.

BLS Healthcare Provider Pediatric Cardiac Arrest Algorithm for the Single Rescuer—2015 Update

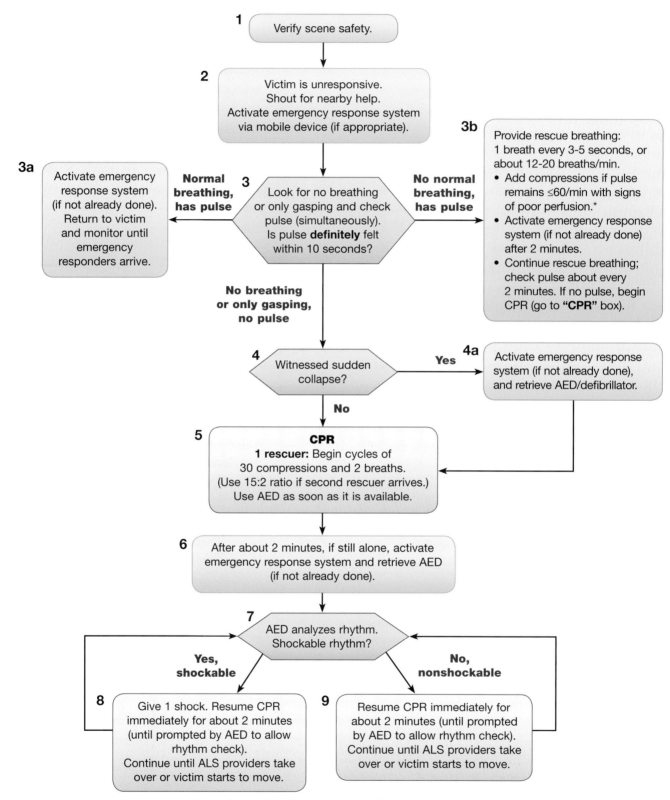

1 Verify scene safety.

2 Victim is unresponsive.
Shout for nearby help.
Activate emergency response system via mobile device (if appropriate).

3a Activate emergency response system (if not already done). Return to victim and monitor until emergency responders arrive.

Normal breathing, has pulse

3 Look for no breathing or only gasping and check pulse (simultaneously). Is pulse **definitely** felt within 10 seconds?

No normal breathing, has pulse

3b Provide rescue breathing:
1 breath every 3-5 seconds, or about 12-20 breaths/min.
• Add compressions if pulse remains ≤60/min with signs of poor perfusion.*
• Activate emergency response system (if not already done) after 2 minutes.
• Continue rescue breathing; check pulse about every 2 minutes. If no pulse, begin CPR (go to "CPR" box).

No breathing or only gasping, no pulse

4 Witnessed sudden collapse?

Yes → **4a** Activate emergency response system (if not already done), and retrieve AED/defibrillator.

No

5 **CPR**
1 rescuer: Begin cycles of 30 compressions and 2 breaths.
(Use 15:2 ratio if second rescuer arrives.)
Use AED as soon as it is available.

6 After about 2 minutes, if still alone, activate emergency response system and retrieve AED (if not already done).

7 AED analyzes rhythm. Shockable rhythm?

Yes, shockable

No, nonshockable

8 Give 1 shock. Resume CPR immediately for about 2 minutes (until prompted by AED to allow rhythm check). Continue until ALS providers take over or victim starts to move.

9 Resume CPR immediately for about 2 minutes (until prompted by AED to allow rhythm check). Continue until ALS providers take over or victim starts to move.

*Signs of poor perfusion may include cool extremities, decrease in responsiveness, weak pulses, paleness, mottling (patchy skin appearance), and cyanosis (turning blue).

© 2015 American Heart Association

Figure 1. The BLS Healthcare Provider Pediatric Cardiac Arrest Algorithm for the Single Rescuer.

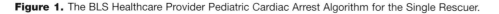

Infant and Child 1-Rescuer BLS Sequence

Introduction

If the rescuer is alone and encounters an unresponsive infant or child, follow the steps outlined in the BLS Healthcare Provider Pediatric Cardiac Arrest Algorithm for the Single Rescuer (Figure 1).

Verify Scene Safety, Check for Responsiveness, and Get Help (Algorithm Boxes 1, 2, 4)

The first rescuer who arrives at the side of an unresponsive infant or child should quickly perform the following steps:

Step	Action
1	Verify that the scene is safe for you and the victim. You do not want to become a victim yourself.
2	Check for responsiveness. Tap the child's shoulder or the heel of the infant's foot and shout, "Are you OK?"
3	If the victim is not responsive, shout for nearby help. Activate the emergency response system via mobile device (if possible).

Assess for Breathing and Pulse (Box 3)

Next, assess the infant or child for normal breathing and a pulse. This will help you determine the next appropriate actions.

To minimize delay in starting CPR, you may assess breathing at the same time as you check the pulse. This should take no more than 10 seconds.

Breathing

To check for breathing, scan the victim's chest for rise and fall for no more than 10 seconds.

- If the victim is breathing, monitor the victim until additional help arrives.
- If the victim is not breathing or is only gasping, the victim has respiratory or (if no pulse is felt) cardiac arrest. (Gasping is not considered normal breathing and is a sign of cardiac arrest.)

Check Pulse

- *Infant:* To perform a pulse check in an infant, palpate a brachial pulse (Figure 2A).
- *Child:* To perform a pulse check in a child, palpate a carotid or femoral pulse (Figures 2B and C).

It can be difficult to determine the presence or absence of a pulse in any victim, particularly in an infant or child. So if you do not definitely feel a pulse within 10 seconds, start CPR, beginning with chest compressions.

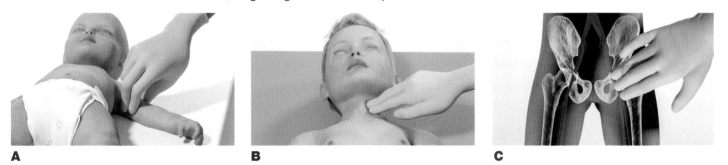

A **B** **C**

Figure 2. Pulse check. To perform a pulse check in an infant, palpate a brachial pulse (**A**). To perform a pulse check in a child, palpate a carotid (**B**) or femoral (**C**) pulse.

Infant: Locating the Brachial Artery Pulse

To perform a pulse check in an infant, palpate for a brachial pulse. Follow the steps below to locate the brachial artery and palpate the pulse. If you do not definitely feel a pulse within 10 seconds, begin high-quality CPR, starting with chest compressions.

Step	Action
1	Place 2 or 3 fingers on the inside of the upper arm, midway between the infant's elbow and shoulder.
2	Then press the fingers to attempt to feel the pulse for *at least 5 but no more than 10 seconds* (Figure 2A).

Child: Locating the Femoral Artery Pulse

To perform a pulse check in a child, palpate a carotid or femoral pulse. If you do not definitely feel a pulse within 10 seconds, begin high-quality CPR, starting with chest compressions.

Follow these steps to locate the femoral artery pulse:

Step	Action
1	Place 2 fingers in the inner thigh, midway between the hipbone and the pubic bone and just below the crease where the leg meets the torso (Figure 2C).
2	Feel for a pulse *for at least 5 but no more than 10 seconds*. If you do not definitely feel a pulse, begin high-quality CPR, starting with chest compressions.

Determine Next Actions (Boxes 3a, 3b)

Determine next actions based on the presence or absence of normal breathing and pulse:

If	Then
If the victim is breathing normally and a pulse is present	Monitor the victim.
If the victim *is not* breathing normally but a pulse *is* present	Provide rescue breathing (see "Rescue Breathing" in Part 7). • Add compressions if pulse remains 60/min or less with signs of poor perfusion (see the Foundational Facts box "Signs of Poor Perfusion" later in this Part). • Confirm that the emergency response system has been activated. • Continue rescue breathing and check pulse about every 2 minutes. Be ready to perform high-quality CPR if you do not feel a pulse or if there is a heart rate less than 60/min with signs of poor perfusion.

(continued)

(continued)

If the victim is not breathing normally or is only gasping and has no pulse	*If you are alone and the arrest was sudden and witnessed:* • Leave the victim to activate the emergency response system in your setting. For example, call 9-1-1 from your phone, mobilize the code team, or notify advanced life support. • Get the AED and emergency equipment. If someone else is available, send that person to get it. *If you are alone and the arrest was not sudden and witnessed:* • Continue to the next step: Begin high-quality CPR for 2 minutes.

Was the Collapse Sudden? (Boxes 4, 4a)

If the victim is not breathing or is only gasping and has no pulse, and the collapse was sudden and witnessed, leave the victim to activate the emergency response system (unless you have already done so by mobile device) and retrieve the AED. If others arrive, send them to activate the system (if not already done) and retrieve the AED while you remain with the child to begin CPR.

Begin High-Quality CPR, Starting With Chest Compressions (Boxes 5, 6)

If the victim is not breathing normally or is only gasping and has no pulse, begin high-quality CPR, starting with chest compressions (see details in "Part 4: Recognition and Management of Cardiac Arrest). Remove or move the clothing covering the victim's chest so that you can locate appropriate hand or finger placement for compression. This will also allow placement of AED pads when the AED arrives.

Single rescuers should use the following compression techniques (see "Infant/Child Chest Compressions" later in this Part for complete details):

- Infant: 2-finger chest compressions
- Child: 1 or 2 hands (whatever is needed to provide compressions of adequate depth)

After about 2 minutes of CPR, if you are still alone and were unable to activate the emergency response system (no mobile phone), leave the victim to activate the emergency response system and get the AED. Use the AED as soon as it is available.

Attempt Defibrillation With the AED (Boxes 7, 8, 9)

Use the AED as soon as it is available and follow the prompts.

Resume High-Quality CPR (Boxes 8, 9)

After shock delivery or if no shock is advised, immediately resume high-quality CPR, starting with chest compressions, when advised by the AED. Continue to provide CPR and follow the AED prompts until advanced life support providers take over or the child begins to breathe, move, or otherwise react.

Signs of Poor Perfusion

Assess the following to determine signs of poor perfusion:

- **Temperature:** Cool extremities
- **Altered mental state:** Continued decline in consciousness/responsiveness
- **Pulses:** Weak pulses
- **Skin:** Paleness, mottling (patchy appearance), and later cyanosis (turning blue)

Infant/Child Chest Compressions

Compression Rate and Compression-to-Ventilation Ratio

The *universal* rate for compressions in all cardiac arrest victims is 100 to 120/min. The compression-to-ventilation ratio for single rescuers is the same (30:2) in adults, children, and infants.

If 2 rescuers are present for the resuscitation attempt of an infant or child, use a compression-to-ventilation ratio of 15:2.

Chest Compression Technique

For most children, either 1 or 2 hands can be used to compress the chest. For most children, the compression technique will be the same as for an adult: 2 hands (heel of one hand with heel of other hand on top of the first hand). For a very small child, 1-handed compressions may be adequate to achieve the desired compression depth. Compress the chest at least one third the anteroposterior (AP) diameter of the chest (about 2 inches, or 5 cm) with each compression.

For infants, single rescuers should use the 2-finger technique. If multiple rescuers are present, the 2 thumb–encircling hands technique is preferred. These techniques are described below.

Infant (1 Rescuer): 2-Finger Technique

Follow these steps to give chest compressions to an infant by using the 2-finger technique:

Step	Action
1	Place the infant on a firm, flat surface.
2	Place 2 fingers in the center of the infant's chest, just below the nipple line, on the lower half of the breastbone. Do not press the tip of the breastbone (Figure 3).
3	Give compressions at a rate of 100 to 120/min.
4	Compress at least one third the AP diameter of the infant's chest (about 1½ inches [4 cm]).
5	At the end of each compression, make sure you allow the chest to fully recoil (reexpand); do not lean on the chest. Chest compression and chest recoil/relaxation times should be about equal. Minimize interruptions in compressions (eg, to give breaths) to less than 10 seconds.
6	After every 30 compressions, open the airway with a head tilt–chin lift and give 2 breaths, each over 1 second. The chest should rise with each breath.

(continued)

(continued)

| 7 | After about 5 cycles or 2 minutes of CPR, if you are alone and the emergency response system has not been activated, leave the infant (or carry the infant with you) to activate the emergency response system and retrieve the AED. |
| 8 | Continue compressions and breaths in a ratio of 30:2, and use the AED as soon as it is available. Continue until advanced providers take over or the infant begins to breathe, move, or otherwise react. |

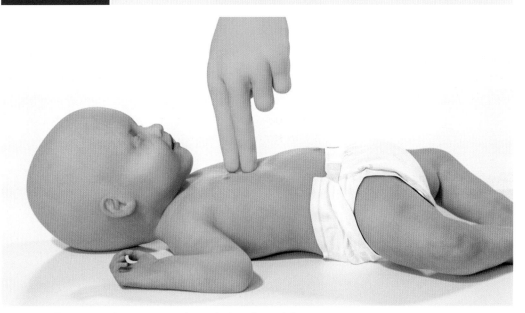

Figure 3. Two-finger chest compression technique for an infant.

Foundational Facts

Chest Recoil

Chest recoil allows blood to flow into the heart. Incomplete chest recoil reduces the filling of the heart between compressions and reduces the blood flow created by chest compressions.

Infant: 2 Thumb–Encircling Hands Technique

The 2 thumb–encircling hands technique is the preferred 2-rescuer chest compression technique because it produces improved blood flow.

Follow these steps to give chest compressions to an infant by using the 2 thumb–encircling hands technique:

Step	Action
1	Place the infant on a firm, flat surface.
2	Place both thumbs side by side in the center of the infant's chest, on the lower half of the breastbone. The thumbs may overlap in very small infants. Encircle the infant's chest and support the infant's back with the fingers of both hands.
3	With your hands encircling the chest, use both thumbs to depress the breastbone (Figure 4) at a rate of 100 to 120/min.
4	Compress at least one third the AP diameter of the infant's chest (about 1½ inches [4 cm]).
5	After each compression, completely release the pressure on the breastbone and allow the chest to recoil completely.
6	After every 15 compressions, pause briefly for the second rescuer to open the airway with a head tilt–chin lift and give 2 breaths, each over 1 second. The chest should rise with each breath. Minimize interruptions in compressions (eg, to give breaths) to less than 10 seconds.
7	Continue compressions and breaths in a ratio of 15:2 (for 2 rescuers). The rescuer providing chest compressions should switch roles with another provider about every 5 cycles or 2 minutes to avoid fatigue so that chest compressions remain effective. Continue CPR until the AED arrives, advanced providers take over, or the infant begins to breathe, move, or otherwise respond.

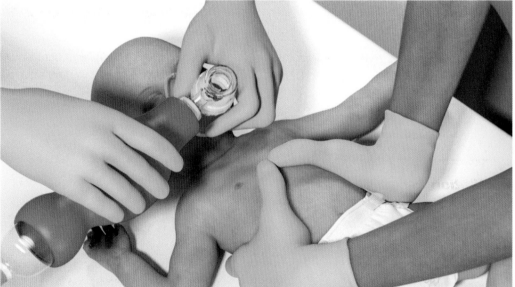

Figure 4. Two thumb–encircling hands technique for an infant (2 rescuers).

Critical Concepts	**The 2 Thumb–Encircling Hands Technique**

The 2 thumb–encircling hands technique is recommended when CPR is provided by 2 rescuers. This technique is preferred over the 2-finger technique because it

- Produces better blood supply to the heart muscle
- Helps ensure consistent depth and force of chest compressions
- May generate higher blood pressures

Foundational Facts	**Compression Depth in Adults vs Children and Infants**

- **Adults and adolescents:** *At least* 2 inches (5 cm)
- **Children:** *At least* one third the AP diameter of the chest or *about* 2 inches (5 cm)
- **Infants:** *At least* one third the AP diameter of the chest or *about* 1½ inches (4 cm)

Infant/Child Breaths

Opening the Airway

For rescue breaths to be effective, the airway must be open. Two methods for opening the airway are the head tilt–chin lift and jaw-thrust maneuvers.

As with adults, if a head or neck injury is suspected, use the jaw-thrust maneuver. If the jaw thrust does not open the airway, use the head tilt–chin lift.

Caution	**Keep Head in Neutral Position**

If you tilt (extend) an infant's head beyond the neutral (sniffing) position, the infant's airway may become blocked. Maximize airway patency by positioning the infant with the neck in a neutral position so that the external ear canal is level with the top of the infant's shoulder.

Why Breaths Are Important for Infants and Children in Cardiac Arrest

When *sudden* cardiac arrest occurs, the oxygen content of the blood is typically adequate to meet oxygen demands of the body for the first few minutes after arrest. So delivering chest compressions is an effective way of distributing oxygen to the heart and brain.

In contrast, infants and children who develop cardiac arrest often have respiratory failure or shock that reduces the oxygen content in the blood even before the onset of arrest. As a result, for most infants and children in cardiac arrest, chest compressions alone are not as effective as compressions and breaths for delivering oxygenated blood to the heart and brain. *For this reason, it is very important to give both compressions and breaths for infants and children during high-quality CPR.*

Ventilation for an Infant or Child With a Barrier Device

Use a barrier device (eg, pocket mask) or a bag-mask device for delivering breaths to an infant or child.

When providing bag-mask ventilation for an infant or child, do the following:

- Select a bag and mask of appropriate size. The mask must cover the victim's mouth and nose completely without covering the eyes or overlapping the chin.
- Perform a head tilt–chin lift to open the victim's airway. Press the mask to the face as you lift the jaw, making a seal between the child's face and the mask.
- Connect supplementary oxygen when available.

BLS Healthcare Provider Pediatric Cardiac Arrest Algorithm for 2 or More Rescuers

Refer to the BLS Healthcare Provider Pediatric Cardiac Arrest Algorithm for 2 or More Rescuers as you read the steps below (Figure 5).

BLS Healthcare Provider Pediatric Cardiac Arrest Algorithm for 2 or More Rescuers—2015 Update

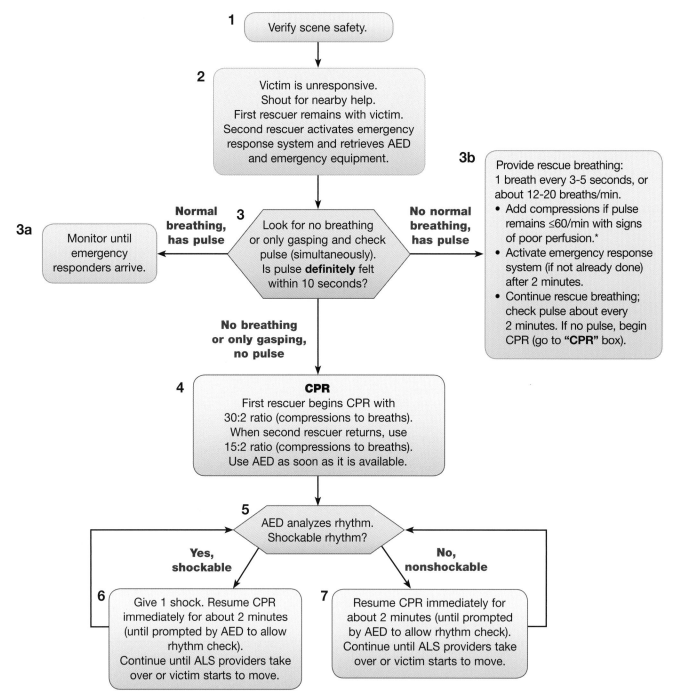

1 Verify scene safety.

2 Victim is unresponsive.
Shout for nearby help.
First rescuer remains with victim.
Second rescuer activates emergency response system and retrieves AED and emergency equipment.

3 Look for no breathing or only gasping and check pulse (simultaneously). Is pulse **definitely** felt within 10 seconds?

Normal breathing, has pulse

3a Monitor until emergency responders arrive.

No normal breathing, has pulse

3b Provide rescue breathing:
1 breath every 3-5 seconds, or about 12-20 breaths/min.
• Add compressions if pulse remains ≤60/min with signs of poor perfusion.*
• Activate emergency response system (if not already done) after 2 minutes.
• Continue rescue breathing; check pulse about every 2 minutes. If no pulse, begin CPR (go to "**CPR**" box).

No breathing or only gasping, no pulse

4 CPR
First rescuer begins CPR with 30:2 ratio (compressions to breaths).
When second rescuer returns, use 15:2 ratio (compressions to breaths).
Use AED as soon as it is available.

5 AED analyzes rhythm.
Shockable rhythm?

Yes, shockable

6 Give 1 shock. Resume CPR immediately for about 2 minutes (until prompted by AED to allow rhythm check).
Continue until ALS providers take over or victim starts to move.

No, nonshockable

7 Resume CPR immediately for about 2 minutes (until prompted by AED to allow rhythm check).
Continue until ALS providers take over or victim starts to move.

*Signs of poor perfusion may include cool extremities, decrease in responsiveness, weak pulses, paleness, mottling (patchy skin appearance), and cyanosis (turning blue).

© 2015 American Heart Association

Figure 5. The BLS Healthcare Provider Pediatric Cardiac Arrest Algorithm for 2 or More Rescuers.

Infant and Child 2-Rescuer BLS Sequence

Introduction

If the rescuer encounters an unresponsive infant or child and other rescuers are available, follow the steps outlined in the BLS Healthcare Provider Pediatric Cardiac Arrest Algorithm for 2 or More Rescuers (Figure 5).

Verify Scene Safety, Check for Responsiveness, and Get Help (Algorithm Boxes 1, 2)

The first rescuer who arrives at the side of an unresponsive infant or child should quickly perform the following steps. As more rescuers arrive, assign roles and responsibilities. When more rescuers are available for a resuscitation attempt, more tasks can be performed simultaneously.

Step	Action
1	Verify that the scene is safe for you and the victim.
2	Check for responsiveness. Tap the child's shoulder or the heel of the infant's foot and shout, "Are you OK?"
3	If the victim is not responsive: • The first rescuer initiates the resuscitation attempt. • The second rescuer activates the emergency response system (Figure 6), retrieves the AED and emergency equipment, and returns to the victim to help with CPR and the use of the AED.

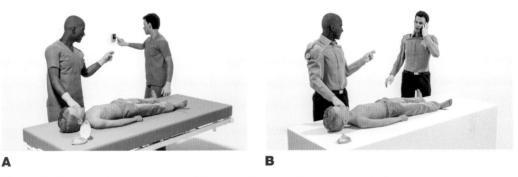

A   **B**

Figure 6. If the arrest of an infant or child was sudden and witnessed, activate the emergency response system in your setting. **A,** In-facility setting. **B,** Prehospital setting.

Assess for Breathing and Pulse (Box 3)

For details on assessing the victim for normal breathing and a pulse, see "Infant and Child 1-Rescuer BLS Sequence" section earlier in this Part.

Determine Next Actions (Boxes 3a, 3b)

For details on determining next actions based on the presence or absence of breathing and pulse, see "Infant and Child 1-Rescuer BLS Sequence" earlier in this Part. If CPR is indicated when the second rescuer is available to assist, use a compression-to-ventilation ratio of 15:2.

Begin High-Quality CPR, Starting With Chest Compressions (Box 4)

If the victim is not breathing normally or is only gasping and has no pulse, immediately do the following:

- The first rescuer begins high-quality CPR, starting with chest compressions (see "Infant/Child Chest Compressions" earlier in this Part for complete details). Remove or move the clothing covering the victim's chest so that you can locate appropriate hand or finger placement for compression. This will also allow placement of the AED pads when the AED arrives.
  - For an infant, use the 2-finger technique until the second rescuer returns to provide 2-rescuer CPR. During 2-rescuer CPR, use the 2 thumb–encircling hands technique.
  - For a child, use 1 or 2 hands (1 hand for a very small child).
- When the second rescuer returns, that rescuer gives breaths.
- Rescuers should switch compressors about every 5 cycles or 2 minutes (or earlier if needed), so that CPR quality is not reduced because of fatigue.

Attempt Defibrillation With the AED (Boxes 5, 6, 7)

Use the AED as soon as it is available and follow the prompts.

Resume High-Quality CPR (Boxes 6, 7)

After shock delivery or if no shock is advised, immediately resume high-quality CPR, starting with chest compressions, when advised by the AED. Continue to provide CPR and follow the AED prompts until advanced life support providers take over or the victim starts to move.

AED for Infants and Children Less Than 8 Years of Age

Be Familiar With the AED Equipment in Your Setting

Although all AEDs operate in basically the same way, AED equipment varies according to model and manufacturer. You must be familiar with the AED used in your particular setting.

Pediatric-Capable AEDs

Some AED models are designed for both pediatric and adult use. These AEDs deliver a reduced shock dose when pediatric pads are used.

Delivering a Pediatric Shock Dose

The AED shock dose may be reduced by pediatric cables, an attenuator, or preprogramming in the device. One commonly used method for reducing a shock dose is a pediatric dose attenuator (Figure 7). When attached to an AED, it reduces the shock dose by about two thirds. Typically, child pads are used to deliver the reduced shock dose.

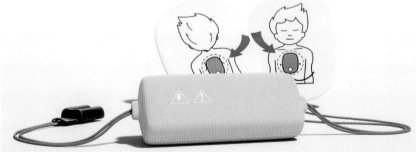

Figure 7. Example of a pediatric dose attenuator, which reduces the shock dose delivered by an AED. Child pads are also used with this attenuator.

Choosing and Placing the AED Pads

Use child pads, if available, for infants and for children less than 8 years of age. If child pads are not available, use adult pads. Make sure the pads do not touch each other or overlap. Adult pads deliver a higher shock dose, but a higher shock dose is preferred to no shock.

Follow the instructions for pad placement provided by the AED manufacturer and the illustrations on the AED pads. Some AEDs require that child pads be placed in a front and back (anteroposterior) position (Figure 8), while others require right-left (anterolateral) placement. Anteroposterior pad placement is commonly used for infants.

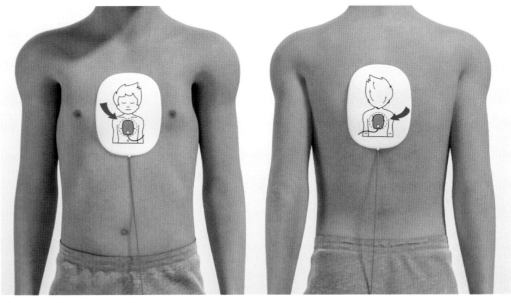

Figure 8. Anteroposterior AED pad placement on a child victim.

Victims 8 Years of Age and Older	Victims Younger Than 8 Years of Age
• Use the AED as soon as it is available. • Use adult pads (Figure 9). Do not use child pads—they will likely give a shock dose that is too low. • Place the pads as illustrated on the pads.	• Use the AED as soon as it is available. • Use child pads (Figure 10) if available. If you do not have child pads, you may use adult pads. Place the pads so that they do not touch each other. • If the AED has a key or switch that will deliver a child shock dose, turn the key or switch. • Place the pads as illustrated on the pads.

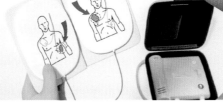

Figure 9. Adult AED pads.   **Figure 10.** Child AED pads.

Use of an AED for Infants

For infants, a manual defibrillator is preferred to an AED for defibrillation. A manual defibrillator has more capabilities than an AED and can provide lower energy doses that are often needed in infants. Advanced training is required to use a manual defibrillator and will not be covered in this course.

- If a manual defibrillator is not available, an AED equipped with a pediatric dose attenuator is preferred.
- If neither is available, you may use an AED without a pediatric dose attenuator.

Foundational Facts

Using Adult Pads or Adult Shock Dose Is Better Than No Attempt at Defibrillation

AED Pads

If you are using an AED for an infant or for a child less than 8 years of age and the AED does not have child pads, you may use adult pads. Pads may need to be placed anterior and posterior so that they do not touch each other or overlap.

Shock Dose

If the AED you are using doesn't have the capability of delivering a pediatric dose, use the adult dose.

Part 3

Systematic Approach to the Seriously Ill or Injured Child

Overview

The PALS provider should use a systematic approach when caring for a seriously ill or injured child. The purpose of this organized approach is to enable you to quickly recognize signs of respiratory distress, respiratory failure, and shock and immediately provide lifesaving interventions.

Learning Objective

After completing this Part, you should be able to

- Differentiate between patients who do and do not require immediate intervention

Preparation for the Course

You need to know all of the concepts presented in this Part to be able to identify the child's clinical condition and target appropriate management in case simulations. The ongoing process of evaluate-identify-intervene is a core component of systematic evaluation and care of a seriously ill or injured child.

Initial Impression to Identify a Life-Threatening Condition

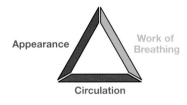

The Systematic Approach Algorithm (Figure 11) outlines the approach to caring for a critically ill or injured child. The initial impression is your first quick "from the doorway" observation of the child's appearance, breathing, and color. It is accomplished within the *first few seconds* of encountering the child. The Pediatric Assessment Triangle (PAT) is the tool used to make the initial impression. The PAT can be used immediately on entering the scene and helps identify the general type of physiologic problem (ie, respiratory, circulatory, or neurologic) and urgency for treatment and transport.

Identify and Intervene

If You Identify a Life-Threatening Problem

If at any time you identify a life-threatening problem, immediately begin appropriate interventions. Activate the emergency response system as indicated in your practice setting.

PALS Systematic Approach Algorithm

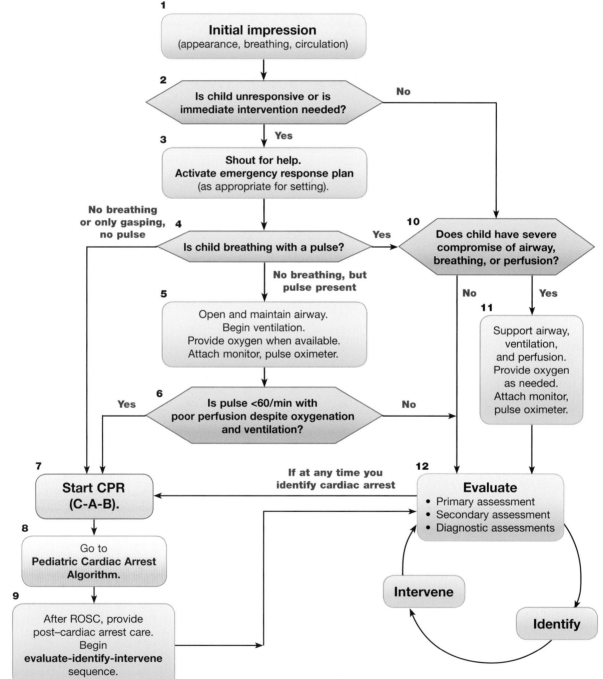

Figure 11. The Systematic Approach Algorithm.

Identify a Life-Threatening Condition and Act

The purpose of the initial impression is to quickly identify a life-threatening condition.

If the child's condition is...	The next action is to...
Life threatening	• Start life support interventions • Get help
Not life threatening	• Continue with the Systematic Approach

Child Who Is Unresponsive and Not Breathing or Only Gasping

Follow Left Side of Algorithm

If the child is unresponsive, shout for help. You will then follow the left side of the Systematic Approach Algorithm (Figure 11). In the text that follows, box numbers refer to the corresponding boxes in this algorithm.

Activate Emergency Response System (Box 3)

If the child is unresponsive and not breathing or only gasping and has no pulse, activate the emergency response system as appropriate for your practice setting (Box 3), and immediately start CPR, beginning with chest compressions (Box 7).

Proceed according to the Pediatric Cardiac Arrest Algorithm. After return of spontaneous circulation, begin the evaluate-identify-intervene sequence (Boxes 10-12) and provide post–cardiac arrest care.

Check Breathing and Pulse (Box 4)

Next, check for breathing and a pulse simultaneously (Box 4).

If No Effective Breathing, But Pulse Is Present, Provide Rescue Breaths (Box 5)

If a pulse is present, open the airway and provide rescue breathing (Box 5). Use oxygen as soon as it is available. See "Rescue Breathing" in Part 7 for more information. For infants and children, give 1 breath every 3 to 5 seconds (about 12 to 20 breaths/min). Give each breath over 1 second. Each breath should result in visible chest rise.

Check the heart rate.

If heart rate is...	Next Steps
<60/min with signs of poor perfusion despite adequate oxygenation and ventilation (Box 6)	Provide chest compressions and ventilation (Box 7). Proceed according to the Pediatric Cardiac Arrest Algorithm.
≥60/min	Continue ventilation as needed. Begin the evaluate-identify-intervene sequence (Boxes 10-12). You should check the pulse about every 2 minutes. Be prepared to intervene according to the Pediatric Cardiac Arrest Algorithm if needed.

If Breathing and Pulse Are Adequate

If unresponsiveness is a new finding and breathing and pulse are adequate, activate the rapid response or the emergency response system as appropriate for your setting. Continue systematic assessment (follow right side of algorithm, Boxes 10-12).

Initial Impression

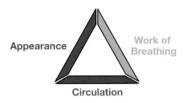

If you do not immediately detect a life-threatening emergency, you can continue forming your initial impression of the child's condition. As noted above, the PAT is the tool used to form your initial impression.

The PAT uses A-B-C, which stands for **a**ppearance, work of **b**reathing, and **c**irculatory status. The PAT begins with evaluation of appearance (A) as an indicator of overall physiologic status, including degree of interactivity, muscle tone, and verbal response or cry. The use of the TICLS (**t**one, **i**nteractiveness, **c**onsolability, **l**ook/gaze, **s**peech/cry) mnemonic can be used as an adjunct. The second component of the PAT is breathing (B), which determines whether a child has increased work of breathing by assessing the patients' position (ie, tripod or sniffing position), work of breathing (ie, retractions), and adventitial breath sounds (eg, stridor, sonorous respirations). The final component of the PAT evaluates the child's overall circulatory status (C) based on general color (eg, pale, mottled, cyanotic). A child with abnormal PAT findings requires prompt evaluation and management. The findings of the PAT may indicate need for immediate intervention (eg, CPR for a patient who is apneic and pulseless, tourniquet use for exsanguinating hemorrhage of an extremity).

Appearance

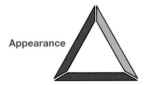

The first part of the PAT is the child's appearance, including level of consciousness and ability to interact. Carefully, but quickly, observe the child's appearance to evaluate the level of consciousness. The level of consciousness may be defined by the child's **t**one, **i**nteractiveness, **c**onsolability, **l**ook/gaze/stare, and **s**peech/cry. If the child is unresponsive, you should shout for nearby help, assess breathing and pulse, and then activate the rapid response or the emergency response system as appropriate for your clinical setting.

If the child is crying or upset, it can be difficult to know if the child is responding appropriately. Try to keep the child as calm as possible. Let her remain with her parent or caregiver if practical. Use distractions such as toys.

Breathing

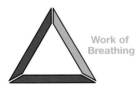

The next part of the PAT is evaluation of work of breathing (Table 1). During the PAT, you evaluate the child's work of breathing, position, and any audible breath sounds (ie, breath sounds or sounds of breathing that can be heard without a stethoscope). Look for signs of absent or increased respiratory effort. Listen for obvious sounds of abnormal breathing, such as grunting, stridor, or wheezing. Note whether the patient's position suggests respiratory distress, such as the tripod position.

Table 1. Evaluation of Work of Breathing

	Normal	**Abnormal**
Respiratory effort*	• Regular breathing, no increased effort • Passive expiration	• Nasal flaring • Retractions or use of accessory muscles • Increased, inadequate, or absent respiratory effort
Lung and airway sounds*	No abnormal respiratory sounds audible	Noisy breathing (eg, wheezing, grunting, stridor)

*See detailed discussion of respiratory effort and lung and airway sounds in the "Primary Assessment" section in this Part.

Circulation (Color)

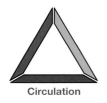

Circulation

To complete the third part of the PAT, assess the child's overall circulatory status. You assess the child's color, which may help you assess how well the child is perfusing. This includes skin color and pattern or obvious significant bleeding. You can often identify important information about circulatory status just by looking at a child.

Pallor (paleness), mottling (an irregular skin color), or cyanosis (bluish/gray skin color) suggests poor perfusion, poor oxygenation, or both. Cyanosis of the lips and fingernails may be present if the child is unable to adequately oxygenate the blood.

Observe the exposed parts of the child, such as the face, arms, and legs. A flushed appearance may suggest fever or distributive shock such as from sepsis, toxins, or anaphylaxis. Inspection of the skin may reveal bruising that suggests injury. You may also see evidence of bleeding within the skin, called *petechiae* or *purpura*. This purplish discoloration of the skin is often a sign of a life-threatening infection.

Evaluate the skin and mucous membranes (Table 2). *Are they normal or abnormal?*

Table 2. Evaluation of Skin and Mucous Membranes

	Normal	**Abnormal**
Skin color*	Appears normal	• Pallor • Mottling • Cyanosis
Petechiae or purpura or visible bleeding wounds	Not normal	• Obvious significant bleeding • Bleeding within the skin (eg, purpura)

*See the discussion of skin color in the "Primary Assessment" section in this Part.

Evaluate-Identify-Intervene

Use the evaluate-identify-intervene sequence (Figure 12) when caring for a seriously ill or injured child. This will help you to determine the best treatment or intervention at any point. From the information gathered during your evaluation, identify the child's clinical condition by type and severity. Intervene with appropriate actions. Then repeat the sequence. This process is ongoing.

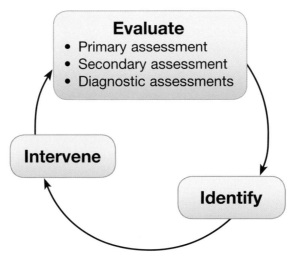

Figure 12. Evaluate-identify-intervene sequence.

Always be alert to a life-threatening problem. If at any point you identify a life-threatening problem, immediately activate the emergency response system (or send someone to do so) while you begin lifesaving interventions.

Evaluate

If no life-threatening condition is present, evaluate the child's condition by using the clinical assessment tools described in Table 3.

Table 3. Clinical Assessment Tools

Clinical Assessment	Brief Description
Primary assessment	A rapid, hands-on ABCDE approach to evaluate respiratory, cardiac, and neurologic function; this step includes assessment of vital signs and pulse oximetry
Secondary assessment	A focused medical history and a focused physical exam
Diagnostic assessments	Laboratory, radiographic, and other advanced tests that help to identify the child's physiologic condition and diagnosis

Providers should be aware of potential environmental dangers when providing care. In out-of-hospital settings, always assess the scene before you evaluate the child.

Identify

Try to identify the type and severity of the child's problem (Table 4).

Table 4. Type and Severity of Potential Problems

	Type	Severity
Respiratory	• Upper airway obstruction • Lower airway obstruction • Lung tissue disease • Disordered control of breathing	• Respiratory distress • Respiratory failure
Circulatory	• Hypovolemic shock • Distributive shock • Cardiogenic shock • Obstructive shock	• Compensated shock • Hypotensive shock

Cardiopulmonary Failure

Cardiac Arrest

The child's clinical condition can result from a combination of respiratory and circulatory problems. As a seriously ill or injured child deteriorates, one problem may lead to others. Note that in the initial phase of your identification, you may be uncertain about the type or severity of problems.

Identifying the problem will help you determine the best initial interventions. Recognition and management are discussed in detail later in this manual.

Intervene

On the basis of your identification of the child's clinical condition, intervene with appropriate actions within your scope of practice. PALS interventions may include

- Positioning the child to maintain an open/patent airway
- Activating the emergency response system
- Starting CPR
- Obtaining the code cart and monitor
- Placing the child on a cardiac monitor and pulse oximeter
- Administering O_2
- Supporting ventilation
- Starting medications and fluids (eg, nebulizer treatment, IV/IO fluid bolus)

Continuous Sequence

The sequence of evaluate-identify-intervene continues until the child is stable. Use this sequence before and after each intervention to look for trends in the child's condition. For example, after you give O_2, reevaluate the child. Is the child breathing a little easier? Are color and mental status improving? After you give a fluid bolus to a child in hypovolemic shock, do heart rate and perfusion improve? Is another bolus needed? Use the evaluate-identify-intervene sequence whenever the child's condition changes.

Critical Concepts

The Evaluate-Identify-Intervene Sequence Is Continuous

Remember to repeat the evaluate-identify-intervene sequence until the child is stable:

- After each intervention
- When the child's condition changes or deteriorates

FYI

Appearance Seems Stable but Condition May Be Life Threatening

Sometimes a child's condition may seem stable despite the presence of a life-threatening problem. An example is a child who has ingested a toxin but is not yet showing effects. Another example is a trauma victim with internal bleeding who may initially maintain blood pressure by increasing heart rate and systemic vascular resistance. Frequent reassessment is key.

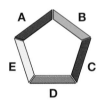

Identify and Intervene

Be Alert for Any Life-Threatening Problem

If at any time you identify a life-threatening problem, immediately begin appropriate interventions. Activate the emergency response system as indicated in your practice setting.

Primary Assessment

The primary assessment (primary survey) uses a hands-on ABCDE approach and includes assessment of the patient's vital signs (including oxygen saturation by pulse oximetry).

- **A**irway
- **B**reathing
- **C**irculation
- **D**isability
- **E**xposure

As the healthcare provider proceeds through each component of the primary assessment, life-threatening abnormalities that are identified should be treated in real time before completing the remainder of the primary assessment (eg, unless the patient is apneic and pulseless or has obvious uncontrolled external hemorrhage). In patients with life-threatening conditions evident in the primary assessment, correction of those conditions takes precedence over establishing baseline vital sign measures such as blood pressure or pulse oximetry. When the primary assessment is completed and after life-threatening problems have been addressed, the healthcare provider proceeds to the secondary assessment.

Airway

Evaluate Airway

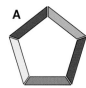

When you assess the airway, you determine if it is patent (open). To assess upper airway openness/patency:

- Look for movement of the chest or abdomen
- Listen for air movement and breath sounds
- Feel for movement of air at the nose and mouth

To check for breathing, scan the victim's chest for rise and fall for no more than 10 seconds.

- If the victim is breathing, monitor the victim until additional help arrives.
- If the victim is not breathing or is only gasping, this is not considered normal breathing and is a sign of cardiac arrest.

To minimize delay in starting CPR, you may assess breathing at the same time as you check the pulse. This should take no more than 10 seconds.

Decide if the upper airway is clear, maintainable, or not maintainable as described in Table 5.

Table 5. Upper Airway Status and Description

Status	Description
Clear	Airway is open and unobstructed for normal breathing.
Maintainable	Airway is obstructed but can be maintained by *simple measures* (eg, head tilt–chin lift).
Not maintainable	Airway is obstructed and cannot be maintained without *advanced interventions (eg, intubation)*.

The following signs suggest that the upper airway is obstructed:

- Increased inspiratory effort with retractions
- Abnormal inspiratory sounds (snoring or high-pitched stridor)
- Episodes where no airway or breath sounds are present despite respiratory effort (ie, complete upper airway obstruction)

If the upper airway is obstructed, determine if you can open and maintain the airway with *simple measures* or if you need *advanced interventions*.

Simple Measures to Maintain the Airway

Simple measures to open and maintain a patent upper airway may include one or more of the following:

Positioning	Allow the child to assume a position of comfort, or position the child to improve airway patency. *For a responsive child:* • Allow the child to assume a position of comfort *or* • Elevate the head of the bed *For an unresponsive child:* • Turn the child on her side if you do not suspect cervical injury *or* • Use a head tilt–chin lift or jaw thrust (below)
Head tilt–chin lift or jaw thrust	• *If you do not suspect cervical spine injury:* Use the head tilt–chin lift maneuver to open the airway. Avoid overextending the head/neck in infants because this may occlude the airway. • *If you suspect cervical spine injury (eg, the child has a head or neck injury):* Open the airway by using a jaw thrust without neck extension. If this maneuver does not open the airway, use a head tilt–chin lift or jaw thrust with neck extension because opening the airway is a priority. During CPR, stabilize the head and neck manually rather than with immobilization devices. Note that the jaw thrust may be used in children without trauma as well.
Suctioning	Suction the nose and oropharynx. Avoid overextending the head/neck in infants because this may occlude the airway.
Relief techniques for foreign-body airway obstruction	If a child is suspected to have aspirated a foreign body, has complete airway obstruction (is unable to make any sound), and is *responsive*, repeat the following as needed: • <1 year of age: give 5 back slaps and 5 chest thrusts • ≥1 year of age: give abdominal thrusts If at any time the child becomes unresponsive, activate (if you have a mobile device) or send someone to activate the emergency response system and begin CPR.
Airway adjuncts	Use airway adjuncts (eg, oropharyngeal airway) to keep the tongue from falling back and obstructing the airway.

Identify and Intervene

Don't Rely on an Adjunct Alone to Maintain an Open Airway

An airway adjunct will help to maintain an open airway, but you may still need to use a head tilt–chin lift. Don't rely only on an airway adjunct alone. Assess the patient!

Advanced Interventions   Advanced interventions to maintain airway openness/patency may include one or more of the following:

- Endotracheal (ET) intubation or placement of a laryngeal mask airway
- Application of continuous positive airway pressure or noninvasive ventilation
- Removal of a foreign body; this intervention may require direct laryngoscopy (ie, visualizing the larynx with a laryngoscope)
- Cricothyrotomy (a needle puncture or surgical opening through the skin and cricothyroid membrane and into the trachea below the vocal cords)

Breathing

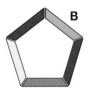

Assessment of breathing includes evaluation of

- Respiratory rate and pattern
- Respiratory effort
- Chest expansion and air movement
- Lung and airway sounds
- O_2 saturation by pulse oximetry

Normal Respiratory Rate   Normal spontaneous breathing is accomplished with minimal work, resulting in quiet breathing with unlabored inspiration and passive expiration. The normal respiratory rate is inversely related to age (Table 6); it is rapid in the neonate and decreases as the child gets older.

Table 6. Normal Respiratory Rates by Age

Age	Breaths per Minute
Infant	30-53
Toddler	22-37
Preschooler	20-28
School-age child	18-25
Adolescent	12-20

Reproduced from Hazinski MF. Children are different. In: Hazinski MF, ed. *Nursing Care of the Critically Ill Child*. 3rd ed. St Louis, MO: Mosby; 2013:1-18, copyright Elsevier.

Critical Concepts

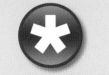

Very Slow or Very Fast Respiratory Rate Is a Warning Sign

A consistent respiratory rate of less than 10 or more than 60 breaths per minute in a child of any age is often abnormal and warrants further assessment for the presence of a potentially serious condition.

Respiratory rate is often best evaluated before your hands-on assessment, because anxiety and agitation commonly alter the baseline rate. If the child has any condition that causes an increase in metabolic demand (eg, excitement, anxiety, exercise, pain, or fever), it is appropriate for the respiratory rate to be higher than normal.

Determine the respiratory rate by counting the number of times the chest rises in 30 seconds and multiplying by 2. Be aware that normal sleeping infants may have irregular (periodic) breathing with pauses lasting up to 10 or even 15 seconds. If you count the number of times the chest rises for less than 30 seconds, you may estimate the respiratory rate inaccurately. Count the respiratory rate several times as you assess and reassess the child to detect changes. Alternatively, the respiratory rate may be displayed continuously on a monitor.

A decrease in respiratory rate from a rapid to a more "normal" rate may indicate overall improvement if it is associated with an improved level of consciousness and reduced signs of air hunger and work of breathing. A decreasing or irregular respiratory rate in a child with a deteriorating level of consciousness, however, often indicates a worsening of the child's clinical condition.

Abnormal Respiratory Rate and Pattern

Abnormal respirations include

- Irregular respiratory pattern
- Fast respiratory rate (tachypnea)
- Slow respiratory rate (bradypnea)
- Apnea

Irregular Respiratory Pattern

Children with neurologic problems may have irregular respiratory patterns. Examples of such irregular patterns are

- A deep gasping breath, followed by a period of apnea (no breathing)
- A rapid respiratory rate, followed by periods of apnea or very shallow breaths

Irregular patterns such as these are serious and require urgent evaluation.

Fast Respiratory Rate

A *fast respiratory rate* (tachypnea) is a breathing rate that is faster than normal for age. This is often the first sign of respiratory distress in infants. Tachypnea can also develop during periods of stress.

A fast respiratory rate may or may not be accompanied by signs of increased respiratory effort. A fast respiratory rate *without* signs of increased respiratory effort (ie, *quiet tachypnea*) may result from

- Conditions that are not primarily respiratory in origin, such as high fever, pain, anemia, cyanotic congenital heart disease, and sepsis (serious infection)
- Dehydration

Slow Respiratory Rate

A slower than normal respiratory rate (bradypnea) may be caused by

- Respiratory muscle fatigue
- A central nervous system injury or problem that affects the respiratory control center
- Severe hypoxia
- Severe shock
- Hypothermia
- Drugs that depress the respiratory drive
- Some muscle diseases that cause muscle weakness

Critical Concepts

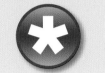

Bradypnea or Irregular Respiratory Rate Often Signal Impending Arrest

Bradypnea or an irregular respiratory rate in an acutely ill infant or child is an ominous clinical sign and often signals impending arrest.

Apnea

Apnea is the cessation of breathing, typically defined as longer than 15 seconds. Apnea may be further classified as **central** or **obstructive.** Central apnea indicates that the child is making no respiratory effort, whereas obstructive apnea is when ventilation is impeded, resulting in hypoxemia, hypercapnia, or both.

FYI

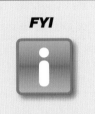

Three Types of Apnea

Apnea is classified into 3 types, depending on whether inspiratory muscle activity is present:

- In *central apnea,* there is no respiratory effort because of an abnormality or suppression of the brain or spinal cord.
- In *obstructive apnea,* there is inspiratory effort without airflow (ie, airflow is partially or completely blocked).
- In *mixed apnea,* there are periods of obstructive apnea and periods of central apnea.

Agonal gasps are common in adults after sudden cardiac arrest and may be confused with normal breathing. They are also present late in the deterioration of a very sick child. Agonal gasps will not produce effective oxygenation and ventilation.

Increased Respiratory Effort

Increased respiratory effort results from conditions that increase resistance to airflow (eg, asthma or bronchiolitis) or that cause the lungs to be stiffer and difficult to inflate (eg, pneumonia, pulmonary edema, or pleural effusion). Nonpulmonary conditions that result in severe metabolic acidosis (eg, shock, DKA, salicylate ingestion, inborn errors of metabolism) can also cause increased respiratory rate and effort. Signs of increased respiratory effort reflect the child's attempt to improve oxygenation, ventilation, or both. Use the presence or absence of these signs to assess the severity of the condition and determine the urgency of intervention. Signs of increased respiratory effort include

- Nasal flaring
- Retractions
- Head bobbing or seesaw respirations

Other signs of increased respiratory effort are prolonged inspiratory or expiratory times, open-mouth breathing, gasping, and use of accessory muscles. Grunting is a serious sign and may indicate respiratory distress or respiratory failure. (See "Grunting" later in this Part.)

Nasal Flaring

Nasal flaring is dilation of the nostrils with each inhalation. The nostrils open more widely to maximize airflow. Nasal flaring is most commonly observed in infants and younger children and is usually a sign of respiratory distress.

Retractions

Retractions are inward movements of the chest wall or tissues or sternum during inspiration. Chest retractions are a sign that the child is trying to move air into the lungs by using the chest muscles, but air movement is impaired by increased airway resistance or stiff lungs. Retractions may occur in several areas of the chest. The severity of the retractions generally corresponds with the severity of the child's breathing difficulty.

Table 7 describes the location of retractions commonly associated with each level of breathing difficulty.

Table 7. Location of Retractions Commonly Associated With Each Level of Breathing Difficulty

Breathing Difficulty	Location of Retraction	Description
Mild to moderate	Subcostal	Retraction of the abdomen, just below the rib cage
	Substernal	Retraction of the abdomen at the bottom of the breastbone
	Intercostal	Retraction between the ribs
Severe (may include the same retractions as seen with mild to moderate breathing difficulty)	Supraclavicular	Retraction in the tissues just above the collarbone
	Suprasternal	Retraction in the chest, just above the breastbone
	Sternal	Retraction of the sternum toward the spine

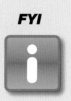

FYI

Combination of Retractions and Other Signs to Identify Type of Respiratory Problem

Retractions accompanied by stridor or an inspiratory snoring sound suggest upper airway obstruction. Retractions accompanied by expiratory wheezing suggest marked lower airway obstruction (asthma or bronchiolitis), causing obstruction during both inspiration and expiration. Retractions accompanied by grunting or labored respirations suggest lung tissue disease. Severe retractions also may be accompanied by head bobbing or seesaw respirations.

Head Bobbing or Seesaw Respirations

Head bobbing and seesaw respirations often indicate that the child has increased risk for deterioration.

- *Head bobbing* is caused by the use of neck muscles to assist breathing. The child lifts the chin and extends the neck during inspiration and allows the chin to fall forward during expiration. Head bobbing is most frequently seen in infants and can be a sign of respiratory failure.

- *Seesaw respirations* are present when the chest retracts and the abdomen expands during inspiration. During expiration, the movement reverses: the chest expands and the abdomen moves inward. Seesaw respirations usually indicate upper airway obstruction. They also may be observed in severe lower airway obstruction, lung tissue disease, and states of disordered control of breathing. Seesaw respirations are characteristic of infants and children with neuromuscular weakness. This inefficient form of ventilation can quickly lead to fatigue.

Foundational Facts

Cause of Seesaw Breathing

The cause of seesaw breathing in most children with neuromuscular disease is weakness of the abdominal and chest wall muscles. Seesaw breathing is caused by strong contraction of the diaphragm that dominates the weaker abdominal and chest wall muscles. The result is retraction of the chest and expansion of the abdomen during inspiration.

Inadequate Respiratory Effort

In your evaluation of respiratory effort, look for signs that respiratory effort is inadequate and be prepared to support airway, oxygenation, and ventilation. These include

- Apnea
- Weak cry or cough
- Bradypnea
- Agonal gasps

Chest Expansion and Air Movement

Evaluate magnitude of chest wall expansion and air movement to assess adequacy of the child's tidal volume. Tidal volume is the volume of air inspired with each breath. Normal tidal volume is approximately 5 to 7 mL/kg of body weight throughout life. Tidal volume is difficult to measure unless a child is mechanically ventilated, so your clinical assessment is very important.

Chest Wall Expansion

Chest expansion (chest rise) during inspiration should be symmetrical. Expansion may be subtle during spontaneous quiet breathing, especially when clothing covers the chest. But chest expansion should be readily visible when the chest is uncovered. In normal infants, the abdomen may move more than the chest. Decreased or asymmetrical chest expansion may result from inadequate effort, airway obstruction, atelectasis, pneumothorax, hemothorax, pleural effusion, mucous plug, or foreign-body aspiration.

Air Movement

Auscultation for air movement is critical. Listen for the intensity of breath sounds and quality of air movement in the following areas:

Area	Location
Anterior	Mid-chest (just to the left and right of the sternum)
Lateral	Under the armpits (the best location for evaluating air movement into the lower parts of the lungs)
Posterior	Both sides of the back

Because the chest is small and the chest wall is thin in infants and children, breath sounds are readily transmitted from one side of the chest to the other. Breath sounds also may be transmitted from the upper airway. To evaluate distal air entry, listen below both axillae. Because these areas are farther from the larger conducting airways, upper airway sounds are less likely to be transmitted.

Listen to the loudness of the air movement:

- Typical inspiratory sounds can be heard distally as soft, quiet noises occurring simultaneously with observed inspiratory effort.
- Normal expiratory breath sounds are often short and quieter; sometimes you may not hear normal expiratory breath sounds.

Decreased chest excursion or decreased air movement observed during auscultation often accompanies poor respiratory effort. In the child with apparently normal or increased respiratory effort, diminished distal air entry suggests airflow obstruction or lung tissue disease. If the child's work of breathing and coughing suggest lower airway obstruction, but no wheezes are heard, the amount and rate of airflow may be insufficient to cause wheezing.

Distal air entry may be difficult to hear in the obese child. As a result, it may be difficult to identify significant airway abnormalities in this population.

FYI

Minute Ventilation

Minute ventilation is the volume of air that moves into or out of the lungs each minute. It is the product of the number of breaths per minute (respiratory rate) and the volume of each breath (tidal volume).

Minute Ventilation = Respiratory Rate × Tidal Volume

Low minute ventilation (hypoventilation) may result from

- Slow respiratory rate
- Small tidal volume (ie, shallow breathing, high airway resistance, stiff lungs)
- Extremely rapid respiratory rate (resulting in very small tidal volumes)

Lung and Airway Sounds

During the primary assessment, listen for lung and airway sounds. Abnormal sounds include stridor, snoring, grunting, gurgling, wheezing, crackles, and change in cry/phonation/cough (including barking cough).

Stridor

Stridor is a coarse, usually higher-pitched breathing sound typically heard on inspiration. It also may be heard during both inspiration and expiration. Stridor is a sign of upper airway (extrathoracic) obstruction and may indicate that the obstruction is critical and requires immediate intervention.

There are many causes of stridor, such as a foreign body in the airway and infection (eg, croup). Congenital airway abnormalities (eg, laryngomalacia) and acquired airway abnormalities (eg, tumor or cyst) also can cause stridor. Upper airway edema (eg, allergic reaction or swelling after a medical procedure) is another cause of this abnormal breathing sound.

Snoring

Although *snoring* may be common during sleep in children, it also can be a sign of airway obstruction. Soft tissue swelling or decreased level of consciousness may cause airway obstruction and snoring.

Grunting

Grunting is typically a short, low-pitched sound heard during expiration. Sometimes it can be misinterpreted as a soft cry. Grunting occurs as the child exhales against a partially closed glottis. Although grunting may accompany the response to pain or fever, infants and children often grunt to help keep the small airways and alveolar sacs in the lungs open. This is an attempt to optimize oxygenation and ventilation.

Grunting is often a sign of lung tissue disease resulting from small airway collapse, alveolar collapse, or both. Grunting may indicate progression of respiratory distress to respiratory failure. Pulmonary conditions that cause grunting include pneumonia, pulmonary contusion, and acute respiratory distress syndrome. It may be caused by cardiac conditions, such as congestive heart failure, that result in pulmonary edema. Grunting may be a sign of pain resulting from abdominal pathology (eg, bowel obstruction, perforated viscus, appendicitis, or peritonitis).

Identify and Intervene

Grunting Is a Sign of Severe Respiratory Distress or Failure

Grunting is typically a sign of severe respiratory distress or failure from lung tissue disease. Identify and treat the cause as quickly as possible. Be prepared to quickly intervene if the child's condition worsens.

Gurgling

Gurgling is a bubbling sound heard during inspiration or expiration. It results from upper airway obstruction due to airway secretions, vomit, or blood.

Wheezing

Wheezing is a high-pitched or low-pitched whistling or sighing sound heard most often during expiration. It is heard less frequently during inspiration. This sound typically indicates lower (intrathoracic) airway obstruction, especially of the smaller airways. Common causes of wheezing are bronchiolitis and asthma. Isolated inspiratory wheezing suggests a foreign body or other cause of partial obstruction of the trachea or upper airway.

Crackles

Crackles, also known as *rales*, are sharp, crackling inspiratory sounds. The sound of dry crackles can be described as the sound made when you rub several hairs together close to your ear. Moist crackles indicate accumulation of alveolar fluid. They are typically associated with lung tissue disease (eg, pneumonia and pulmonary edema) or interstitial lung disease. Dry crackles are more often heard with atelectasis (small airway collapse) and interstitial lung disease. Note that you may not hear crackles despite the presence of pulmonary edema.

Change in Cry/Phonation/Cough (Including Barking Cough)

If an infant's cry becomes very soft with only short sounds during expiration (ie, so the cry sounds more like the soft "mewing" of a cat) or an older child begins to talk in short phrases or single words instead of sentences, this may indicate severe respiratory distress and shortness of breath. If an infant or child develops a "barking" cough or change in pitch of cry or voice, this may indicate upper airway obstruction.

Oxygen Saturation by Pulse Oximetry

Pulse oximetry is a tool to monitor the percentage of the child's hemoglobin that is fully saturated with oxygen. The pulse oximeter consists of a probe linked to a monitor. The probe is attached to the child's finger, toe, or earlobe, and it must detect a consistent pulsatile signal. The unit displays the calculated percentage of saturated hemoglobin. Most units make an audible sound for each pulse beat and display the heart rate. Some models display the quality of the pulse signal as a waveform or with bars.

Foundational Facts

O₂ Saturation

The O₂ saturation is the percent of total hemoglobin that is fully saturated with oxygen (ie, the oxyhemoglobin saturation).

This oxyhemoglobin saturation does not indicate the amount of O₂ delivered to the tissues. O₂ delivery is the product of arterial O₂ content (oxygen bound to hemoglobin plus dissolved O₂) and cardiac output.

It is also important to note that O₂ saturation does not provide information about effectiveness of ventilation (CO_2 elimination).

Pulse oximetry can indicate low O₂ saturation (hypoxemia) before it causes cyanosis or bradycardia. Providers can use pulse oximetry to monitor trends in O₂ saturation in response to treatment. If available, continuously monitor pulse oximetry for a child in respiratory distress or failure during stabilization, transport, and post–cardiac arrest care.

Identify and Intervene

Need for O₂ Administration or Additional Intervention

An O₂ saturation (SpO₂) of 94% or more while a child is breathing room air usually indicates that oxygenation is adequate; conversely, an SpO₂ less than 94% when the child is breathing room air indicates hypoxemia. Consider administration of supplementary O₂ if the O₂ saturation is below this value in a critically ill or injured child. An SpO₂ of less than 90% in a child receiving 100% O₂ is an indication for additional intervention.

FYI

Function of a Pulse Oximeter

The pulse oximeter probe has 2 parts that must be placed opposite each other, so they are located on either side of a pulsatile tissue bed. Lights of different wavelengths originate from one side of the probe, and the light is captured on the other side of the tissue by the other side of the probe. A processor in the oximeter calculates the percent of each light that has been absorbed by the tissues. Hemoglobin that is fully saturated with oxygen absorbs light differently than hemoglobin that is not fully saturated with oxygen. By determining the absorption of the different wavelengths of light, the pulse oximeter can estimate the percent of hemoglobin that is fully saturated with blood.

Errors in pulse oximetry can occur if the probe is not placed across an area of pulsatile blood flow (ie, the pulses are very weak or poorly perfused, or the probe is placed so the side emitting light is not directly across from the side that captures the light). Bright light in the room can interfere with accurate detection of light absorption. In addition, because hemoglobin bound by carbon monoxide (as in carbon monoxide poisoning) absorbs light in a way that is very similar to hemoglobin that is fully saturated with oxygen, a pulse oximeter will not differentiate between carboxyhemoglobin and hemoglobin that is fully saturated with oxygen. As a result, the pulse oximeter will report falsely high values in the presence of carbon monoxide poisoning.

For additional information, see "Caution in Interpreting Pulse Oximetry Readings" in this Part.

Caution in Interpreting Pulse Oximetry Readings

Be careful to interpret pulse oximetry readings in conjunction with your clinical assessment, including consideration of signs such as respiratory rate, respiratory effort, and level of consciousness. A child may be in respiratory distress yet maintain normal O_2 saturation by increasing respiratory rate and effort, especially if supplementary O_2 is administered.

If the heart rate displayed by the pulse oximeter is not the same as the heart rate determined by electrocardiographic (ECG) monitoring, the displayed O_2 saturation is not reliable. *When the pulse oximeter does not detect a consistent pulse or there is an irregular or poor waveform, the child may have poor distal perfusion and the pulse oximeter may not be accurate—check the child and intervene as needed.* The pulse oximeter may not be accurate if the child develops severe shock and won't be accurate during cardiac arrest.

As noted above, pulse oximetry only indicates O_2 saturation and does not indicate O_2 delivery. For example, if the child is profoundly anemic (hemoglobin is very low), the saturation may be 100%, but O_2 content in the blood and O_2 delivery may be low.

The pulse oximeter does not accurately recognize methemoglobin or carboxyhemoglobin (hemoglobin bound to carbon monoxide). If carboxyhemoglobin (from carbon monoxide poisoning) is present, the pulse oximeter will reflect a falsely high O_2 saturation, because it counts the carboxyhemoglobin as fully saturated hemoglobin. If methemoglobin concentrations are above 5%, the pulse oximeter will read approximately 85% regardless of the degree of methemoglobinemia. If you suspect either of these conditions, obtain a blood gas and send it for laboratory analysis of O_2 saturation measurement by co-oximeter.

Signs of probable respiratory failure include

- Very rapid or inadequate respiratory rate; possible apnea
- Significant, inadequate, or absent respiratory effort
- Absent distal air movement
- Extreme tachycardia; bradycardia often indicates life-threatening deterioration
- Low oxygen saturation (hypoxemia) despite high-flow supplementary oxygen
- Decreased level of consciousness
- Cyanosis

Circulation

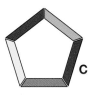

Circulation is assessed by the evaluation of

- Heart rate and rhythm
- Pulses (both peripheral and central)
- Capillary refill time
- Skin color and temperature
- Blood pressure

Urine output and level of consciousness also reflect adequacy of circulation. See the Foundational Facts box "Assessment of Urine Output" later in this Part. For more information on assessing level of consciousness, see the section "Disability" later in this Part.

Heart Rate and Rhythm

To determine heart rate, check the pulse rate, listen to the heart, or view a monitor display of the ECG or pulse oximeter waveform. The heart rate should be appropriate for the child's age, level of activity, and clinical condition (Table 8). Note that there is a wide range of normal heart rates. For example, a child who is sleeping or is athletic may have a heart rate lower than the normal range for age.

Table 8. Normal Heart Rates*

Age	Awake Rate (/min)	Sleeping Rate (/min)
Neonate	100-205	90-160
Infant	100-180	90-160
Toddler	98-140	80-120
Preschooler	80-120	65-100
School-age child	75-118	58-90
Adolescent	60-100	50-90

*Always consider the patient's normal range and clinical condition. Heart rate will normally increase with fever or stress.
Reproduced from Hazinski MF. Children are different. In: Hazinski MF, ed. *Nursing Care of the Critically Ill Child*. 3rd ed. St Louis, MO: Mosby; 2013:1-18, copyright Elsevier.

The heart rhythm is typically regular with only small fluctuations in rate. When checking the heart rate, assess for abnormalities in the monitored ECG. Cardiac rhythm disturbances (arrhythmias) result from abnormalities in, or insults to, the cardiac conduction system or heart tissue. Arrhythmias also can result from shock or hypoxia. In the advanced life support setting, an arrhythmia in a child can be broadly classified according to the observed heart rate or effect on perfusion:

Heart Rate	Classification
Slow	Bradycardia
Fast	Tachycardia
Absent	Cardiac arrest

Bradycardia is a heart rate slower than normal for a child's age and clinical condition. Slight bradycardia may be normal in athletic children, but a very slow rate in a child with other symptoms is a worrisome sign and may indicate that cardiac arrest is imminent. Hypoxia is the most common cause of bradycardia in children. If a child with bradycardia has signs of poor perfusion (decreased responsiveness, weak peripheral pulses, cool mottled skin), immediately support ventilation with a bag and mask and administer supplementary O_2. Be prepared to start chest compressions if the heart rate remains less than 60/min with signs of poor perfusion despite adequate oxygenation and ventilation. If the child with bradycardia is alert and has no signs of poor perfusion, consider other causes of a slow heart rate, such as heart block or drug overdose.

Tachycardia is a resting heart rate that is faster than the normal range for a child's age and clinical condition. Sinus tachycardia is a common, nonspecific response to a variety of conditions. It is often appropriate when the child is anxious, crying, febrile, or seriously ill or injured. To determine if the tachycardia is a sinus tachycardia or represents a cardiac rhythm disturbance, evaluate the child's history, clinical condition, and ECG. Any tachycardia that is associated with signs of circulatory compromise, including hypotension, altered mental status or signs of shock requires immediate evaluation and intervention.

Critical Concepts

Tachycardia Can Be a Sign of a Serious Condition

A heart rate that is greater than 180/min in an infant or toddler and greater than 160/min in a child older than 2 years of age warrants further assessment and may be a serious condition.

For more information, see "Part 10: Recognition of Arrhythmias."

FYI

Evaluating Heart Rate and Rhythm

Consider the following when evaluating the heart rate and rhythm in any seriously ill or injured child:

- The child's typical heart rate and baseline rhythm
- The child's level of activity and clinical condition
- The child's cardiac function and perfusion

Children with congenital heart disease may have conduction abnormalities. Consider the child's baseline ECG when interpreting heart rate and rhythm. Children with poor cardiac function are more likely to be symptomatic from arrhythmias than are children with normal cardiac function.

FYI

Relationship of Breathing to Heart Rhythm

In healthy children, the heart rate may fluctuate with the respiratory cycle, increasing with inspiration and slowing down with expiration. This condition is called *sinus arrhythmia*. Note if the child has an irregular rhythm that is not related to breathing. An irregular rhythm may indicate an underlying rhythm disturbance, such as premature ventricular or atrial contractions or an atrioventricular block.

Pulses

Evaluation of pulses is critical to the assessment of systemic perfusion in an ill or injured child. Palpate both central and peripheral pulses. Central pulses are ordinarily stronger than peripheral pulses because they are present in vessels of larger size that are located closer to the heart. Exaggeration of the difference in quality between central and peripheral pulses occurs when peripheral vasoconstriction is associated with shock. The following pulses are easily palpable in healthy infants and children (unless the child is obese or the ambient temperature is cold).

Central Pulses	Peripheral Pulses
• Femoral	• Radial
• Brachial (in infants)	• Dorsalis pedis
• Carotid (in older children)	• Posterior tibial
• Axillary	

Weak central pulses are worrisome and indicate the need for very rapid intervention to prevent cardiac arrest.

Weakening of Pulses as Perfusion Decreases

When cardiac output decreases in shock, systemic perfusion decreases incrementally. The decrease in perfusion starts in the extremities with a decrease in intensity of pulses and then an absence of peripheral pulses. As cardiac output and perfusion decrease further, there is eventual weakening of central pulses.

A cold environment can cause vasoconstriction and a discrepancy between peripheral and central pulses. However, if cardiac output remains adequate, central pulses should remain strong.

Beat-to-beat fluctuation in pulse volume may occur in children with arrhythmias (eg, premature atrial or ventricular contractions). Fluctuation in pulse volume with the respiratory cycle (pulsus paradoxus) can occur in children with severe asthma and pericardial tamponade. In an intubated child receiving positive-pressure ventilatory support, a reduction in pulse volume with each positive-pressure breath may indicate hypovolemia.

Capillary Refill Time

Capillary refill time is the time it takes for blood to return to tissue blanched by pressure. Capillary refill time increases as skin perfusion decreases. A prolonged capillary refill time may indicate low cardiac output. Normal capillary refill time is 2 seconds or less.

It is best to evaluate capillary refill in a neutral thermal environment (ie, room temperature). To evaluate capillary refill time, lift the extremity slightly above the level of the heart, press on the skin, and rapidly release the pressure. Note how many seconds it takes for the area to return to its baseline color.

Common causes of sluggish, delayed, or prolonged capillary refill (a refill time of greater than 2 seconds) are dehydration, shock, and hypothermia. Note that shock can be present despite a normal (or even brisk) capillary refill time. Children with septic shock (see "Part 8: Recognition of Shock") may have warm skin and extremities with very rapid (ie, less than 2 seconds) capillary refill time (often called *flash capillary refill*) despite the presence of shock.

Skin Color and Temperature

Monitor changes in skin color, temperature, and capillary refill time to assess a child's perfusion and response to therapy. Normal skin color and temperature should be consistent over the trunk and extremities. The mucous membranes, nail beds, palms of the hands, and soles of the feet should be pink. When perfusion deteriorates and O_2 delivery to the tissues becomes inadequate, the hands and feet are typically affected first. They may become cool, pale, dusky, or mottled. If perfusion becomes worse, the skin over the trunk and extremities may undergo similar changes.

Foundational Facts

Evaluating Skin Temperature

Consider the temperature of the child's surroundings (ie, ambient temperature) when evaluating skin color and temperature. If the ambient temperature is cool, peripheral vasoconstriction may produce mottling or pallor with cool skin and delayed capillary refill, particularly in the extremities. These changes develop despite normal cardiovascular function.

To assess skin temperature, use the back of your hand. The back of the hand is more sensitive to temperature changes than the palm, which has thicker skin. Slide the back of your hand up the extremity to determine if there is a point where the skin changes from cool to warm. Monitor this line of demarcation between warm and cool skin over time to determine the child's response to therapy. The line should move distally as the child improves.

Carefully monitor for the following skin findings (Table 9), which may indicate inadequate O_2 delivery to the tissues:

- Pallor
- Mottling
- Cyanosis

Table 9. Skin Findings, Location, and Causes

Skin Color	Location	Causes
Pallor (paleness; lack of normal color)	Skin or mucous membranes	• Normal skin color • Decreased blood supply to the skin (cold; stress; shock, especially hypovolemic and cardiogenic) • Decreased number of red blood cells (anemia) • Decreased skin pigmentation
Central pallor	Mucous membranes	• Anemia • Poor perfusion
Mottling (irregular or patchy discoloration)	Skin	• Normal distribution of skin melanin • Intense vasoconstriction from irregular supply of oxygenated blood to the skin due to hypoxemia, hypovolemia, or shock
Cyanosis (blue discoloration)	Skin or mucous membranes	
Acrocyanosis	Hands and feet and around the mouth (ie, the skin around the lips)	Normal in the newly born

(continued)

(continued)

Peripheral cyanosis	Hands and feet (beyond newborn period)	• Shock • Congestive heart failure • Peripheral vascular disease • Conditions causing venous stasis
Central cyanosis	Lips and other mucous membranes	• Low ambient O_2 tension (eg, high altitude) • Alveolar hypoventilation (eg, traumatic brain injury, drug overdose) • Diffusion defect (eg, pneumonia) • Ventilation/perfusion imbalance (eg, asthma, bronchiolitis, acute respiratory distress syndromes) • Intracardiac shunt (eg, cyanotic congenital heart disease)

Pallor, or paleness, is a lack of normal color in the skin or mucous membrane. Pallor must be interpreted within the context of other signs and symptoms. It is not necessarily abnormal and can result from lack of exposure to sunlight or inherited paleness. Pallor is often difficult to detect in a child with dark skin. Thick skin and variation in the vascularity of subcutaneous tissue also can make detection of pallor difficult. Family members often can tell you if a child's color is abnormal. Central pallor (ie, pale color of the lips and mucous membranes) strongly suggests anemia or poor perfusion. Pallor of the mucous membranes (the lips, lining of the mouth, tongue, lining of the eyes) and pale palms and soles are more likely to be clinically significant.

Mottling is an irregular or patchy discoloration of the skin. Areas may appear as an uneven combination of pink, bluish gray, or pale skin tones.

Cyanosis is a blue discoloration of the skin and mucous membranes. Blood saturated with O_2 is bright red, whereas unoxygenated blood is dark bluish-red. The location of cyanosis is important.

Acrocyanosis is a bluish discoloration of the hands and feet and of the skin around the mouth. It is a common normal finding during the newborn period.

Peripheral cyanosis (ie, bluish discoloration of the hands and feet seen beyond the newborn period) can be caused by diminished O_2 delivery to the tissues.

Central cyanosis is a blue color of the lips and other mucous membranes.

Critical Concepts

Variability in Appearance of Central Cyanosis

Cyanosis is not apparent until at least 5 g/dL of hemoglobin are desaturated (not bound to O_2). The O_2 saturation at which a child will appear cyanotic depends on the child's hemoglobin concentration. For example, in a child with a hemoglobin concentration of 16 g/dL, cyanosis will appear at an O_2 saturation of approximately 70% (ie, 30% of the hemoglobin, or 4.8 g/dL, is desaturated). If the hemoglobin concentration is low (eg, 8 g/dL), a very low O_2 saturation (eg, less than 40%) is required to produce cyanosis. Thus, cyanosis may be apparent with a milder degree of hypoxemia in a child with cyanotic congenital heart disease and polycythemia (increased amount of hemoglobin and red blood cells) but may not be apparent despite significant hypoxemia if the child is anemic.

Cyanosis may be more obvious in the mucous membranes and nail beds than in the skin, particularly if the skin is dark. It also can be seen on the soles of the feet, tip of the nose, and earlobes. As noted in the Critical Concepts box "Variability in Appearance of Central Cyanosis," children with different hemoglobin levels will be cyanotic at different levels of O_2 saturation; cyanosis is more readily detected at higher O_2 saturations if the hemoglobin level is high. The development of central cyanosis typically indicates the need for emergency intervention, such as O_2 administration and ventilatory support.

Blood Pressure

Accurate blood pressure measurement requires a properly sized cuff. The cuff bladder should cover about 40% of the mid–upper arm circumference. The blood pressure cuff should extend at least 50% to 75% of the length of the upper arm (from the axilla to the antecubital fossa). For more details, see National High Blood Pressure Education Program Working Group on High Blood Pressure in Children and Adolescents, *The Fourth Report on the Diagnosis, Evaluation, and Treatment of High Blood Pressure in Children and Adolescents*, 2005 (full reference in the Suggested Reading List on the Student Website).

Normal Blood Pressures

Table 10 lists normal blood pressures by age. This table summarizes the range of systolic and diastolic blood pressures according to age from 1 standard deviation below to 1 standard deviation above the mean in the first year of life and from the 50th to 95th percentile (assuming the 50th percentile for height) for children 1 year or older. As with heart rates, there is a wide range of values within the normal range, and normal blood pressures may fall outside the ranges listed here.

Table 10. Normal Blood Pressures

Age	Systolic Pressure (mm Hg)*	Diastolic Pressure (mm Hg)*	Mean Arterial Pressure (mm Hg)[†]
Birth (12 hours, <1000 g)	39-59	16-36	28-42[‡]
Birth (12 hours, 3 kg)	60-76	31-45	48-57
Neonate (96 hours)	67-84	35-53	45-60
Infant (1-12 months)	72-104	37-56	50-62
Toddler (1-2 years)	86-106	42-63	49-62
Preschooler (3-5 years)	89-112	46-72	58-69
School-age child (6-9 years)	97-115	57-76	66-72
Preadolescent (10-12 years)	102-120	61-80	71-79
Adolescent (12-15 years)	110-131	64-83	73-84

*Systolic and diastolic blood pressure ranges assume 50th percentile for height for children 1 year and older.
[†]Mean arterial pressures (diastolic pressure + [difference between systolic and diastolic pressure/3]) for 1 year and older, assuming 50th percentile for height.
[‡]Approximately equal to postconception age in weeks (may add 5 mm Hg).
Reproduced from Hazinski MF. Children are different. In: Hazinski MF, ed. *Nursing Care of the Critically Ill Child.* 3rd ed. St Louis, MO: Mosby; 2013:1-18, copyright Elsevier. Data from Gemelli M, Manganaro R, Mamì C, De Luca F. Longitudinal study of blood pressure during the 1st year of life. *Eur J Pediatr.* 1990;149(5):318-320; Versmold HT, Kitterman JA, Phibbs RH, Gregory GA, Tooley WH. Aortic blood pressure during the first 12 hours of life in infants with birth weight 610 to 4,220 grams. *Pediatrics.* 1981;67(5):607-613; Haque IU, Zaritsky AL. Analysis of the evidence for the lower limit of systolic and mean arterial pressure in children. *Pediatr Crit Care Med.* 2007;8(2):138-144; and National High Blood Pressure Education Program Working Group on High Blood Pressure in Children and Adolescents. *The Fourth Report on the Diagnosis, Evaluation, and Treatment of High Blood Pressure in Children and Adolescents.* Bethesda, MD: National Heart, Lung, and Blood Institute; 2005. NIH publication 05-5267.

Hypotension

Hypotension is defined by the thresholds of systolic blood pressure shown in Table 11.

Table 11. Definition of Hypotension by Systolic Blood Pressure and Age

Age	Systolic Blood Pressure (mm Hg)
Term neonates (0-28 days)	<60
Infants (1-12 months)	<70
Children 1-10 years	<70 + (age in years × 2) **(this estimates systolic blood pressure that is less than the fifth blood pressure percentile for age)***
Children >10 years	<90

*This fifth percentile is a systolic blood pressure that is lower than all but 5% of normal children (ie, it will be hypotensive for 95% of normal children).

Note that these blood pressure thresholds approximate just above the fifth percentile systolic blood pressures for age, so they will overlap with normal blood pressure values for 5% of healthy children. An observed decrease in systolic blood pressure of 10 mm Hg from baseline should prompt serial evaluations for additional signs of shock. In addition, remember that these threshold values were established in normal, resting children. Children with injury and stress typically have increased blood pressure. A blood pressure in the low-normal range may be abnormal in a seriously ill child.

Foundational Facts

Hypotension: An Ominous Sign of Impending Arrest

When hypotension develops in a child with shock, physiologic compensatory mechanisms (eg, tachycardia and vasoconstriction) have failed. Hypotension with hemorrhage is thought to be consistent with an acute loss of 20% to 25% of circulating blood volume. Hypotension in septic shock can occur from loss of intravascular volume and inappropriate vasodilation or severe vasoconstriction and inadequate cardiac output/cardiac index.

The development of bradycardia in a child with hypotension and poor perfusion is an ominous sign. Management of airway and breathing and support of adequate intravascular volume, cardiac function, and perfusion are needed to prevent cardiac arrest.

Foundational Facts

Assessment of Urine Output

Urine output can be an indirect indication of kidney perfusion. Normal urine output requires adequate blood flow and hydration. Normal values for urine output are age dependent:

Age	Normal Urine Output
Infants and young children	1.5 to 2 mL/kg per hour
Older children and adolescents	1 mL/kg per hour

Children with shock typically have decreased urine output.

Accurate measurement of urine output in all critically ill or injured children requires an indwelling catheter. Initial urine output is not a reliable indicator of the child's clinical condition because much of the urine may have been produced before the onset of symptoms. An increase in urine output is a good indicator of positive response to therapy.

Disability

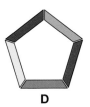

D

The disability assessment is a quick evaluation of neurologic function. Rapid assessment can use one of several tools to evaluate responsiveness and level of consciousness. Perform this evaluation at the end of the primary assessment. Repeat it during the secondary assessment to monitor for changes in the child's neurologic status.

Clinical factors that reflect brain perfusion can provide indirect evidence of circulatory function in the ill or injured pediatric patient. These signs include level of consciousness and TICLS (muscle **t**one, **i**nteractiveness, **c**onsolability, **l**ook/gaze/stare, and **s**peech/cry). Signs of inadequate O_2 delivery to the brain correlate with the severity and duration of cerebral hypoxia.

Sudden and severe cerebral hypoxia may cause the following neurologic signs:

- Decreased level of consciousness
- Loss of muscular tone
- Generalized seizures
- Pupil dilation

You may observe other neurologic signs when cerebral hypoxia develops gradually. These signs can be subtle and are best detected if repeated measurements are performed over time:

- Decreased level of consciousness with or without confusion
- Irritability
- Lethargy
- Agitation alternating with lethargy

Standard evaluations include

- AVPU (**A**lert, Responsive to **V**oice, Responsive to **P**ain, **U**nresponsive) Pediatric Response Scale
- Glasgow Coma Scale (GCS)
- Pupil response to light
- Blood glucose test

AVPU Pediatric Response Scale

To rapidly evaluate cerebral cortex function, use the AVPU Pediatric Response Scale. This scale is a system for rating a child's level of consciousness, an indicator of cerebral cortex function. The scale consists of 4 ratings:

Alert	The child is awake, active, and appropriately responsive to caregivers and external stimuli. "Appropriate response" is assessed in terms of the anticipated response based on the child's age and/or developmental level and the setting or situation.
Voice	The child responds only to voice (eg, calling the child's name or speaking loudly).
Painful	The child responds only to a painful stimulus, such as a sternal rub or pinching the trapezius
Unresponsive	The child does not respond to any stimulus.

Causes of decreased level of consciousness in children include

- Poor cerebral perfusion
- Severe shock
- Traumatic brain injury
- Seizure activity
- Encephalitis, meningitis
- Hypoglycemia
- Drugs
- Hypoxemia
- Hypercarbia

In a pediatric patient with altered mental status, hypoglycemia should be considered and blood glucose evaluated as soon as possible. *Altered mental status* refers to the range of mental states from agitation to coma. The previous terminology, *altered level of consciousness*, was felt to be confusing because it often is used to suggest and describe a depressed level of consciousness or a loss of consciousness.

Identify and Intervene

Decreased Responsiveness

If an ill or injured child has decreased responsiveness, immediately assess oxygenation, ventilation, perfusion, and blood glucose.

Glasgow Coma Scale Overview

The GCS is the most widely used method of evaluating a child's level of consciousness and neurologic status. The *best* eye opening (E), verbal (V), and motor (M) responses are individually scored (Table 12). The individual scores are then added together to produce the GCS score.

For example, a person who has spontaneous eye opening (E=4), is fully oriented (V=5), and is able to follow commands (M=6) is assigned a GCS score of 15, the highest possible score. A person with no eye opening (E=1), no verbal response (V=1), and no motor response (M=1) to a painful stimulus is assigned a GCS score of 3, the lowest possible score.

Severity of head injury is categorized into 3 levels based on GCS score after initial resuscitation:

- Mild head injury: GCS score 13 to 15
- Moderate head injury: GCS score 9 to 12
- Severe head injury: GCS score 3 to 8

Table 12. Glasgow Coma Scale

	Eye Opening		Best Motor Response		Best Verbal Response
4	Spontaneous	6	Obeys commands	5	Oriented
3	To speech	5	Localizes pain	4	Confused
2	To pain	4	Withdraws from pain	3	Inappropriate words
1	No response	3	Abnormal flexion	2	Incomprehensible words
		2	Abnormal extension	1	No response
		1	No response		

From Jennett B, Teasdale G, et al. Severe head injuries in three countries. *J Neurol Neurosurg Psychiatry.* 1977:40(3):291-298.

Glasgow Coma Scale Scoring

The GCS has been modified for preverbal or nonverbal children (Table 13). Scores for eye opening are essentially the same as in the standard GCS. The best motor response score (of a possible 6) requires that a child follow commands, so this section was adapted to accommodate the preverbal or nonverbal child. The verbal score was also adapted to assess age-appropriate responses.

Important: When using the GCS or its pediatric modification, record the individual components of the score. If the patient is intubated, unconscious, or preverbal, the most important part of this scale is motor response. Providers should carefully evaluate this component.

Table 13. Pediatric Glasgow Coma Scale*

Score	Child	Infant
Eye Opening		
4	Spontaneously	Spontaneously
3	To verbal command	To shout, speech
2	To pain	To pain
1	No response	No response
Best Motor Response		
6	Obeys commands	Spontaneous movements
5	Localizes pain	Withdraws to touch
4	Flexion-appropriate withdraw	Flexion-appropriate withdraw
3	Flexion-abnormal (decorticate rigidity)	Flexion-abnormal (decorticate rigidity)
2	Extension (decerebrate rigidity)	Extension (decerebrate rigidity)
1	No response	No response
Best Verbal Response		
5	Oriented and converses	Smiles, coos, and babbles
4	Disoriented, confused	Cries but is consolable
3	Inappropriate words	Persistent, inappropriate crying and/or screaming
2	Incomprehensible sounds	Moans, grunts to pain
1	No response	No response
Total = 3 to 15		

*Score is the sum of the individual scores from eye opening, best motor response, and best verbal response, using age-specific criteria. GCS score of 13 to 15 indicates mild head injury; GCS score of 9 to 12 indicates moderate head injury; and GCS score of ≤8 indicates severe head injury.

Modified from James HE, Trauner DA. The Glasgow Coma Score and Modified Coma Score for Infants. In: James HE, Anas NG, Perkin RM, eds. *Brain Insults in Infants and Children: Pathophysiology and Management.* Orlando, FL: Grune & Stratton Inc; 1985:179-182, copyright Elsevier.

The best disability scale for an individual child may be site specific. For example, the AVPU scale may be appropriate in the prehospital setting, whereas the GCS (particularly the motor component) or pediatric GCS may be better in the emergency department and hospital. The differences between the AVPU scale and GCS or pediatric GCS do not appear significant when associated with neurologic outcome. Each component of the AVPU scale generally correlates with the GCS scores shown in Table 14.

Table 14. AVPU Scale and Glasgow Coma Scale Equivalents

Response	GCS Score
Alert	15
Verbal	13
Painful stimulation	8
Unresponsive to noxious stimulation	6

Pupil Response to Light

Healthcare providers also should assess and record the pupillary size and response to light for each eye in any patient with altered level of consciousness. The response of pupils to light is a useful indicator of brainstem function. Normally pupils constrict in response to light and dilate in a dark environment. If the pupils fail to constrict in response to direct light (eg, flashlight directed at the eyes), suspect that brainstem injury is present. The pupils are typically equal in size, although slight variations are normal. Irregularities in pupil size or response to light may occur as a result of ocular trauma or other conditions, such as increased intracranial pressure. See Table 15 for examples of abnormal pupil responses and their possible causes.

Table 15. Abnormal Pupil Responses and Possible Causes

Abnormal Pupil Response	Possible Cause
Pinpoint pupils	• Narcotic ingestion (eg, opioid)
Dilated pupils	• Predominant sympathetic autonomic activity • Sympathomimetic ingestion (eg, cocaine) • Anticholinergic ingestion (eg, local or systemic atropine) • Increased intracranial pressure
Unilaterally dilated pupils	• Inadvertent topical absorption of a breathing treatment (eg, ipratropium) • Dilating eye drops
Unilaterally dilated pupils with altered mental status	• Ipsilateral (same side) uncal herniation (lateral herniation of the temporal lobe, caused by increased intracranial pressure)

During the disability assessment, assess and record the following for each eye:

- Size of pupils (in millimeters)
- Equality of pupil size
- Constriction of pupils to light (ie, the magnitude and rapidity of the response to light)

The acronym PERRL (**P**upils **E**qual, **R**ound, **R**eactive to **L**ight) describes the normal pupil responses to light.

Blood Glucose Test

Hypoglycemia refers to blood glucose less than or equal to 45 mg/dL in the newly born and less than or equal to 60 mg/dL in a child. It may result in brain injury if not recognized and effectively treated. Treatment decisions should be based on patient symptoms and can include oral glucose. You should monitor the blood glucose concentration of any seriously ill infant or child. A low blood glucose concentration may cause altered level of consciousness and other signs. It can cause brain injury if it is not quickly identified and adequately treated. Measure the blood glucose concentration with a point-of-care glucose test.

For more information about the recognition and treatment of hypoglycemia, see "Glucose" section in Part 9.

Exposure

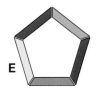

Exposure is the final component of the primary assessment. Undress the seriously ill or injured child as necessary to perform a focused physical examination. Remove clothing one area at a time to carefully observe the child's face and head, trunk (front and back), extremities, and skin. Maintain cervical spine precautions when turning any child with a suspected neck or spine injury. Keep the child comfortable and warm. If necessary, use blankets and, if available, heating lamps to prevent cold stress or hypothermia. Be sure to include an assessment of core temperature. Note any difference in warmth between trunk and extremities. Identify the presence of fever, which may indicate infection and early need for antibiotics (eg, sepsis).

During this part of the examination, look for evidence of trauma, such as bleeding, burns, or unusual markings that suggest nonaccidental trauma. Such signs include bruises in different stages of healing, injuries that don't correlate with the child's history, and delay from time of injury until the child receives medical attention.

Look for the presence and progression of petechiae and purpura (nonblanching purple discolorations in the skin caused by bleeding from capillaries and small vessels). Petechiae appear as tiny red dots and suggest a low platelet count. Purpura appears as larger areas. Both petechiae and purpura may be signs of septic shock. Also look for other rashes that may be suggestive of shock (eg, hives in anaphylactic shock).

Look for signs of injury to the extremities, including deformities or bruising. Palpate the extremities and note the child's response. If there is tenderness, suspect injury; if necessary, immobilize the extremity.

Secondary Assessment

Secondary assessment consists of a focused history and detailed physical examination with ongoing reassessment of physiologic status and response to treatment. Components of the secondary assessment are

- Focused history
- Focused physical examination
- Ongoing reassessment

Focused History

Obtain a focused history to gather information about the patient and the incident. Try to gain information that might help explain impaired respiratory or cardiovascular function. One memory aid for obtaining a focused history is the SAMPLE mnemonic. The SAMPLE mnemonic helps you gather information on a sick child in a systematic manner. Obtain an accurate timeline for all signs, symptoms, and events leading up to the current presentation. See below for details on what information to gather for each category.

Signs and symptoms	Signs and symptoms at onset of illness, such as - Breathing difficulty (eg, cough, rapid breathing, increased respiratory effort, breathlessness, abnormal breathing pattern, chest pain on deep inhalation) - Wheezing - Tachypnea - Tachycardia - Diaphoresis - Decreased level of consciousness - Agitation, anxiety - Fever - Headache - Decreased oral intake - Diarrhea, vomiting - Abdominal pain - Bleeding - Fatigue - Time course of symptoms
Allergies	- Medications, foods, latex, etc - Associated reactions
Medications	- Patient medications, including over-the-counter, vitamins, inhalers, and herbal supplements - Last dose and time of recent medications - Medications that can be found in the child's environment
Past medical history	- Health history (eg, premature birth, previous illnesses, hospitalizations) - Significant underlying medical problems (eg, asthma, chronic lung disease, congenital heart disease, arrhythmia, congenital airway abnormality, seizures, head injury, brain tumor, diabetes, hydrocephalus, neuromuscular disease) - Past surgeries - Immunization status

| **L**ast meal | • Time and nature of last intake of liquid or food (including breast or bottle feeding in infants)
• Elapsed time between last meal and presentation of current illness can affect treatment and management of the condition (eg, possible anesthesia, possible intubation) |
| **E**vents | • Events leading to current illness or injury (eg, onset sudden or gradual, type of injury)
• Hazards at scene
• Treatment during interval from onset of disease or injury until evaluation
• Estimated time of onset (if out-of-hospital onset) |

Focused Physical Examination

Next, perform a focused physical examination. The severity of the child's illness or injury should determine the extent of the physical examination. This should include careful assessment of the primary area of concern of the illness or injury (ie, respiratory assessment with respiratory distress) as well as a brief head-to-toe evaluation. Some examples of areas to assess for certain illnesses are outlined in Table 16.

Table 16. Some Examples of Areas to Assess During Physical Examination for Certain Illnesses and Injuries

Illness	Areas to Evaluate
Respiratory distress	• Nose/mouth (signs of obstruction, nasal congestion, stridor, mucosal edema) • Chest/lungs • Heart (tachycardia, gallop, or murmur) • Level of consciousness (somnolence secondary to hypercardia, anxiety secondary to hypoxia)
Suspected heart failure and/or arrhythmias	• Heart (gallop or murmur) • Lungs (crackles, difficulty breathing, intolerance of supine position) • Abdomen (evidence of hepatomegaly consistent with right heart failure) • Extremities (peripheral edema)
Trauma	• Abdomen • Back

Ongoing Reassessment

Ongoing reassessment of all patients is essential to evaluate the response to treatment and to track the progression of identified physiologic and anatomic problems. This reassessment should be applied in real time as needed based on the child's clinical condition through all phases of assessment. It should not be limited to the last part of the assessment sequence. New problems also may be identified on reassessment. Data from the reassessment will guide ongoing treatment. The elements of ongoing reassessment are

• The PAT
• The ABCDE of the primary assessment with repeat vital signs, including pulse oximetry
• Assessment of abnormal anatomic and physiologic findings
• Review of the effectiveness of treatment interventions, which may then be reviewed by returning to the PAT in a cyclic manner

Diagnostic Assessments

Diagnostic assessments help detect and identify the presence and severity of respiratory and circulatory problems. Some of these assessments (such as rapid bedside glucose or point-of-care laboratory testing) may be used early in your evaluation. The timing of diagnostic assessments is dictated by the clinical situation.

The following diagnostic assessments help assess respiratory and circulatory problems:

- Arterial blood gas (ABG)
- Venous blood gas (VBG)
- Capillary blood gas
- Hemoglobin concentration
- Central venous O_2 saturation
- Arterial lactate
- Central venous pressure monitoring
- Invasive arterial pressure monitoring
- Chest x-ray
- ECG
- Echocardiogram
- Peak expiratory flow rate (PEFR)

Arterial Blood Gas

An ABG analysis measures the partial pressure of arterial O_2 (PaO_2) and CO_2 ($PaCO_2$) dissolved in the blood plasma (ie, the liquid component of blood). An additional tool to assess the adequacy of arterial oxygenation is the pulse oximeter, a device that estimates hemoglobin saturation with O_2.

Critical Concepts	**Normal PaO_2 Does Not Confirm Adequate Blood O_2 Content**
	PaO_2 reflects only the O_2 dissolved in the arterial blood plasma. If the child's hemoglobin is only 3 g/dL, the PaO_2 may be normal or high, but O_2 delivery to the tissues will be inadequate. Because most O_2 is carried by hemoglobin in the red blood cells rather than the plasma, a hemoglobin of 3 g/dL is inadequate to carry sufficient O_2. In this case, the pulse oximeter may reflect 100% saturation despite inadequate O_2 content and delivery.

FYI	**Measurement of Arterial O_2 Saturation**
	The arterial O_2 saturation can be estimated by using a pulse oximeter, or it may be calculated from the PaO_2 and pH (by using an oxyhemoglobin dissociation curve). It may also be directly measured by using a co-oximeter. Obtain co-oximeter measurement if there is uncertainty about the calculated O_2 saturation and to rule out the presence of carbon monoxide intoxication or methemoglobinemia.

Identify respiratory failure on the basis of inadequate oxygenation (hypoxemia) or inadequate ventilation (hypercarbia). Use an ABG analysis to confirm your clinical impression and evaluate the child's response to therapy. An ABG analysis, however, is not required to initiate therapy. The following chart will help you interpret an ABG:

Diagnosis	ABG Result
Hypoxemia	Low PaO_2
Hypercarbia	High $PaCO_2$
Acidosis	pH <7.35
Alkalosis	pH >7.45

Critical Concepts

ABG and Treatment Decisions in Seriously Ill or Injured Children

Don't wait for an ABG analysis to start treatment or guide therapy. Limitations of ABG analysis in pediatric critical care include

- An ABG analysis may not be available (eg, during transport); you should not delay initiation of therapy.
- A single ABG analysis provides only information at the time the sample was obtained. It does not provide information about trends in the child's condition. Monitoring clinical response to therapy by using serial ABG analyses is often more valuable than any single ABG analysis.

Interpretation of ABG results requires consideration of the child's clinical appearance and condition. For example, an infant with bronchopulmonary dysplasia (a form of chronic lung disease) is likely to have chronic hypoxemia and hypercarbia. Diagnosis of acute respiratory failure in this infant relies heavily on clinical examination and evaluation of the arterial pH. The infant will compensate for chronic hypercarbia by renal retention of bicarbonate, and, as a result, the child's arterial pH is likely to be normal or nearly normal at baseline. Deterioration will be apparent if the child's respiratory status (ie, hypercarbia) is significantly worse than the baseline status and acidosis develops.

Hyperoxia is an increased arterial oxygen saturation detected by direct measurement of oxygen saturation in an ABG sample. This has been associated with worse outcomes, such as after return of spontaneous circulation, in the newly born and in some forms of cyanotic heart disease. Because of the uncertainty of measuring hyperoxia without ABGs, administering oxygen to achieve a displayed pulse oximetry of 100% is not recommended in these conditions.

The arterial pH and bicarbonate (HCO_3^-) concentrations obtained with ABG analysis may be useful in the diagnosis of acid-base imbalances. Note that ABG values do not reliably reflect O_2, CO_2, or acid-base status in the tissues. However, it is useful to monitor these values over time as an index of improving or worsening tissue oxygenation, as reflected by an increasing base deficit (accumulation of acid in the blood).

Venous Blood Gas

A venous blood pH, measured by VBG analysis, typically correlates well with the pH on ABG analysis. A VBG analysis is not as useful for monitoring ABG status (PaO_2 and $PaCO_2$) in acutely ill children. If the child is well perfused, the venous PCO_2 is usually within 4 to 6 mm Hg of the arterial PCO_2. If the child is poorly perfused, however, the gradient between arterial and venous PCO_2 increases. In general, venous PO_2 is not useful in the assessment of arterial oxygenation.

When interpreting a VBG, also consider the source of the venous specimen. A peripheral specimen that is free flowing from a well-perfused extremity may give results similar to the ABG, but if a tourniquet is used and the specimen is from a poorly perfused extremity, it often shows a much higher PCO_2 and lower pH than an arterial specimen. For this reason, a central venous specimen, if available, is preferred to a peripheral venous specimen. A VBG may be used if an arterial sample is unavailable. There is generally adequate correlation with ABG samples to make venous pH useful in the detection of acid-base imbalance.

Capillary Blood Gas

If arterial collection is not practical, CBG analysis can be used. Arterialization of the capillary bed yields pH and $PaCO_2$ comparable to arterial blood. A CBG analysis is not as useful for estimating arterial oxygenation (PaO_2).

Hemoglobin Concentration

Hemoglobin concentration determines the O_2-carrying capacity of the blood. O_2 content is the total amount of O_2 bound to hemoglobin plus the unbound (dissolved) O_2 in arterial blood. O_2 content is determined chiefly by the hemoglobin concentration (in grams per deciliter) and its saturation with O_2 (SaO_2). At normal hemoglobin concentrations, the amount of O_2 dissolved in the blood represents a very small part of total O_2 content. The amount of O_2 dissolved in the blood is determined by the partial pressure of arterial O_2 (PaO_2), also referred to as the *arterial oxygen tension*. For more information on the determination of the arterial oxygen content, see "Impairment of Oxygenation and Ventilation in Respiratory Problems" in Part 6.

Central Venous Oxygen Saturation

VBGs may provide a useful indicator of changes in the balance between O_2 delivery to the tissues and tissue O_2 consumption. Trends in venous O_2 saturation (SvO_2) may be used as a surrogate for monitoring trends in O_2 delivery (ie, the product of cardiac output and arterial O_2 content). Such trending assumes that O_2 consumption remains stable (an assumption that is not always correct).

Normal SvO_2 is about 70% to 75%, assuming arterial O_2 saturation is 100%. If the arterial O_2 saturation is not normal, the SvO_2 should be about 25% to 30% below the arterial O_2 saturation. For example, if the child has cyanotic heart disease and the arterial O_2 saturation is 80%, the SvO_2 should be about 55%.

When O_2 delivery to the tissues is low, the tissues consume proportionately more O_2, so the difference between arterial O_2 saturation and SvO_2 is more substantial when shock is present. For more information about SvO_2, see "Part 9: Management of Shock."

Arterial Lactate

The arterial concentration of lactate reflects the balance between lactate production and metabolism or breakdown. In a seriously ill or injured child, the arterial lactate can rise as a result of increased production of lactate (metabolic acidosis) associated with tissue hypoxia and resultant anaerobic metabolism. Arterial lactate is easy to measure, is a good prognostic indicator, and may be followed sequentially to assess the child's response to therapy. However, the potential for sampling error with lactate should be noted; it can be falsely elevated if not drawn with a free-flowing sample. Delayed testing of the sample can also affect accuracy.

An elevated lactate concentration does not always represent tissue ischemia, especially when there is no accompanying metabolic acidosis. For example, lactate concentration also can be elevated in conditions associated with increased glucose production, such as stress hyperglycemia. In general, it is more helpful to monitor trends in lactate concentration over time than any single measurement. If treatment of shock is effective, the lactate concentration should decrease. Lack of response to therapy (ie, the lactate concentration does not decrease) is more predictive of poor outcome than the initial elevated lactate concentration.

Central venous lactate concentration can be monitored if arterial blood samples are not readily available. Again, the trend in lactate concentration over time is more predictive than the initial concentration.

Invasive Arterial Pressure Monitoring

Invasive arterial pressure monitoring enables continuous evaluation and display of the systolic and diastolic blood pressures. The arterial waveform pattern may provide information about systemic vascular resistance and visual indication of a compromised cardiac output (eg, pulsus paradoxus, an exaggerated decrease in the systolic blood pressure during inspiration). Invasive arterial pressure monitoring requires an arterial catheter, monitoring (noncompliant) tubing, a transducer, and a monitoring system. Accurate measurements require that the transducer is appropriately zeroed, leveled, and calibrated. For more detailed information, see the "Hemodynamic Monitoring" section in the Suggested Reading List on the Student Website.

Near-Infrared Spectroscopy

Near-infrared spectroscopy is a noninvasive optical technique to monitor tissue oxygenation in the brain and other tissues. The monitors measure the concentrations of oxyhemoglobin and desaturated hemoglobin to determine cerebral oxygen saturation, which can be followed as an idea of central venous oxygenation trends. The cerebral oximeter electrode is placed on the forehead below the hairline. It contains 2 light-emitting diodes and light receivers that will detect light reflected from both shallow and deep tissue, and a computer analyzes the data to provide continuous measurements. Near-infrared spectroscopy monitoring has wide interpatient variability but is used to trend cerebral and other tissue oxygenation in the critical care settings.

Chest X-Ray

A chest x-ray is useful in respiratory illness to aid in the diagnosis of the following conditions:

- Airway obstruction (upper airway or lower airway)
- Lung tissue disease
- Barotrauma (pneumothorax, pneumomediastinum)
- Pleural disease (pleural effusion/pneumothorax)

A chest x-ray will show the depth of ET tube placement, but an anteroposterior (or posterior-anterior) x-ray will *not* help determine tracheal vs esophageal placement.

Use the chest x-ray in combination with clinical assessment to evaluate circulatory abnormalities. The chest x-ray may be helpful to assess heart size and presence or absence of congestive heart failure (pulmonary edema).

- A small heart is often present with reduced cardiac preload or severe lung hyperinflation.
- A large heart may be associated with normal or increased cardiac preload, pericardial effusion, congestive heart failure, or when the patient is unable to take a deep breath (eg, with severe abdominal distension).
- An x-ray taken from the front (anteroposterior view) of the heart will appear larger as compared with the heart size when taken from a posterior-anterior view.

Electrocardiogram

Obtain a 12-lead ECG to assess for cardiac arrhythmias. For more information, see "Part 11: Management of Arrhythmias."

Echocardiogram

Echocardiography is a valuable noninvasive tool for determining

- Cardiac chamber size
- Ventricular wall thickness
- Ventricular wall motion (contractility)
- Valve configuration and motion
- Pericardial space
- Estimated ventricular pressures
- Interventricular septal position
- Congenital anomalies

It can be useful in the diagnosis and evaluation of cardiac disease. Technical expertise in performing and interpreting the echocardiogram is essential.

Peak Expiratory Flow Rate

The PEFR represents the maximum flow rate generated during forced expiration. Measurement of the PEFR requires cooperation, so it can only be evaluated in children who are alert, can follow directions, and can provide a maximum effort. The PEFR decreases in the presence of airway obstruction, such as asthma. Evaluate the child's PEFR by comparing measurements with the child's personal best and also with normal values predicted from the child's height and gender. The PEFR measurement should improve in response to therapy. An asthmatic child in severe distress may not be able to cooperate with PEFR measurements. This suggests that the child has very significant respiratory distress.

Life Is Why

Science Is Why

Cardiovascular diseases claim more lives than all forms of cancer combined. This unsettling statistic drives the AHA's commitment to bring science to life by advancing resuscitation knowledge and research in new ways.

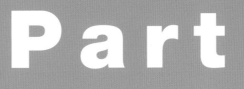
Recognition and Management of Cardiac Arrest

Overview

This section will discuss how to recognize and promptly intervene in life-threatening emergencies and cardiac arrest in infants and children. It will cover reversible causes, as well as treatments, and the Pediatric Cardiac Arrest Algorithm.

Learning Objective

By the end of this Part, you should be able to

- Recognize cardiopulmonary arrest immediately and begin CPR within 10 seconds

Preparation for the Course

During the course, you will have the opportunity to practice and be tested on CPR skills. Your performance will also be tested in 2 case scenarios.

Rapid Intervention to Prevent Cardiac Arrest

If not appropriately treated, children with respiratory failure and shock can quickly develop cardiopulmonary failure and even cardiac arrest (Figure 13). In infants and children, most cardiac arrests result from progressive respiratory failure, shock, or both. Less commonly, pediatric cardiac arrests can occur without warning (ie, with sudden collapse) secondary to an arrhythmia (ventricular fibrillation [VF] or ventricular tachycardia [VT]).

Once cardiac arrest occurs, even with optimal resuscitation efforts, the outcome is generally poor. In the out-of-hospital setting, only about 8% of children who experience cardiac arrest survive to hospital discharge. The outcome is better for children who experience cardiac arrest in the hospital, although only about 43% of those children survive to hospital discharge. For this reason, it is important to learn the concepts presented in the PALS Provider Course so that you can identify signs of respiratory failure and shock and rapidly intervene to prevent progression to cardiac arrest.

Identify and Intervene

Rapid, Systematic Intervention Is Key

Rapid, systematic intervention for seriously ill or injured infants and children is key to preventing progression to cardiac arrest. Such rapid intervention can save lives.

Pathways to Pediatric Cardiac Arrest

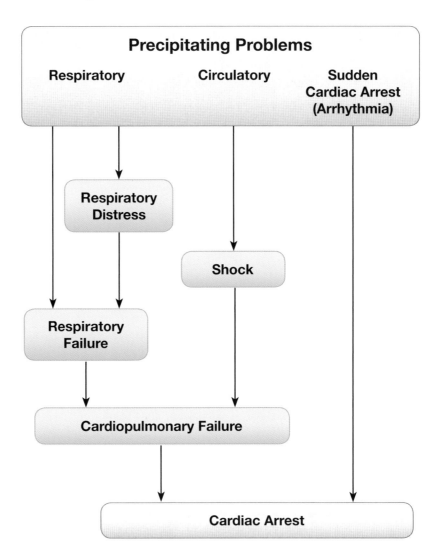

Figure 13. Pathways to pediatric cardiac arrest.

Note that respiratory conditions may progress to respiratory failure with or without signs of respiratory distress. Respiratory failure without respiratory distress occurs when the child fails to maintain an open airway or adequate respiratory effort and is typically associated with a decreased level of consciousness. Sudden cardiac arrest in children is less common than in adults, and typically results from arrhythmias such as VF or VT. During sports activities, sudden cardiac arrest can occur in children with underlying cardiac conditions that may or may not have been previously recognized. Look for fever or cooling of the extremities (or a difference between the temperature of the trunk and the extremities). Note the color of the extremities.

Life-Threatening Problems

Signs of a life-threatening condition are listed in Table 17.

Table 17. Signs of a Life-Threatening Condition

Airway	Complete or severe airway obstruction
Breathing	Apnea, significant increased work of breathing, bradypnea
Circulation	Weak or absent pulses, poor perfusion, hypotension, bradycardia
Disability	Unresponsiveness, decreased level of consciousness
Exposure	Significant hypothermia, significant bleeding, petechiae, or purpura consistent with septic shock or coagulation problem

Interventions

Activate the emergency response system as indicated in your practice setting and begin lifesaving interventions in the following circumstances:

- If the child has a life-threatening condition
- If you are uncertain or "something feels wrong"

If the child does not have a life-threatening condition, begin the secondary assessment and diagnostic assessments.

Cardiac Arrest in Infants and Children

In contrast to adults, cardiac arrest in infants and children does not usually result from a primary cardiac cause (ie, sudden cardiac arrest). It is typically the end result of progressive respiratory failure or shock. This form of arrest is referred to as a *hypoxic, asphyxial,* or a *hypoxic-ischemic arrest*; the term *hypoxic/asphyxial arrest* will be used in this Part. It occurs most often in infants and young children, especially those with underlying disease. Respiratory failure and shock can generally be reversed if identified and treated early. If they progress to cardiac arrest, the outlook is generally poor.

Sudden cardiac arrest from ventricular arrhythmia occurs in about 5% to 15% of all pediatric in-hospital cardiac arrests (IHCAs) and out-of-hospital cardiac arrests (OHCAs). Although a shockable rhythm (ie, VF or pulseless ventricular tachycardia [pVT]) is the presenting rhythm in only about 14% of pediatric in-hospital arrests, it is present in up to 27% of such arrests at some point during the resuscitation. For more details, see Nadkarni et al. *JAMA.* 2006;295:50-57 in the Suggested Reading List on the Student Website and the FYI box below. The incidence of cardiac arrest from VF/pVT increases with age and should be suspected in any patient with a sudden collapse. Increasing evidence suggests that sudden unexpected death in young people is often associated with underlying cardiac conditions.

FYI

Survival Rates From Pediatric Cardiac Arrest

Survival rates from pediatric cardiac arrest vary according to the location of the arrest and the presenting rhythm. Information about in-hospital pediatric arrests is now available from Get With The Guidelines®-Resuscitation (formerly the National Registry of Cardiopulmonary Resuscitation).

Rate of survival to hospital discharge is higher if the arrest occurs in-hospital (43%) compared with out-of-hospital (8%). Intact neurologic survival is also much higher if the arrest occurs in-hospital.

Survival is higher (about 25% to 34%) when the presenting rhythm is shockable (VF or pVT) compared with asystole (about 7% to 24%). Survival for a presenting rhythm of pulseless electrical activity (PEA) is about 38% for in-hospital arrest. Conversely, when VF/pVT develops as a secondary rhythm during a resuscitation attempt (ie, not as the initial arrest rhythm) in hospitalized children, survival is lower than that observed in cardiac arrests with nonshockable rhythms (11% vs 27% survival to discharge). The highest survival rate (64%) occurs when there is bradycardia and poor perfusion, and chest compressions and ventilation are provided before pulseless arrest develops.

 For more details, see the "Epidemiology and Outcome" and "CPR Quality" sections in the Suggested Reading List on the Student Website. For additional information about in-hospital resuscitation outcomes, see the Get With The Guidelines-Resuscitation website: **www.heart.org/resuscitation.**

Despite the improved outcome of in-hospital CPR, a majority of children with IHCA, and an even larger percentage of children with OHCA, do not survive or they survive with significant neurologic impairment. Because outcome from cardiac arrest is so poor, focus should be placed on prevention of cardiac arrest through

- Prevention of disease processes and injuries that can lead to cardiac arrest
- Early recognition and management of respiratory distress, respiratory failure, and shock before they cause cardiac arrest

Definition of Cardiac Arrest

Cardiac arrest is the cessation of blood circulation resulting from absent or ineffective cardiac mechanical activity. Clinically, the child is unresponsive and not breathing or only gasping. There is no detectable pulse. Cerebral hypoxia causes the child to lose consciousness and stop breathing, although agonal gasps may be observed during the first minutes after sudden arrest. When circulation stops, the resulting organ and tissue ischemia can cause cell, organ, and patient death if not rapidly reversed.

Pathways to Cardiac Arrest

The 2 pathways to cardiac arrest in children are

- Hypoxic/asphyxial
- Sudden cardiac arrest

Hypoxic/Asphyxial Arrest

Hypoxic/asphyxial arrest is the most common cause of cardiac arrest in infants, children, and adolescents. It is the end result of progressive tissue hypoxia and acidosis caused by respiratory failure or hypotensive shock. Regardless of the initiating event or disease process, the final common pathway preceding cardiac arrest is cardiopulmonary failure (Figure 13).

Critical Concepts

Prioritize Airway and Breathing in Children in Cardiac Arrest

In contrast to adults, infants and children usually arrest as the result of progression of respiratory failure or shock. As a result, the child's arterial oxygen content and oxygen delivery to the tissues are often low by the time of arrest. Although C-A-B sequence for CPR is used for both adults and children, establishment of adequate airway, oxygenation, and ventilation should be a particularly high priority in children during CPR.

Identify and Intervene

Stop Progression to Cardiac Arrest

It is important to identify and treat respiratory distress, respiratory failure, and shock before progression to cardiopulmonary failure and cardiac arrest. Early identification and treatment are crucial to saving the lives of seriously ill or injured children.

Sudden Cardiac Arrest

Sudden cardiac arrest is less common in children than in adults. It is most often caused by the sudden development of VF or pVT. Predisposing conditions or causes for sudden cardiac arrest may include

- Hypertrophic cardiomyopathy
- Anomalous coronary artery
- Long QT syndrome or other channelopathies
- Myocarditis
- Drug intoxication (eg, digoxin, ephedra, cocaine)
- Commotio cordis (ie, sharp blow to the chest)

Primary prevention of some episodes of pediatric cardiac arrest may be possible with cardiovascular screening (eg, for hypertrophic cardiomyopathy or long QT syndrome) and treatment of predisposing problems (eg, myocarditis or anomalous coronary artery). Some cases of sudden cardiac arrest in children and young adults are associated with genetic mutations that cause cardiac ion channelopathies. A *channelopathy* is a disorder of the ion channels in myocardial cells that predisposes the heart to arrhythmias. These genetic mutations are present in 2% to 10% of victims and 14% to 20% of young adults with sudden cardiac death when no cause of death is found in a routine autopsy. Because these mutations can be genetically inherited, a careful family history to identify syncopal episodes, seizures, sudden and unexplained death (including sudden infant death syndrome [SIDS], drowning, and even a motor vehicle crash) might indicate the presence of a familial channelopathy.

Secondary prevention of death from sudden cardiac arrest requires prompt and effective resuscitation, including timely defibrillation. Most episodes of sudden cardiac arrest in children occur during athletic activity. Prompt treatment of sudden cardiac arrest in children will be possible only if coaches, trainers, parents, and the general public are aware that sudden cardiac arrest can occur in children. Bystanders must be prepared and willing to activate the emergency response system, provide high-quality CPR, and use an AED as soon as one is available.

Causes of Cardiac Arrest

Causes of cardiac arrest in children vary based on the child's age and underlying health. Causes also vary based on event location (in-hospital vs out-of-hospital).

Most OHCA in infants and children occur at or near the home. SIDS is a leading cause of death in infants younger than 6 months of age. The frequency of SIDS has decreased with the "Back to Sleep" campaign, which instructs parents to place infants on their backs to sleep. See the "SIDS" section of the Suggested Reading List on the Student Website for a reference on SIDS.

Co-bedding is an increasing cause of death in the infant population. Therefore, it is important that parents also be instructed that infants should have their own sleep space. Trauma is the predominant cause of death in children 6 months of age through young adulthood. Causes of traumatic cardiac arrest include airway compromise, tension pneumothorax, hemorrhagic shock, and brain injury.

Cardiac arrest in children may be associated with a reversible condition. Review of the H's and T's (see the Identify and Intervene box "H's and T's" later in this Part) will help you identify reversible causes. The most common immediate causes of pediatric cardiac arrest are respiratory failure and hypotensive shock. Arrhythmia is a less common cause of arrest.

Identify and Intervene

H's and T's

Cardiac arrest in children may be associated with a reversible condition. If you don't think about reversible causes or complicating factors, you are likely to miss them. Review the following H's and T's to help you identify potentially reversible causes of cardiac arrest or factors that may be complicating resuscitative efforts.

H's	T's
Hypovolemia	**T**ension pneumothorax
Hypoxia	**T**amponade (cardiac)
Hydrogen ion (acidosis)	**T**oxins
Hypoglycemia	**T**hrombosis, pulmonary
Hypo-/Hyperkalemia	**T**hrombosis, coronary
Hypothermia	

Also consider unrecognized trauma (eg, abdominal injury and hemorrhage) as a cause of cardiac arrest, especially in infants and young children.

Identifying a Child at Risk for Cardiac Arrest

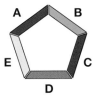

Children with the combination of severe respiratory failure and shock will likely develop cardiac arrest within minutes unless you intervene immediately. Be alert for signs of inadequate oxygenation, ventilation, and tissue perfusion.

Identify and Intervene

Respiratory Failure and Shock

Detect and treat respiratory failure and shock before the child deteriorates to cardiopulmonary failure and cardiac arrest.

Recognition of Cardiac Arrest

Signs of cardiac arrest are

- Unresponsiveness
- No breathing or only gasping
- No pulse (assess for no more than 10 seconds)

Arrest rhythm may be noted on the cardiac monitor. However, monitoring is not mandatory for recognition of cardiac arrest.

If a child is unresponsive and not breathing (agonal gasps aren't effective breathing), try to palpate a central pulse (brachial in an infant, carotid or femoral in a child). Because even healthcare providers are unable to reliably detect a pulse, take no more than 10 seconds to try to palpate the pulse. If there is no pulse or you are not sure if a pulse is present, start CPR, beginning with chest compressions.

Arrest Rhythms

Cardiac arrest is associated with one of the following rhythms, also known as *arrest rhythms* or *states*:

- Asystole
- PEA
- VF
- pVT, including torsades de pointes

Asystole and PEA are the most common initial rhythms seen in both in-hospital and out-of-hospital pediatric cardiac arrest, especially in children younger than 12 years of age. Slow wide QRS complex rhythms that immediately precede asystole are often referred to as *agonal rhythms* (Figure 14). VF and pVT are more likely terminal rhythms in older children with sudden collapse or in children with underlying cardiovascular conditions.

Asystole

Asystole is cardiac standstill without discernable electrical activity. It is represented by a straight (flat) line on the electrocardiogram (ECG). Do not rely on the ECG for a diagnosis of cardiac arrest; always confirm it clinically because a "flat line" on the ECG also can be caused by a loose ECG lead.

You can recall potentially reversible causes of asystole by remembering the H's and T's (see the Identify and Intervene box "H's and T's" earlier in this Part).

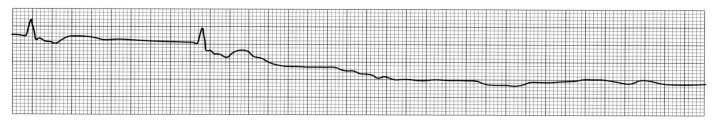

Figure 14. Agonal rhythm (slow ventricular rhythm progressing to asystole).

Pulseless Electrical Activity

PEA is not a specific rhythm. It is a term describing any organized electrical activity (ie, not VF or asystole) on an ECG or cardiac monitor that is associated with no *palpable* pulses; pulsations may be detected by an arterial waveform or Doppler study, but pulses are not palpable. The rate of electrical activity may be slow (most common), normal, or fast. Very slow PEA may be referred to as *agonal*.

In PEA, the ECG may display normal or wide QRS complexes or other abnormalities, including

- Low- or high-amplitude T waves
- Prolonged PR and QT intervals
- Atrioventricular dissociation, complete heart block, or ventricular complexes without P waves

Assess the monitored rhythm and note the rate and width of the QRS complexes.

PEA may be caused by reversible conditions easily recalled by remembering the H's and T's. (See the Identify and Intervene box "H's and T's" earlier in this Part.) Unless you can quickly identify and treat the cause of PEA, the rhythm will likely deteriorate to asystole.

Ventricular Fibrillation

When VF is present, the heart has no organized rhythm and no coordinated contractions (Figure 15). Electrical activity is chaotic. The heart quivers and does not pump blood. Therefore, pulses are not palpable. VF may be preceded by a brief period of VT with or without pulses.

Primary VF is uncommon in children. In studies of pediatric cardiac arrest, VF was the initial rhythm in 5% to 15% of both OHCAs and IHCAs. Overall prevalence may be higher because VF may occur early during an arrest and quickly deteriorate to asystole. VF has been reported in up to 27% of pediatric in-hospital arrests at some point during the resuscitation.

VF without a previously known underlying cause may occasionally occur in otherwise healthy teens during sports activities. The cause of VF may be an undiagnosed cardiac abnormality or channelopathy, such as long QT syndrome. Sudden impact to the chest from a collision or moving object may result in commotio cordis, leading to VF. Consider the H's and T's for other potential reversible causes.

Survival and outcome of patients with VF or pVT as the *initial* arrest rhythm are generally better than those of patients presenting with asystole or PEA. Outcome may be improved by prompt recognition and provision of CPR and defibrillation.

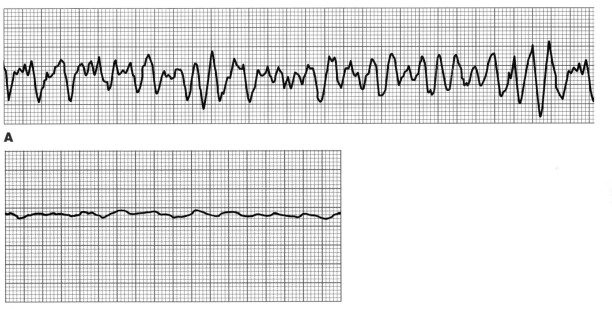

A

B

Figure 15. Ventricular fibrillation. **A,** Coarse VF. High-amplitude electrical activity varies in size and shape, representing chaotic ventricular electrical activity with no identifiable P, ORS, or T waves. **B,** Fine VF. Electrical activity is reduced as compared with previous (**A**) rhythm strip.

Part 4

Pulseless Ventricular Tachycardia

VT may produce pulses or may be a form of pulseless arrest of ventricular origin. Because the treatment of pVT differs from the treatment of VT with a pulse, pulse assessment is needed to determine appropriate treatment. Almost any cause of VT can present without detectable pulses. Unlike VF, pVT is characterized by organized, wide QRS complexes (Figure 16A). This form of pulseless arrest is usually of brief duration before it deteriorates into VF. See "Part 10: Recognition of Arrhythmias" for more information.

pVT is treated exactly the same as VF. See the Pediatric Cardiac Arrest Algorithm in the Management of Cardiac Arrest section (Figure 18).

Torsades de Pointes (Turning on a Point)

pVT may be monomorphic (ventricular complexes appear uniform) or polymorphic (ventricular complexes do not look alike). Torsades de pointes is a distinctive form of polymorphic VT (Figure 16B). This arrhythmia is seen in conditions distinguished by a prolonged QT interval, including congenital long QT syndrome, drug toxicity, and electrolyte abnormalities (eg, hypomagnesemia). See "Part 10: Recognition of Arrhythmias" for more information.

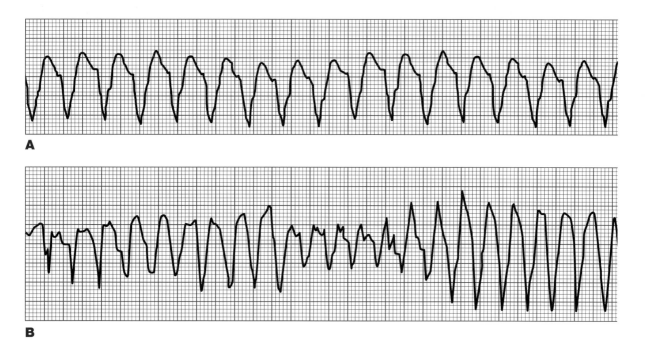

A

B

Figure 16. Ventricular tachycardia (VT). **A,** VT in a child with muscular dystrophy and known cardiomyopathy. The ventricular rhythm is rapid and regular at a rate of 158/min (greater than the minimum 120/min characteristic of VT). The QRS is wide (greater than 0.09 second), and there is no evidence of atrial depolarization. The complexes are uniform in appearance, so the VT is monomorphic. **B,** Torsades de pointes in a child with hypomagnesemia. The complexes differ in appearance, so this is a form of polymorphic VT. With this form of VT, the complexes appear to be "turning on a point."

Management of Cardiac Arrest

High-Quality CPR

High-quality CPR is the foundation of basic and advanced life support for the management of cardiac arrest. BLS focuses on preparing providers to perform CPR skills. CPR is a lifesaving procedure for a victim who has signs of cardiac arrest (ie, unresponsive, no normal breathing, and no pulse). Components of CPR are chest compressions and breaths.

High-quality CPR improves a victim's chances of survival. Study and practice the characteristics of high-quality CPR so that you can perform each skill effectively.

The *2010 AHA Guidelines for CPR and ECC* recommended a change in the CPR sequence from A-B-C (Airway-Breathing-Circulation/Compressions) to C-A-B (Compressions-Airway-Breathing). After a review of the literature, the C-A-B sequence for BLS was reaffirmed. Consistency in the order of compressions, airway, and breathing for CPR in victims of all ages may be easiest for rescuers who treat people of all ages to remember and perform. Maintaining the same sequence for adults and children offers consistency in teaching.

Foundational Facts

Minimize Interruptions in Chest Compressions

Chest compressions should be minimally interrupted. Attempt to limit any interruptions (eg, for ventilation [until an advanced airway is placed], rhythm check, and shock delivery) to less than 10 seconds if at all possible.

FYI

Hands-Only (Compression-Only) CPR

Hands-Only (compression-only) CPR is easy for an untrained rescuer to perform and can be readily guided by dispatchers over the telephone for adult victims of cardiac arrest. In addition, adult survival rates from sudden witnessed cardiac arrest are similar with either Hands-Only CPR or CPR with both compressions and rescue breathing. However, for the trained lay rescuer who is able and for all healthcare providers, the recommendation remains for the rescuer to perform both compressions and ventilation. Ventilation is a critical part of resuscitation from hypoxic/asphyxial arrest, such as occurs in most pediatric arrest as well as with drowning and drug overdose.

Critical Concepts

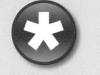

CPR in Hypoxic/Asphyxial Arrest

Conventional CPR (chest compressions and rescue breaths) should be provided for pediatric cardiac arrests. The asphyxial nature of the majority of pediatric cardiac arrests necessitates ventilation as part of effective CPR. However, because compression-only CPR is effective in patients with sudden, witnessed cardiac arrest, if rescuers are unwilling or unable to deliver breaths, we recommend rescuers perform compression-only CPR.

Please review the fundamentals of BLS in Table 18. These recommendations are based on the *2015 AHA Guidelines Update for CPR and ECC*.

Table 18. Summary of High-Quality CPR Components for BLS Providers

Component	Adults and Adolescents	Children (Age 1 Year to Puberty)	Infants (Age Less Than 1 Year, Excluding Newborns)
Scene safety	Make sure the environment is safe for rescuers and victim		
Recognition of cardiac arrest	Check for responsiveness No breathing or only gasping (ie, no normal breathing) No definite pulse felt within 10 seconds (Breathing and pulse check can be performed simultaneously in less than 10 seconds)		
Activation of emergency response system	If you are alone with no mobile phone, leave the victim to activate the emergency response system and get the AED before beginning CPR Otherwise, send someone and begin CPR immediately; use the AED as soon as it is available	*Witnessed collapse* Follow steps for adults and adolescents on the left *Unwitnessed collapse, single rescuer* Give 2 minutes of CPR Leave the victim to activate the emergency response system and get the AED Return to the child or infant and resume CPR; use the AED as soon as it is available	
Compression-ventilation ratio *without advanced airway*	*1 or 2 rescuers* 30:2	*1 rescuer* 30:2 *2 or more rescuers* 15:2	
Compression-ventilation ratio *with advanced airway*	Continuous compressions at a rate of 100-120/min Give 1 breath every 6 seconds (10 breaths/min)		
Compression rate	100-120/min		
Compression depth	At least 2 inches (5 cm)*	At least one third AP diameter of chest About 2 inches (5 cm)	At least one third AP diameter of chest About 1½ inches (4 cm)
Hand placement	2 hands on the lower half of the breastbone (sternum)	2 hands or 1 hand (rescuer can use either method on a small child) on the lower half of the breastbone (sternum)	*1 rescuer* 2 fingers in the center of the chest, just below the nipple line *2 or more rescuers* 2 thumb–encircling hands in the center of the chest, just below the nipple line
Chest recoil	Allow full recoil of chest after each compression; do not lean on the chest after each compression		
Minimizing interruptions	Limit interruptions in chest compressions to less than 10 seconds		

*Compression depth should be no more than 2.4 inches (6 cm).

Monitoring for CPR Quality

During the resuscitation attempt, the team leader as well as team members should monitor CPR quality. Use good team communication to ensure that chest compressions are the appropriate depth and rate, that the chest is allowed to fully recoil after each compression, and that ventilation is not excessive (Table 19).

Table 19. High-Quality CPR

Push fast	• Push at a rate of 100 to 120 compressions per minute for infants, children, and adults
Push hard	• Push with enough force to depress the chest at least one third the anteroposterior diameter of the chest in pediatric patients (infants [younger than 1 year] to children up to the onset of puberty). This equates to approximately 1½ inches (4 cm) in infants and 2 inches (5 cm) in children. Once children have reached puberty (ie, adolescents), the recommended adult compression depth of at least 2 inches (5 cm), but no greater than 2.4 inches (6 cm), is used.
Allow complete chest recoil	• Allow complete chest recoil after each compression; this allows the heart to refill with blood.
Minimize interruptions	• Try to limit interruptions in chest compressions to 10 seconds or less or as needed for interventions (eg, defibrillation). Ideally, compressions are interrupted only for ventilation (until an advanced airway is placed), rhythm check, and actual shock delivery. • Once an advanced airway is in place, provide continuous chest compressions and asynchronous ventilation (ie, without pausing compressions for ventilation).
Avoid excessive ventilation	• Each rescue breath should be given over about 1 second. • Each breath should result in visible chest rise. • After an advanced airway is in place, deliver 10 breaths per minute (1 breath every 6 seconds), being careful to avoid excessive ventilation.

Many in-hospital patients, especially if they are in an intensive care unit, have advanced monitoring in place; some have advanced airways and are receiving mechanical ventilation. Continuous monitoring of the child's end-tidal CO_2 ($PETCO_2$) can provide indirect evidence of the quality of chest compressions (Figure 17). If $PETCO_2$ is less than 10 to 15 mm Hg, cardiac output during CPR is probably low and not much blood is being delivered to the lungs. Efforts should be made to verify that cardiac compressions are effective, with a goal of increasing the $PETCO_2$ to greater than 10 to 15 mm Hg. If the child has an indwelling arterial catheter, use the waveform as feedback to evaluate hand position and chest compression depth. A minor adjustment of hand position or depth of compression can significantly improve the amplitude of the arterial waveform, reflecting better chest compression–induced stroke volume and cardiac output. Verify that ventilation is not excessive. Both the $PETCO_2$ and arterial waveform may be useful in identification of return of spontaneous circulation (ROSC).

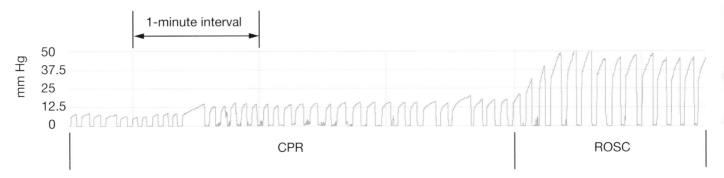

Figure 17. Capnography to monitor effectiveness of resuscitative efforts.

This capnography tracing displays the P_{ETCO_2} in mm Hg on the vertical axis over time (time is depicted horizontally). This patient is intubated and receiving CPR. Note that the ventilation rate is approximately 8 to 10/min. Chest compressions in this patient were given continuously at a rate slightly faster than 100/min but are not visible with this tracing. The initial P_{ETCO_2} is less than 12.5 mm Hg during the first minute, indicating very low blood flow. The P_{ETCO_2} increases to between 12.5 and 25 mm Hg during the second and third minutes, consistent with the increase in blood flow with ongoing resuscitation. ROSC occurs during the fourth minute. ROSC is identifiable by the abrupt increase in the P_{ETCO_2} (visible just after the fourth vertical line) to over 40 mm Hg, which is consistent with a substantial improvement in blood flow with ROSC.

Life Is Why

Saving Lives Is Why

Cardiac arrest remains a leading cause of death, so the AHA trains millions of people each year to help save lives both in and out of the hospital. This course is a key part of that effort.

PALS in Cardiac Arrest

The immediate goal of therapeutic interventions for cardiac arrest is ROSC. ROSC has occurred when there is resumption of an organized cardiac electrical rhythm on the monitor plus palpable central pulses. Corresponding clinical evidence of perfusion will also be apparent (eg, sudden increase in P_{ETCO_2}, measurable blood pressure, improved color).

PALS to treat cardiac arrest may include the following:

- Rhythm assessment (shockable vs nonshockable)
- Establishment of vascular access
- Defibrillation
- Medication therapy
- Advanced airway management

Foundational Facts

Factors of a Successful Resuscitation

Remember that the success of any resuscitation is built on a strong base of high-quality CPR, timely shock delivery for any shockable rhythm, and good teamwork.

Arrest Rhythm Assessment

Identifying the arrest rhythm as shockable or nonshockable determines the applicable pathway of the Pediatric Cardiac Arrest Algorithm. The algorithm outlines the recommended sequence of CPR, shocks, and medication administration for both shockable and nonshockable pediatric cardiac arrest rhythms. Although the algorithm depicts actions sequentially, many actions (eg, compressions and medication administration) are typically performed simultaneously when multiple rescuers are present.

Vascular Access

Priorities for drug delivery routes during PALS are (in order of preference)

1. Intravenous

2. Intraosseous

3. Endotracheal

When the critically ill child develops cardiac arrest, vascular access may already be established. If vascular access is not present, it should be established immediately. Peripheral IV access is the first choice during resuscitation if it can be placed rapidly, but placement may be difficult in critically ill or injured children. Limit the time you spend trying to obtain IV access in a seriously ill or injured child. If IV access is not already present and you cannot achieve reliable IV access immediately, establish IO access. *IO access is useful as the initial vascular access in cases of cardiac arrest.* If neither IV nor IO access is available for delivery of medications, the endotracheal (ET) route is a third option.

Intravenous Route

Although a central venous catheter provides a more secure route of vascular access than a peripheral catheter, central venous access is not needed during most resuscitation attempts and its placement requires interruptions in chest compressions. Complications of central catheter placement attempts that are made during chest compressions may include vascular lacerations, hematomas, pneumothorax, and bleeding. If a central venous catheter is already in place, it is the preferred route for drug and fluid administration. Central venous administration of medications provides more rapid onset of action and higher peak concentration than peripheral venous delivery.

Establishing peripheral venous access does not require interruption of CPR, but drug delivery to the central circulation may be delayed. To improve drug delivery to the central circulation, do the following when administrating drugs into a peripheral IV catheter infusion system:

- Give the drug by bolus injection
- Give the drug while chest compressions are being performed
- Follow with a 5-mL flush of normal saline to move the drug from the peripheral to the central circulation

Intraosseous Route

If IV access is not available, drugs and fluids can be delivered safely and effectively via the IO route. In fact, the IO route is useful as the initial route of vascular access in cases of cardiac arrest. Important points about IO access are

- IO access can be established in all age groups
- IO access can often be achieved in 30 to 60 seconds
- The IO route is preferred over the ET route
- Any drug or fluid that can be administered IV can be administered IO

IO cannulation provides access to a noncollapsible marrow venous plexus, which serves as a rapid, safe, and reliable route for administration of resuscitation drugs and fluids. The technique uses a rigid needle, preferably a specially designed IO or bone marrow needle. Although an IO needle with a stylet is preferred to prevent obstruction of the needle with cortical bone during insertion, butterfly needles, standard hypodermic needles, and spinal needles can be inserted successfully and used effectively. Powered IO insertion devices are commercially available and are widely used in the United States. See the "Resources for Management of Circulatory Emergencies" at the end of Part 9 for more information on IO access.

Endotracheal Route

The IV and IO routes are preferable to the ET route for administration of drugs. Lipid-soluble drugs can be given by the ET route. These include lidocaine, epinephrine, atropine, and naloxone (LEAN) and vasopressin. However, there are limited human studies about ET vasopressin administration and limited studies to provide dosing guidelines for most drugs given by the ET route.

When considering administration of drugs via the ET route during CPR, keep these concepts in mind:

- Drug absorption from the tracheobronchial tree is unpredictable, so drug concentrations and drug effects will be unpredictable.
- The optimal dose of most drugs given by the ET route is unknown.
  - Drug administration into the trachea results in lower blood concentrations than the same dose given via IV or IO routes.
  - Animal data suggest that the lower epinephrine concentrations achieved when the drug is delivered by the ET route may produce transient but detrimental β-adrenergic–mediated vasodilation.
- Recommended drug doses administered by the ET route are higher than for the IV/IO route.
  - The recommended ET dose of epinephrine is 10 times the IV/IO dose.
  - The typical ET dose of other drugs is 2 to 3 times the IV/IO dose.

Foundational Facts

Technique for Administering Medication by ET Route

If a drug is given by the ET route, administer it as follows:

- Instill the drug into the ET tube (briefly pause compressions during instillation).
- Follow with a minimum of 5 mL normal saline flush; a smaller volume may be used in neonates.
- Provide 5 rapid positive-pressure breaths after the drug is instilled.

Defibrillation

A defibrillation shock "stuns" the heart by depolarizing a critical mass of the myocardium. If a shock is successful, it terminates VF. This allows the heart's natural pacemaker cells to resume an organized rhythm. The return of an organized rhythm alone, however, does not ensure survival. The organized rhythm must ultimately produce effective cardiac mechanical activity that results in ROSC, defined by the presence of palpable central pulses. If the child's P_{ETCO_2} or intra-arterial pressure is being monitored, it also can be used to provide an indication of ROSC (Figure 17).

When attempting defibrillation, provide compressions until the defibrillator is charged, deliver 1 shock, and immediately resume CPR, starting with chest compressions. Chest compressions are needed to maintain blood flow to the heart (the coronary circulation) and brain until effective cardiac contractility resumes. There is no evidence that performance of chest compressions in a child with spontaneous cardiac activity is harmful. If VF is not eliminated by a shock, the heart is probably ischemic. Resumption of chest compressions is likely to be of greater value to the child than immediate delivery of a second shock.

In an out-of-hospital or unmonitored setting, do not waste time looking for a shockable rhythm or palpating a pulse immediately after shock delivery; neither is likely to be present. Resume high-quality CPR, beginning with chest compressions. This sequence may be modified at a provider's direction in hospital units with invasive arterial monitoring. In in-hospital settings with invasive monitoring in place, return of an arterial waveform or a sudden increase in P_{ETCO_2} suggests ROSC. When evidence of ROSC is indicated by monitored parameters, confirm by palpating a central pulse.

For more information about the manual defibrillation procedure, see the Critical Concepts box "Manual Defibrillation (for VF or pVT)" later in this Part.

Critical Concepts

Defibrillation and CPR

If a shock eliminates VF, continue CPR because most victims have asystole or PEA immediately after shock delivery.

Medication Therapy

The objectives for medication administration during cardiac arrest are to

- Increase coronary and cerebral perfusion pressures and blood flow
- Stimulate spontaneous or more forceful myocardial contractility
- Accelerate heart rate
- Correct and treat the possible cause of cardiac arrest
- Suppress or treat arrhythmias

Medications that may be used during treatment of pediatric cardiac arrest are listed in Table 20.

Table 20. Pediatric Cardiac Arrest Medications

Agent	Indication	Mechanism(s) of Action	Clinical Data
Vasopressors			
Epinephrine	• Used for cardiac arrest associated with VF/pVT as well as asystole/PEA • High doses may be considered for special resuscitation circumstances, such as β-blocker overdose	• Causes α-adrenergic–mediated vasoconstriction that increases aortic diastolic pressure and coronary perfusion pressure, a critical determinant of successful resuscitation	• Both beneficial and toxic physiologic effects during CPR have been demonstrated in animal and human studies • No adult or pediatric studies have demonstrated improved survival with use of epinephrine • High doses may be harmful, particularly in hypoxic/asphyxial arrest • No survival benefit from routine use of high-dose IV/IO epinephrine
Antiarrhythmics			
Amiodarone	• May be used for shock-refractory VF or pVT	• α-Adrenergic and β-adrenergic blocking activity • Affects sodium, potassium, and calcium channels • Slows atrioventricular conduction • Prolongs the atrioventricular refractory period and QT interval • Slows ventricular conduction (widens the QRS)	• Increased survival to hospital admission but not to hospital discharge compared with placebo or lidocaine for shock-resistant VF in adults • No association between amiodarone use and ROSC, 24-hour survival, or survival to hospital discharge in pediatric observational study
Lidocaine	• May be used for treatment of shock-refractory VF or pVT in children	• Decreases automaticity and suppresses ventricular arrhythmias	Pediatric observational data showed improved ROSC with the use of lidocaine as compared with no lidocaine No association between lidocaine use and survival to hospital discharge
Magnesium sulfate	• Used for the treatment of torsades de pointes • Used for hypomagnesemia	• Used for treatment of arrhythmias associated with hypomagnesemia	• Insufficient evidence to recommend for or against routine use in pediatric cardiac arrest not associated with torsades de pointes or hypomagnesemia

Agent	Indication	Mechanism(s) of Action	Clinical Data
Other Agents			
Atropine	• Indicated for treatment of bradycardia, especially if it results from excessive vagal tone, cholinergic drug toxicity (eg, organophosphates), or complete atrioventricular block	• Increases heart rate	• No published studies suggesting efficacy for treatment of cardiac arrest in pediatric patients • See complete discussion in "Part 11: Management of Arrhythmias"
Calcium	• Routine use in cardiac arrest is not recommended • Indicated for documented ionized hypocalcemia (relatively common in critically ill children, particularly during sepsis or after cardiopulmonary bypass) and hyperkalemia, particularly in children with hemodynamic compromise • May also be considered for hypermagnesemia or calcium channel blocker overdose	• Restores calcium • Helps maintain the cell membrane action potential threshold • Helps maintain the gradient between intracellular potassium and extracellular sodium	• Does not improve survival in cardiac arrest and may be harmful
Sodium bicarbonate	• Routine administration in cardiac arrest is not recommended • Recommended for symptomatic patients with hyperkalemia, tricyclic antidepressant overdose, or an overdose of other sodium channel blocking agents	• Helpful in the treatment of arrhythmias in tricyclic overdose • Rapidly reduces potassium concentrations in hyperkalemia	• Does not improve survival in cardiac arrest

Advanced Airway Management

In managing the airway and ventilation in pediatric victims of cardiac arrest, consider the following:

- Avoid excessive ventilation during resuscitation.
  - Excessive ventilation can be harmful because it impedes venous return and decreases cardiac output.
  - Increased intrathoracic pressure from positive-pressure ventilation also elevates right atrial pressure and thus reduces coronary perfusion pressure.
  - When providing ventilation with a bag and mask (in cycles of 15 compressions and 2 breaths for 2 rescuers), give each breath over 1 second and provide just enough volume to make the chest rise.
  - Excessive tidal volume or pressure during bag-mask ventilation may distend the stomach; gastric distention impedes ventilation and increases the risk of regurgitation and aspiration.
- Avoid routine use of cricoid pressure if it interferes with intubation or ventilation.
- Use waveform capnography or capnometry with clinical examination to confirm and monitor ET tube placement.

- Colorimetric exhaled CO_2 devices may fail to detect the presence of exhaled CO_2 (ie, lack of a color change indicates no CO_2 detected) during cardiac arrest despite correct placement of the ET tube. Use direct laryngoscopy to confirm tube placement if exhaled CO_2 is not detected and there is evidence that the tube is in the trachea (eg, chest rise and bilateral breath sounds).

- When providing ventilation via an advanced airway during CPR, provide 1 breath every 6 seconds (10 breaths/min) without pausing chest compressions. Chest compressions are delivered without interruption at a rate of 100 to 120/min. For more details, see "Insertion of an Advanced Airway During CPR" section later in this Part.

An advanced airway (eg, ET tube) can be placed during CPR. However, in a study of OHCA when emergency medical services transport time was short and providers had limited ongoing experience in pediatric intubation, there was no demonstrated survival advantage of ET intubation over effective bag-mask ventilation. This study does not address ET intubation in the in-hospital setting but suggests that immediate intubation may not be necessary. For more details, see Gausche et al. *JAMA*. 2000;283:783-790 in the Suggested Reading List on the Student Website.

Pediatric Cardiac Arrest Algorithm

The Pediatric Cardiac Arrest Algorithm (Figure 18) outlines assessment and management steps for an infant or child in cardiac arrest who does not respond to BLS interventions. The Pediatric Cardiac Arrest Algorithm is based on expert consensus. It is designed to maximize uninterrupted periods of CPR while enabling efficient delivery of electrical therapy and medications as appropriate. Although the actions are listed sequentially, when several rescuers are involved, some actions will occur simultaneously.

Critical Concepts

Coordination of Team Members During Resuscitation

Using the Pediatric Cardiac Arrest Algorithm, providers should structure assessments and interventions around 2-minute periods of uninterrupted high-quality CPR. This requires organization so that every member of the team knows his or her responsibilities. When all team members are familiar with the algorithm, they can anticipate and prepare for the next steps, getting equipment ready and drawing up the proper doses of medications. Chest compressors should rotate about every 2 minutes.

Step numbers in the text below refer to the corresponding steps in the algorithm. The algorithm consists of 2 pathways, depending on the cardiac rhythm as identified on a monitor or interpreted by an AED:

- A shockable rhythm (VF/pVT) pathway is displayed on the left side of the algorithm.
- A nonshockable rhythm (asystole/PEA) pathway is displayed on the right side of the algorithm.

Pediatric Cardiac Arrest Algorithm—2015 Update

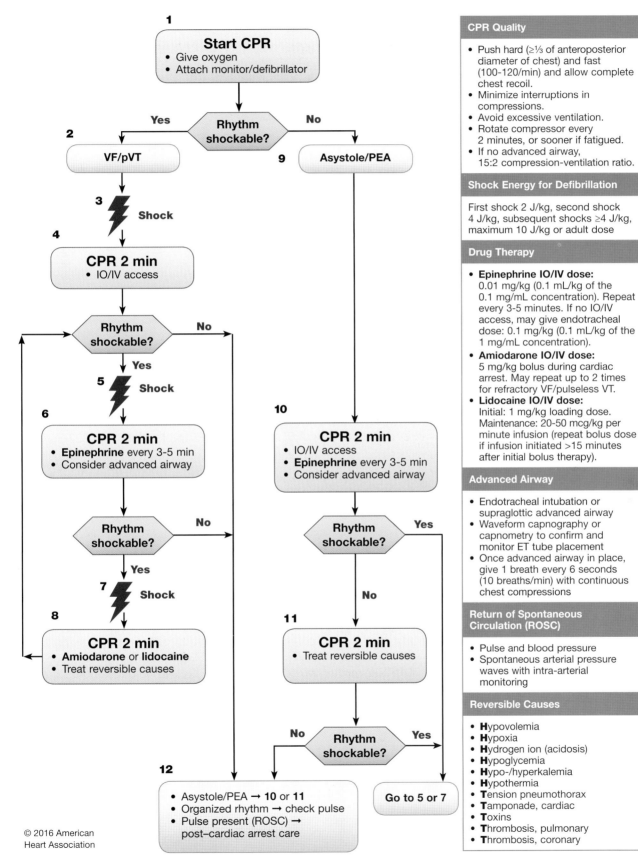

CPR Quality

- Push hard (≥⅓ of anteroposterior diameter of chest) and fast (100-120/min) and allow complete chest recoil.
- Minimize interruptions in compressions.
- Avoid excessive ventilation.
- Rotate compressor every 2 minutes, or sooner if fatigued.
- If no advanced airway, 15:2 compression-ventilation ratio.

Shock Energy for Defibrillation

First shock 2 J/kg, second shock 4 J/kg, subsequent shocks ≥4 J/kg, maximum 10 J/kg or adult dose

Drug Therapy

- **Epinephrine IO/IV dose:** 0.01 mg/kg (0.1 mL/kg of the 0.1 mg/mL concentration). Repeat every 3-5 minutes. If no IO/IV access, may give endotracheal dose: 0.1 mg/kg (0.1 mL/kg of the 1 mg/mL concentration).
- **Amiodarone IO/IV dose:** 5 mg/kg bolus during cardiac arrest. May repeat up to 2 times for refractory VF/pulseless VT.
- **Lidocaine IO/IV dose:** Initial: 1 mg/kg loading dose. Maintenance: 20-50 mcg/kg per minute infusion (repeat bolus dose if infusion initiated >15 minutes after initial bolus therapy).

Advanced Airway

- Endotracheal intubation or supraglottic advanced airway
- Waveform capnography or capnometry to confirm and monitor ET tube placement
- Once advanced airway in place, give 1 breath every 6 seconds (10 breaths/min) with continuous chest compressions

Return of Spontaneous Circulation (ROSC)

- Pulse and blood pressure
- Spontaneous arterial pressure waves with intra-arterial monitoring

Reversible Causes

- **H**ypovolemia
- **H**ypoxia
- **H**ydrogen ion (acidosis)
- **H**ypoglycemia
- **H**ypo-/hyperkalemia
- **H**ypothermia
- **T**ension pneumothorax
- **T**amponade, cardiac
- **T**oxins
- **T**hrombosis, pulmonary
- **T**hrombosis, coronary

© 2016 American Heart Association

Figure 18. The Pediatric Cardiac Arrest Algorithm.

Start CPR (Step 1)

As soon as the child is found to be unresponsive with no breathing (or only gasping), shout for nearby help and activate the emergency response system, send for a defibrillator (manual or AED), check a pulse, and start CPR, beginning with chest compressions. Attach the ECG monitor or AED pads as soon as they are available. Throughout resuscitation, provide high-quality CPR (give chest compressions of adequate rate and depth, allow complete chest recoil after each compression, minimize interruptions in compressions, and avoid excessive ventilation). Use a compression-to-ventilation ratio of 30:2 for 1 rescuer and 15:2 for 2 rescuers. Administer O_2 with ventilation as soon as it is available.

Once the monitor/defibrillator is attached, check the rhythm. Determine whether the rhythm is shockable (VF/pVT) or nonshockable (asystole/PEA). If the rhythm is shockable, follow the left side of the algorithm.

Shockable Rhythm: VF/pVT (Step 2)

If the rhythm is shockable, deliver 1 unsynchronized shock (Step 3). Perform CPR while the defibrillator is charging, if possible. The shorter the interval is between the last compression and shock delivery, the higher the potential shock success (elimination of VF). Therefore, try to keep that interval as short as possible, ideally less than 10 seconds. Immediately after shock delivery, resume high-quality CPR, beginning with chest compressions. In a monitored setting, this approach may be modified at the provider's discretion.

If the resuscitation takes place in a critical care setting and the child has intra-arterial monitoring in place, the presence of a waveform with an adequate arterial pressure can be useful in identifying ROSC. In other settings, that determination will be made after about 2 minutes of CPR during the next rhythm check. A sharp increase in the exhaled CO_2 pressure ($PETCO_2$) can also indicate ROSC.

Defibrillation devices for children are the

- AED (able to distinguish pediatric shockable from nonshockable rhythms and ideally equipped with a pediatric dose attenuator)
- Manual cardioverter/defibrillator (capable of variable shock doses)

Institutions that care for children at risk for arrhythmias and cardiac arrest (eg, hospitals, emergency departments) ideally should have defibrillators available that are capable of energy adjustment appropriate for children.

Manual Defibrillator

The optimal electrical energy dose for pediatric defibrillation is unknown. For manual defibrillation, an initial dose of 2 to 4 J/kg is acceptable, and for ease of teaching, a 2 J/kg (biphasic or monophasic waveform) may be considered. If VF or pVT persists at the next rhythm check, deliver a dose of 4 J/kg for the second shock. If VF persists after the second shock, use at least 4 J/kg or higher, not to exceed 10 J/kg or the maximum adult dose. Successful resuscitation using shock doses up to 9 J/kg have been reported in children.

Either self-adhesive electrode pads or paddles can be used to deliver shocks with a manual defibrillator. Self-adhesive pads are preferred because they are easy to apply and reduce the risk of current arcing. They also can be used to monitor the heart rhythm. If you use paddles, apply a conducting gel, cream, or paste, or place an electrode pad between the paddle and the child's chest to reduce transthoracic impedance. Do not use saline-soaked gauze pads, sonographic gels, or alcohol pads. Alcohol pads may pose a fire hazard and cause chest burns.

See the Critical Concepts box "Manual Defibrillation (for VF or pVT)" later in this Part for the universal steps for operating a manual defibrillator.

Pads/Paddles

Use the largest self-adhering electrode pads that will fit on the chest wall without contact between the pads. Recommended paddle sizes are based on the child's weight/age (Table 21).

Table 21. Paddle Sizes

Weight/Age	Paddle Size
>10 kg (approximately 1 year or older)	Large "adult" paddles (8-13 cm)
<10 kg (<1 year)	Small "infant" paddles (4.5 cm)

The selection of pediatric pads vs adult pads is manufacturer specific. Refer to package instructions to determine the appropriate size.

Place the electrode pads/paddles so that the heart is between them. Place 1 electrode pad/paddle on the upper right side of the victim's chest below the right clavicle and the other to the left of the left nipple in the anterior axillary line directly over the heart. Place pads so they don't touch. Allow at least 3 cm between paddles, and apply firm pressure to create good contact with the skin.

FYI

Anteroposterior Pad Placement

Some defibrillator manufacturers recommend placement of self-adhesive electrode pads in an anteroposterior position, with one over the victim's heart and the other over the back. Anteroposterior placement may be necessary in an infant, particularly if only large electrode pads are available.

Place the electrode pads according to the recommendations of the defibrillator manufacturer. These are typically illustrated on the pads themselves.

Modifications may be required in special situations (eg, if the child has an implanted defibrillator).

Clearing for Defibrillation

To ensure the safety of rescuers during defibrillation, perform a visual check of the child and the resuscitation team just before you deliver a shock. Make sure that high-flow O_2 is not directed across the child's chest. Warn others that you are about to deliver a shock and that everyone must stand clear. State a "warning chant" firmly and in a forceful voice before delivering each shock (this entire sequence should take less than 5 seconds). See the Critical Concepts box "Manual Defibrillation (for VF or pVT)."

Critical Concepts

Manual Defibrillation (for VF or pVT)

Continue CPR without interruption during all steps until step 8 in this box. Minimize interval between the last compression and shock delivery (do not deliver breaths between last compression and shock delivery).

1. Turn on the defibrillator.

2. Set *lead switch* to *paddles* (or lead I, II, or III if monitor leads are used).

3. Select adhesive pads or paddles; use the largest pads or paddles that can fit completely on the patient's chest without touching each other.

4. If using paddles, apply conductive gel or paste. Be sure cables are attached to the defibrillator.

5. Position the adhesive pads on the patient's chest: right anterior chest wall and left axillary positions. If using paddles, apply firm pressure. If the patient has an implanted pacemaker, do not position the pads/paddles directly over the device. Be sure that oxygen is not directed over the patient's chest.

6. Select energy dose:

   Initial dose: 2 J/kg (acceptable range 2-4 J/kg)
   Subsequent doses: 4 J/kg or higher (not to exceed 10 J/kg or standard adult dose)

7. Announce "Charging defibrillator," and press *charge* on the defibrillator controls or apex paddle. Chest compressions should resume/continue during charging unless charging occurs immediately.

8. When the defibrillator is fully charged, state firm chant, such as "I am going to shock on 3." Then count. The chant can be shortened to "Clear for shock." (Chest compressions should continue until this announcement.)

9. After confirming all personnel are clear of the patient, press the *shock* button on the defibrillator or press the 2 paddle *discharge* buttons simultaneously.

10. Immediately after shock delivery, resume CPR beginning with compressions for 5 cycles (about 2 minutes), and then recheck rhythm. Interruption of compressions should be minimized.

Resume CPR, Establish IV/IO Access (Step 4)

Immediately after the shock, resume CPR, beginning with chest compressions. Give about 2 minutes of CPR. (For 2 rescuers, this will be about 10 cycles of 15 compressions followed by 2 breaths.) While CPR is being performed, if vascular access (IO or IV) is not already present, another member of the resuscitation team should establish vascular access in anticipation of the need for medications.

Before the rhythm check, the team leader should ensure that the team is prepared to do the following:

- Rotate compressors
- Calculate appropriate shock dose to administer if VF/pVT persists
- Prepare drugs for administration if indicated

Check Rhythm (Step 4)

After 2 minutes of CPR, check the rhythm. *Try to limit interruptions in CPR to less than 10 seconds for a rhythm check.*

This rhythm check may indicate the following outcomes from the previous shock and CPR:

- Termination of VF/pVT to a "nonshockable" rhythm (asystole, PEA) or to an organized rhythm with a pulse
- Persistence of a shockable rhythm (VF/pVT)

Termination of VF/pVT (ie, Rhythm Is "Nonshockable") (Step 12)

If the rhythm is nonshockable, check for an "organized" rhythm (ie, one with regular complexes [Figure 19]). If the rhythm is organized, palpate for a central pulse. If a pulse is present, begin post–cardiac arrest care. If the rhythm is not organized, do not take the time to perform a pulse check; instead, immediately resume CPR (Step 10).

Foundational Facts

Rhythm and Pulse Checks

Remember, rhythm and pulse checks should be brief (less than 10 seconds). Pulse checks are unnecessary unless an organized rhythm (or other evidence of a perfusing rhythm, such as an arterial waveform or an abrupt and sustained increase in P_{ETCO_2}) is present. In specialized environments (eg, an intensive care unit) with intra-arterial or other hemodynamic monitoring in place, providers may alter this sequence.

If PEA (an organized rhythm without a palpable pulse) or asystole is present at the rhythm check, resume CPR beginning with compressions and proceed to the right side of the algorithm (Step 10 or 11).

If there is any doubt about the presence of a pulse, immediately resume CPR (Step 10). Chest compressions are unlikely to be harmful to a child with a spontaneous rhythm and weak pulses. *If there is no pulse or you are not sure, resume CPR.*

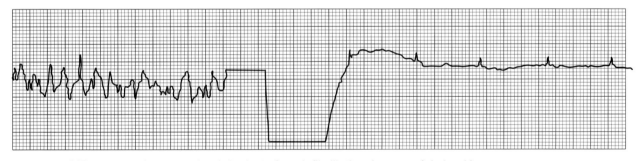

Figure 19. VF converted to organized rhythm after defibrillation (successful shock).

Persistent VF/pVT (Step 5)

If the rhythm check reveals a shockable rhythm (ie, persistent VF/pVT), prepare to deliver a second shock with a manual defibrillator (4 J/kg) or AED. Resume chest compressions while the defibrillator is charging. If IV/IO access is established, administer epinephrine while compressions continue. Consider insertion of an advanced airway if one is not in place. Once the defibrillator is charged, "clear" the patient and deliver the shock (Step 5).

Resume CPR with chest compressions immediately after the shock delivery (Step 6). A different compressor should be performing the compressions (ie, compressors should rotate every 2 minutes). Give about 2 minutes of CPR. (For 2 rescuers, this will be about 10 cycles of 15 compressions followed by 2 breaths.)

Give Epinephrine (Step 6)

If VF/pVT persists, administer epinephrine as soon as IO/IV access is available while compressions continue (Table 22).

Table 22. Epinephrine Doses

Epinephrine	
Route	**Dose**
IO/IV	0.01 mg/kg (0.1 mL/kg) bolus
ET	0.1 mg/kg (0.1 mL/kg) bolus
Repeat epinephrine about every 3-5 minutes of cardiac arrest. This will generally result in epinephrine delivery after every second (ie, every other) rhythm check.	

The Pediatric Cardiac Arrest Algorithm and the *2015 AHA Guidelines Update for CPR and ECC* do not state a specific time for delivery of the first dose of epinephrine because there is no published evidence to guide recommendations for the timing of drug administration. In addition, some patients will have early IO/IV access and hemodynamic monitoring and others will not. Epinephrine administration is not suggested earlier (immediately after the *first* shock) because it might not be necessary if the first shock is successful (ie, elimination of VF and an organized rhythm may be observed at the rhythm check that follows the first shock and 2 minutes of CPR).

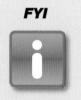

FYI

Timing of Epinephrine Administration

In a monitored setting, a provider may choose to administer epinephrine before or after the second shock. When VF/pVT is identified during the rhythm check, the administration of epinephrine can occur during the CPR that precedes (during charging) or immediately follows the shock delivery. Conversely, if, in a monitored setting, an organized rhythm is present during the rhythm check, it is reasonable to check for a pulse to avoid an unnecessary dose of epinephrine because it can produce adverse effects. For example, if the initial VF/pVT was related to a cardiomyopathy, myocarditis, or drug toxicity, epinephrine administration immediately after elimination of VF/pVT could induce recurrent VF/pVT.

Medication Administration During CPR

Ideally, administer IO/IV medications *during compressions* because blood flow generated by compressions helps to circulate the drugs. By consensus, the *2015 AHA Guidelines Update for CPR and ECC* recommend medication administration during compressions immediately *before* (if compressions are performed while the defibrillator is charging) or *after* shock delivery so that the drugs have time to circulate before the next rhythm check (and shock delivery, if needed).

Team members responsible for resuscitation drugs should anticipate and prepare the *next* drug dose that might be needed after the next rhythm check. All team members should be familiar with the Pediatric Cardiac Arrest Algorithm and refer to it during the resuscitation attempt to anticipate the next interventions. Drug tables, charts, or other references should be readily available to expedite the calculation of drug doses. Use of a color-coded length-based resuscitation tape facilitates rapid estimation of appropriate drug doses.

ET administration of resuscitation drugs results in lower blood concentrations than the same dose given intravascularly or by IO route. Studies also suggest that the lower epinephrine concentration achieved when the drug is delivered by the ET route may produce transient β-adrenergic effects (rather than the desired α-adrenergic vasoconstrictive effects). The β-adrenergic effects can be detrimental and cause hypotension, lower coronary artery perfusion pressure and flow, and reduce potential for ROSC. Another disadvantage of ET drug delivery is that chest compressions must be interrupted for drug delivery by this route.

Insertion of an Advanced Airway During CPR

The team leader will determine the best time for ET intubation or insertion of another advanced airway. Because insertion of an advanced airway is likely to require interruption of chest compressions, the team leader must weigh the relative benefits of the advanced airway vs benefits of minimizing interruptions in compressions. If insertion of an advanced airway is necessary, careful planning and organization of supplies and personnel will minimize the time that compressions are interrupted. Once the advanced airway is inserted, confirm that it is in the correct position.

When an advanced airway is in place during CPR, continuous chest compressions can be provided. See the Critical Concepts box "CPR With an Advanced Airway."

Critical Concepts

CPR With an Advanced Airway

Once an advanced airway (eg, ET tube) is in place, the CPR sequence changes from "cycles" to *continuous* chest compressions and a regular ventilation rate. One team member compresses the chest at a rate of 100 to 120/min. Another team member ventilates with 1 breath every 6 seconds (a rate of about 10 breaths per minute).

Team members performing chest compressions should rotate every 2 minutes to reduce rescuer fatigue and ensure that high-quality chest compressions are provided throughout the resuscitation. Limit interruptions of chest compressions to the minimum required for rhythm checks and shock delivery. This sequence may be modified in special settings (eg, an intensive care unit) with continuous ECG and hemodynamic monitoring in place.

Check Rhythm (Step 7)

After 2 minutes of CPR and epinephrine administration, recheck the rhythm. Try to limit interruptions in chest compressions for rhythm checks to less than 10 seconds. Actions to take based on the rhythm present are listed in the box:

If the rhythm check reveals...	Then...

Termination of VF/pVT	Check for an organized rhythm:
	• No organized rhythm (asystole/PEA): Go to Step 11
	• Organized rhythm: Check pulse.
	  – If pulse is present, begin post–cardiac arrest care.
	  – If no pulse is present (PEA), go to Step 11.

Persistence of VF/pVT	Go to Step 7.

For Persistent VF/pVT (Step 7)

Deliver Shock

If VF/pVT persists, deliver 1 shock by manual defibrillator (4 J/kg or more, up to 10 J/kg or the maximum adult dose) or AED. Perform chest compressions, if possible, while the defibrillator is charging. When the defibrillator is charged, "clear" the victim and deliver the shock.

Immediately after the shock, resume CPR, beginning with chest compressions. Give about 2 minutes of CPR. (For 2 rescuers, this will be about 10 cycles of 15 compressions followed by 2 breaths.)

Antiarrhythmic Medications (Step 8)

Immediately after resuming chest compressions, administer amiodarone or lidocaine (Table 23). If torsades de pointes is present, give magnesium.

Table 23. Doses for Antiarrhythmic Agents

Drug	Dose
Amiodarone	5 mg/kg IV/IO bolus (maximum single dose 300 mg); may repeat 5 mg/kg IV/IO bolus up to total dose of 15 mg/kg (maximum dose 2.2 g) IV per 24 hours
Lidocaine	1 mg/kg IO/IV
Magnesium	25 to 50 mg/kg IO/IV bolus, maximum dose 2 g

Administer IO/IV drugs during chest compressions.

Summary of the VF/pVT Sequence

Figure 20 summarizes the recommended sequence of CPR, rhythm checks, shocks, and administration of drugs for VF/pVT based on expert consensus.

Think of the management of pulseless arrest with VF/pVT as a provision of nearly continuous CPR. Ideally, CPR is interrupted for only brief periods, for rhythm checks and shock delivery. Drug preparation and administration do not require interruption of CPR and should not delay shock delivery.

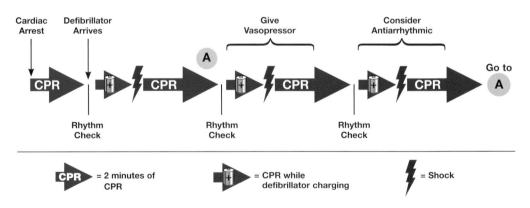

Figure 20. Summary of the VF/pVT cardiac arrest sequence.

Prepare next drug before rhythm check. Administer drug during chest compressions, as soon as possible after the rhythm check confirms VF/pVT. Do not delay shock. Continue CPR while the drugs are prepared and administered and the defibrillator is charging. Ideally, chest compressions should be interrupted only for ventilation (until advanced airway is placed), rhythm check, and actual shock delivery.

Nonshockable Rhythm (Asystole/PEA, Step 9)

If the rhythm is nonshockable, asystole or PEA may be present. The management of this rhythm is outlined in the pathway on the right side of the Pediatric Cardiac Arrest Algorithm (Figure 18). Note that 25% of hospitalized children in the National Registry of CPR developed a shockable rhythm at some point during the resuscitation attempt. If VF develops during the resuscitation attempt, return to the left side of the Pediatric Cardiac Arrest Algorithm (Step 5 or 7).

Establish Vascular Access (Step 10)

For treatment of asystole or PEA, provide high-quality CPR, deliver epinephrine as appropriate, and try to identify and treat potentially reversible causes of the arrest.

Continue high-quality CPR for about 2 minutes. During this time, establish vascular (IO or IV) access and consider advanced airway placement. As soon as vascular access is established, give a bolus of epinephrine during chest compressions (Table 24).

Table 24. Epinephrine Doses

Epinephrine	
Route	**Dose**
IO/IV	0.01 mg/kg (0.1 mL/kg) bolus
ET	0.1 mg/kg (0.1 mL/kg) bolus

Repeat epinephrine administration about every 3-5 minutes if cardiac arrest persists. This generally results in the administration of epinephrine after every second (ie, every other) rhythm check.

Check Rhythm

After about 2 minutes of CPR, check the rhythm.

If the rhythm is...	Then...
Shockable	Go to Step 7 and proceed through the steps on the left side of the algorithm.
Nonshockable	Go to Step 11.

Nonshockable Rhythm (Step 11)

If the rhythm check reveals a nonshockable rhythm, resume CPR immediately, beginning with chest compressions, and treat potentially reversible causes of cardiac arrest. These can be recalled by remembering the H's and T's mnemonic (Table 25). After another 2 minutes of CPR, check the rhythm. If it is organized, check for a pulse. If a pulse is present, proceed with post–cardiac arrest care. If a pulse is not palpable or the rhythm is not organized, go to Step 10. If a shockable rhythm is present at any time, go to the left side of the algorithm (Step 5 or 7).

Summary of Asystole/ PEA Treatment Sequence

Figure 21 summarizes the recommended sequence of CPR, based on expert consensus, of rhythm checks, shocks, and delivery of drugs for asystole and PEA.

The management of any pulseless arrest includes provision of nearly continuous CPR, interrupted ideally by only brief rhythm checks. Do not interrupt CPR for drug preparation and administration. Administer IO/IV drugs during chest compressions. See the Critical Concepts box "CPR With an Advanced Airway" earlier in this Part.

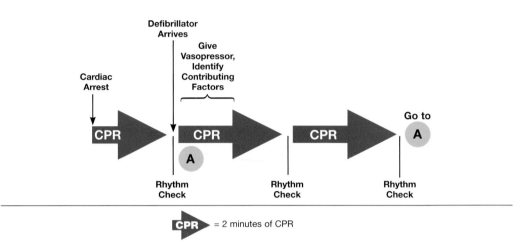

Figure 21. Cardiac arrest treatment sequence: asystole and PEA.

If, at any rhythm check, a shockable rhythm is detected, see Figure 20.

Identifying and Treating Potentially Reversible Causes of Cardiac Arrest

The outcome of hypoxic-ischemic pediatric cardiac arrest is generally poor. Rapid recognition, immediate high-quality CPR, and correction of contributing factors and potentially reversible causes offer the best chance for a successful resuscitation. Some cardiac arrests may be associated with a potentially reversible condition. If you can quickly identify the condition and treat it, your resuscitative efforts may be successful.

In a search for potentially reversible causes or contributing factors, do the following:

- Ensure that high-quality CPR is being provided.
- Check that the advanced airway is open/patent and effective.
- Verify that the bag-mask device is connected to a source of high-flow O_2.
- Ensure that ventilation produces visible chest rise without excessive volume or rate.
- Consider potentially reversible causes by recalling the H's and T's.

H's and T's

Cardiac arrest in children may be associated with the following underlying, and potentially reversible, conditions (Table 25).

Table 25. Possible Causes of Cardiac Arrest

H's	**T's**
Hypovolemia	**T**ension pneumothorax
Hypoxia	**T**amponade (cardiac)
Hydrogen ion (acidosis)	**T**oxins
Hypoglycemia	**T**hrombosis, coronary
Hypo-/Hyperkalemia	**T**hrombosis, pulmonary
Hypothermia	

Also consider unrecognized trauma as a cause of cardiac arrest, particularly in infants and young children.

ROSC

If resuscitative efforts successfully restore an organized rhythm (or there is other evidence of ROSC, such as an abrupt and sustained increase in P_{ETCO_2} or visible pulsations on an arterial waveform), check the child's pulse to determine if a perfusing rhythm is present. If a pulse is present, continue with post–cardiac arrest care.

Pediatric Cardiac Arrest: Special Circumstances

The following special circumstances resulting in pediatric cardiac arrest require specific management:

- Trauma
- Drowning
- Anaphylaxis
- Poisoning
- Congenital heart disease: single ventricle
- Pulmonary hypertension

Cardiac Arrest due to Trauma

Cardiac arrest associated with trauma in children represents a significant subgroup of pediatric OHCAs. An improper resuscitation (including inadequate volume resuscitation) is a major cause of preventable pediatric trauma deaths. Despite rapid and effective out-of-hospital and trauma center response, survival of children with traumatic OHCA is low. Survival from pediatric OHCAs due to blunt trauma is very low. Factors that may improve outcome from traumatic OHCA include treatable penetrating injuries and prompt transport (typically 10 minutes or less) to a trauma care facility. For more details, see Sasser et al. *MMWR Recomm Rep.* 2009;58:1-35 in the Suggested Reading List on the Student Website.

Traumatic cardiac arrest in children has multiple possible causes, including

- Hypoxia secondary to respiratory arrest, airway obstruction, or tracheobronchial injury
- Injury to vital structures (eg, heart, aorta, pulmonary arteries)
- Severe brain injury with secondary cardiovascular collapse
- Upper cervical spinal cord injury with respiratory arrest, which may be accompanied by spinal shock, progressing to cardiac arrest
- Diminished cardiac output or PEA from tension pneumothorax, cardiac tamponade, or massive hemorrhage

Basic and advanced life support techniques for the pediatric trauma victim in cardiac arrest are fundamentally the same as for the child with nontraumatic cardiac arrest: support of circulation, airway, and breathing. The focus of a resuscitation attempt in an out-of-hospital setting is to

- Provide high-quality CPR, if needed
- Maintain adequate airway, ventilation, and circulation
- Anticipate airway obstruction by dental fragments, blood, or other debris (use a suction device, if necessary)
- Minimize motion of the cervical spine (if indicated), while assuring airway and ventilation
- Control external bleeding with pressure with a tourniquet and/or hemostatic dressings as indicated
- Minimize interventions that delay transport to definitive care
- Transport infants and children with multisystem trauma to a trauma center with pediatric expertise
- Establish IO/IV access and initiate volume resuscitation as needed

The following is a summary of key management principles for traumatic cardiac arrest in children (Table 26).

Table 26. Management of Traumatic Cardiac Arrest

CPR	• Perform high-quality CPR. • Attach a monitor/defibrillator. • Control visible hemorrhage with direct pressure or tourniquet.
Airway	• Open and maintain the airway by using a jaw-thrust maneuver. • Restrict cervical spine motion by manual stabilization of the head and neck if the mechanism of the injury or physical findings suggests cervical spine injury.
Breathing	• Ventilate with a bag-mask device using 100% O_2; a 2-person bag-mask ventilation technique is preferable to maintain manual stabilization of the head and neck (if spinal motion restriction is indicated). • If an advanced airway is inserted, 1 rescuer should stabilize the head and neck in a neutral position (if spinal motion restriction is indicated). • Avoid excessive ventilation. • Perform unilateral or bilateral needle decompressions for suspected tension pneumothoraxes. • Seal any significant open pneumothorax and insert a thoracotomy tube.
Circulation	• Assume that the patient is hypovolemic; establish IO/IV access and replace fluids rapidly *(do not place an IO in any bone in which there is a concern for fracture)*. Consider noncrosshatched type O-negative blood for females (and either O-negative or O-positive for males). • Consider pericardiocentesis for possible cardiac tamponade (if suspected). • Consider spinal shock (ie, loss of sympathetic innervation) resulting in fluid-refractory hypotension and bradycardia. Vasopressor therapy is indicated if spinal shock is suspected.

Cardiac Arrest due to Drowning

Immediate high-quality CPR is the single most important factor influencing survival in drowning (Table 27). Chest compressions may be difficult to perform while the victim is still in the water, but you can initiate ventilation immediately. Start chest compressions as soon as you can do so safely, and when the child is lying faceup on a firm surface.

No modifications of the standard pediatric BLS sequence are necessary for drowning victims other than consideration of cervical spine injury and the possibility of hypothermia as contributing factors. Rescuers should remove drowning victims from the water by the fastest means available and should begin the resuscitation attempt as quickly as possible.

Table 27. Management of Cardiac Arrest due to Drowning

CPR	• Perform high-quality CPR. • Attach a monitor/defibrillator; provide rapid defibrillation if needed. • If defibrillation is indicated and the chest is covered with water, quickly wipe the child's chest to minimize electrical arcing between the defibrillation pads or paddles.
Airway	• Open the airway. • If there is reason to suspect a cervical spine injury (eg, diving injury), restrict spinal motion.
Breathing	• Ventilate with a bag-mask device by using 100% O_2. • Be prepared to suction the airway, because drowning victims often vomit swallowed water; decompress the stomach with a nasogastric/orogastric tube after the advanced airway is inserted.
Circulation	• Continue high-quality CPR if needed.
Exposure	• Evaluate core body temperature and attempt rewarming if the child is severely hypothermic (core temperature <30°C).

In cardiac arrest associated with hypothermia, it is often difficult to know when to terminate resuscitative efforts. In victims of drowning in icy water, survival is possible after submersion times of as long as 40 minutes and prolonged duration of CPR (greater than 2 hours). When drowning occurs in ice water, rewarming to a core temperature of at least 30°C is recommended before CPR efforts are abandoned. The heart may be unresponsive to resuscitative efforts until this core temperature is achieved.

Extracorporeal circulation is the most rapid and effective technique for rewarming severely hypothermic cardiac arrest victims after submersion in icy water. Although the patient may be rewarmed with passive techniques or body cavity irrigation in the out-of-hospital or community hospital setting, rapid transfer to a facility that is capable of performing pediatric ECPR/extracorporeal membrane oxygenation is preferred.

Cardiac Arrest due to Anaphylaxis

Near-fatal anaphylaxis produces airway edema and obstruction and profound vasodilation, which significantly increases intravascular capacity and produces relative hypovolemia. Anaphylaxis is often accompanied by bronchoconstriction, which compromises oxygenation and further impairs tissue O_2 delivery. If cardiac arrest develops, primary therapy is CPR with attention to establishment and maintenance of an adequate airway, bolus fluid administration, and epinephrine. Children with anaphylaxis are often young with healthy hearts and cardiovascular systems. They may respond to establishment of an airway with adequate oxygenation and ventilation and rapid correction of vasodilation and low intravascular volume. Effective CPR may maintain sufficient O_2 delivery until the catastrophic effects of the anaphylactic reaction resolve.

If cardiac arrest results from anaphylaxis, management may include the following critical therapies (Table 28).

Table 28. Management of Cardiac Arrest due to Anaphylaxis

CPR	• Perform high-quality CPR and rapid defibrillation as needed.
Airway	• Open and maintain the airway by using manual maneuvers. • If ET intubation is performed, be prepared for the possibility of airway edema and the need to use a smaller ET tube than predicted by the child's age or length.
Breathing	• Perform bag-mask ventilation until insertion of advanced airway, and then provide bagged tube ventilation by using 100% O_2.
Circulation	• Administer boluses of isotonic crystalloid as needed to treat shock. Insert 2 IO catheters or 2 large-bore IVs. • Administer epinephrine in standard doses (0.01 mg/kg IO/IV [0.1 mL/kg of 0.1 mg/mL concentration) or via the ET tube if no vascular access can be obtained (0.1 mg/kg [0.1 mL/kg of 1 mg/mL concentration] every 3 to 5 minutes during cardiac arrest). • Provide epinephrine infusion as needed. • Manage according to the Pediatric Cardiac Arrest Algorithm if the arrest rhythm is asystole or PEA (which is often the case).

There are sparse data about the value of antihistamines in anaphylactic cardiac arrest, but it is reasonable to assume that administration of antihistamines would result in little harm. Steroids given during cardiac arrest have little effect, but they may have potential value in the management of anaphylaxis before or after cardiac arrest. Therefore, administer steroids such as methylprednisolone 1 to 2 mg/kg IV/IO as soon as possible in the post–cardiac arrest resuscitation period.

Cardiac Arrest Associated With Poisoning

Drug overdose or poisoning may cause cardiac arrest as a result of direct cardiac toxicity or the secondary effects of respiratory depression, airway obstruction and possible respiratory arrest, peripheral vasodilation, arrhythmias, and hypotension. The myocardium of the poisoning victim is often healthy, but temporary cardiac dysfunction may be present until the effects of the drug or toxin have been reversed or metabolized. This will require a variable amount of time, often several hours, depending on the nature of the toxin, drug, or poison. Because the toxicity may be temporary, prolonged resuscitation efforts and use of advanced support techniques such as extracorporeal life support may result in good long-term survival.

Initiate advanced life support measures according to the Pediatric Cardiac Arrest Algorithm. Check glucose as soon as possible. If the patient is in cardiac arrest and hypoglycemic (eg, from a β-blocker or alcohol overdose), glucose must be normalized as soon as possible to improve the chances of a successful cardiac and neurologic outcome. PALS treatment for victims of a suspected poisoning should include a search for and treatment of reversible causes. Early consultation with a poison control center or toxicologist is recommended.

Congenital Heart Disease: Single Ventricle

The prevalence of complex cyanotic congenital heart disease in children is low. Nevertheless, the patient with single ventricle (tricuspid/pulmonary atresia, hypoplastic left heart syndrome, and their variants) represents a large proportion of children who suffer cardiac arrest, particularly in the in-hospital setting. An increasing number of infants and children survive after palliative surgical procedures; these children may require resuscitation postoperatively or during readmission for critical illness.

Single-ventricle physiology is complex and varies with the specific lesion and stage of surgical repair. Therefore, it is important to obtain a history from the caretakers to determine the child's baseline hemodynamic status and arterial O_2 saturation. During cardiac arrest, standard resuscitation care is indicated for all infants with single-ventricle anatomy after stage I (Norwood) palliation or those with a univentricular heart and aortopulmonary shunt to provide pulmonary blood flow. In addition to standard resuscitation, specific measures include

- Heparin administration may be considered for children with aortopulmonary or right ventricular-pulmonary artery shunt if shunt openness/patency is a concern.
- After resuscitation, titrate administered O_2 to achieve an O_2 saturation appropriate to maintain the optimum pulmonary-to-systemic blood flow ratio and adequate systemic profusion and oxygenation (must be individualized for each patient).
- PETCO2 may not be a reliable indicator of CPR quality in a single-ventricle patient because pulmonary blood flow in these patients does not always reflect cardiac output (ie, it is influenced by additional factors).
- Consider permissive hypoventilation strategies or even negative-pressure ventilation in the periarrest state to improve cardiac output.
- Extracorporeal life support or extracorporeal membrane oxygenation may be considered for patients in cardiac arrest who have undergone stage I palliation (Norwood) or Fontan-type procedures.

Pulmonary Hypertension

In pulmonary hypertension, cardiac output may be impaired by increased resistance to blood flow through the lungs. Standard PALS recommendations should be followed during cardiac arrest. Other measures include

- Correct hypercarbia and acidosis if present.
- A bolus of isotonic crystalloid (eg, normal saline) may be useful to maintain ventricular preload.
- If the patient was receiving pulmonary vasodilators such as nitric oxide or prostacyclin immediately before the arrest, be sure that drug administration continues.
- Consider administration of inhaled nitric oxide or prostacyclin (or IV prostacyclin) to reduce pulmonary vascular resistance.
- ECPR may be useful if instituted early during resuscitation.

FYI

Extracorporeal CPR

ECPR may be considered for pediatric patients with cardiac diagnoses who have IHCA in settings with existing extracorporeal membrane oxygenation protocols, expertise, and equipment. While evidence has shown no overall benefit to the use of ECPR, observational data from a registry of pediatric IHCA showed improved survival to hospital discharge with the use of ECPR in patients with surgical cardiac diagnoses. For children with underlying cardiac disease, when ECPR is initiated in a critical care setting, long-term survival has been reported after prolonged CPR. When ECPR is used during cardiac arrest, the outcome for children with underlying cardiac disease is better than for those with noncardiac disease.

For more details, see the references under "Extracorporeal Life Support (ECLS)/ Extracorporeal Cardiopulmonary Resuscitation (ECPR)" in the Suggested Reading List on the Student Website.

Effective Resuscitation Team Dynamics

Overview

Successful resuscitation attempts often require healthcare providers to simultaneously perform a variety of interventions. Although a CPR-trained bystander working alone can resuscitate a patient within the first moments after collapse, most attempts require the concerted efforts of multiple healthcare providers. Effective teamwork divides the tasks while multiplying the chances of a successful outcome.

Successful high-performance teams not only have medical expertise and mastery of resuscitation skills, but they also demonstrate effective communication and team dynamics. Part 5 of this manual discusses the importance of team roles, behaviors of effective team leaders and team members, and elements of effective high-performance team dynamics.

During the course, you will have an opportunity to practice performing different roles as a member and as a leader of a simulated high-performance team.

Learning Objective

By the end of this Part, you should be able to

- Apply team dynamics

Preparation for the Course

During the course you will participate as both the team leader and a team member during case simulations. You will be expected to model the behaviors discussed in this Part.

Critical Concepts	Understanding Team Roles

Understanding Team Roles

Whether you are a team member or team leader during a resuscitation attempt, you should understand your role and the roles of other team members. This awareness will help you anticipate

- The actions that will be performed next
- How to communicate and work as a member or leader of the team

Roles of the Team Leader and Team Members

Role of the Team Leader

The role of the team leader is multifaceted. The team leader

- Organizes the group
- Monitors individual performance of team members
- Backs up team members
- Models excellent team behavior
- Trains and coaches
- Facilitates understanding
- Focuses on comprehensive patient care

Every high-performance team needs a leader to organize the efforts of the group. The team leader is responsible for making sure everything is done at the right time in the right way by monitoring and integrating individual performance of team members. The role of the team leader is similar to that of an orchestra conductor directing individual musicians. Like a conductor, the team leader does not play the instruments but instead knows how each member of the orchestra fits into the overall music.

The role of the team leader also includes modeling excellent team behavior and leadership skills for the team and other people involved or interested in the resuscitation attempt. The team leader should serve as a teacher or guide to help train future team leaders and improve team effectiveness. After resuscitation, the team leader can facilitate analysis, critique, and practice in preparation for the next resuscitation attempt. The team leader also helps team members understand why they must perform certain tasks in a specific way.

The team leader should be able to explain why it is essential to

- Push hard and fast in the center of the chest
- Ensure complete chest recoil
- Minimize interruptions in chest compressions
- Avoid excessive ventilation

Whereas members of a high-performance team should focus on their individual tasks, the team leader must focus on comprehensive patient care.

Role of Each Team Member

Team members must be proficient in performing the skills authorized by their scope of practice. It is essential to the success of the resuscitation attempt that members of a high-performance team are

- Clear about role assignments
- Prepared to fulfill their role responsibilities
- Well practiced in resuscitation skills
- Knowledgeable about the algorithms
- Committed to success

Roles

Clear Roles and Responsibilities

Every member of the team should know his or her role and responsibilities. Just as different-shaped pieces make up a jigsaw puzzle, each team member's role is unique and critical to the effective performance of the team. Figure 22A identifies 6 team roles for resuscitation. When fewer than 6 people are present, these tasks must be prioritized and assigned to the healthcare providers present. Figure 22B shows how multiple providers can take on high-priority tasks seamlessly as more team members get to the patient.

When roles are unclear, team performance suffers. Signs of unclear roles include

- Performing the same task more than once
- Missing essential tasks
- Team members having multiple roles even if there are enough providers

To avoid inefficiencies, the team leader must clearly delegate tasks. Team members should communicate when and if they can handle additional responsibilities. The team leader should encourage team members to participate in leadership and not simply follow directions blindly.

Do	
Team leader	• Clearly define all team member roles in the clinical setting
Team members	• Seek out and perform clearly defined tasks appropriate to your level of competence

Don't	
Team leader	• Neglect to assign tasks to all available team members • Assign tasks to team members who are unsure of their responsibilities • Distribute assignments unevenly, leaving some with too much to do and others with too little
Team members	• Avoid taking assignments • Take assignments beyond your level of competence or expertise

Knowing Your Limitations

Not only should everyone on the team know his or her own limitations and capabilities, but the team leader should also be aware of them. This allows the team leader to evaluate team resources and call for backup of team members when assistance is needed. High-performance team members should anticipate situations in which they might require assistance and inform the team leader.

During the stress of an attempted resuscitation, do not practice or explore a new skill. If you need extra help, request it early. It is not a sign of weakness or incompetence to ask for help; it is better to have more help than needed rather than not enough help, which might negatively affect patient outcome.

Do	
Team leader and team members	• Call for assistance early rather than waiting until the patient deteriorates to the point that help is critical • Seek advice from more experienced personnel when the patient's condition worsens despite primary treatment

Don't	
Team leader and team members	• Reject offers from others to carry out an assigned task you are unable to complete, especially if task completion is essential to treatment
Team members	• Use or start an unfamiliar treatment or therapy without seeking advice from more experienced personnel • Take on too many assignments at a time when assistance is readily available

Constructive Interventions

During a resuscitation attempt, the leader or a member of a high-performance team may need to intervene if an action that is about to occur may be inappropriate at the time.

Although constructive intervention is necessary, it should be tactful. Team leaders should avoid confrontation with team members. Instead, conduct a debriefing afterward if constructive criticism is needed.

Do	
Team leader	• Ask that a different intervention be started if it has a higher priority
Team members	• Suggest an alternative drug or dose in a confident manner • Question a colleague who is about to make a mistake

Don't	
Team leader	• Fail to reassign a team member who is trying to function beyond his or her level of skill
Team members	• Ignore a team member who is about to administer a drug incorrectly

What to Communicate

Knowledge Sharing

Sharing information is a critical component of effective team performance. Team leaders may become trapped in a specific treatment or diagnostic approach; this common human error is called a *fixation error*. Examples of 3 common types of fixation errors are

- "Everything is OK."
- "This and only this is the correct path."
- "Do anything but this."

When resuscitative efforts are ineffective, go back to the basics and talk as a team, with conversations like, "Well, we've observed the following on the Primary Assessment… Have we missed something?" Members of a high-performance team should inform the team leader of any changes in the patient's condition to ensure that decisions are made with all available information.

Do	
Team leader	• Encourage an environment of information sharing and ask for suggestions if uncertain of the next best interventions • Ask for ideas for differential diagnoses • Ask if anything has been overlooked (eg, IV access should have been obtained or drugs should have been administered)
Team members	• Share information with other team members

Don't	
Team leader	• Ignore others' suggestions for treatment • Overlook or fail to examine clinical signs that are relevant to the treatment
Team members	• Ignore important information to improve your role

Summarizing and Reevaluating

An essential role of the team leader is monitoring and reevaluating

- The patient's status
- Interventions that have been performed
- Assessment findings

A good practice is for the team leader to summarize this information out loud in a periodic update to the team. Review the status of the resuscitation attempt and announce the plan for the next few steps. Remember that the patient's condition can change. Remain flexible to changing treatment plans and revisiting the initial differential diagnosis. Ask for information and summaries from the timer/recorder as well.

Do	
Team leader	• Draw continuous attention to decisions about differential diagnoses • Review or maintain an ongoing record of drugs and treatments administered and the patient's response
Team leaders and team members	• Clearly draw attention to significant changes in the patient's clinical condition • Increase monitoring (eg, frequency of respirations and blood pressure) when the patient's condition deteriorates

Don't	
Team leader	• Fail to change a treatment strategy when new information supports such a change • Fail to inform arriving personnel of the current status and plans for further action

Positions for 6-Person High-Performance Teams*

Resuscitation Triangle Roles

Compressor

- Assesses the patient
- Does 5 cycles of chest compressions
- Alternates with AED/Monitor/ Defibrillator every 5 cycles or 2 minutes (or earlier if signs of fatigue set in)

AED/Monitor/ Defibrillator

- Brings and operates the AED/monitor/defibrillator
- Alternates with Compressor every 5 cycles or 2 minutes (or earlier if signs of fatigue set in), ideally during rhythm analysis
- If a monitor is present, places it in a position where it can be seen by the Team Leader (and most of the team)

Airway

- Opens the airway
- Provides bag-mask ventilation
- Inserts airway adjuncts as appropriate

The team owns the code. No team member leaves the triangle except to protect his or her safety.

A

Leadership Roles

Team Leader

- **Every resuscitation team must have a defined leader**
- Assigns roles to team members
- Makes treatment decisions
- Provides feedback to the rest of the team as needed
- Assumes responsibility for roles not assigned

IV/IO/Medications

- An ACLS provider role
- Initiates IV/IO access
- Administers medications

Timer/Recorder

- Records the time of interventions and medications (and announces when these are next due)
- Records the frequency and duration of interruptions in compressions
- Communicates these to the Team Leader (and the rest of the team)

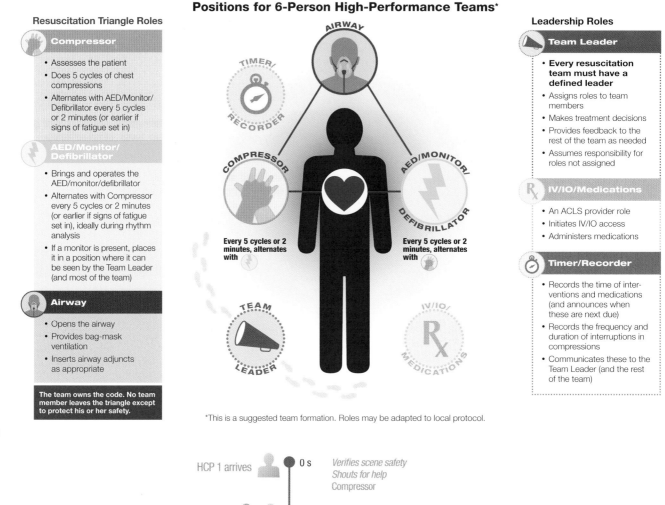

*This is a suggested team formation. Roles may be adapted to local protocol.

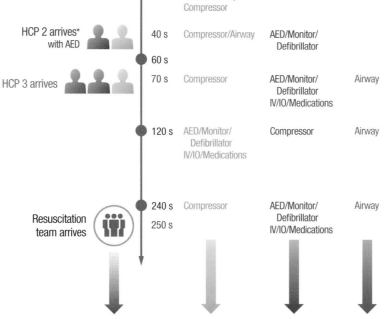

B

*With 2 or more rescuers, 1 healthcare provider should assume the role of team leader.

Figure 22. A, Suggested locations of team leader and team members during case simulations and clinical events. **B,** Priority-based multiple-rescuer response. This figure illustrates a potential seamless, time-sensitive, integrated team-based approach to resuscitation where roles and interventions are prioritized and distributed as more resources arrive to the patient. Times (in seconds) may vary based on circumstances, response times, and local protocols.

How to Communicate

Closed-Loop Communications

When communicating with high-performance team members, the team leader should use closed-loop communication by taking these steps:

1. The team leader gives a message, order, or assignment to a team member.

2. By receiving a clear response and eye contact, the team leader confirms that the team member heard and understood the message.

3. The team leader listens for confirmation of task performance from the team member before assigning another task.

Do	
Team leader	• Assign another task after receiving oral confirmation that a task has been completed, such as, "Now that the IV is in, give 1 mg of epinephrine"
Team members	• Close the loop: Inform the team leader when a task begins or ends, such as, "The IV is in"

Don't	
Team leader	• Give more tasks to a team member without asking or receiving confirmation of a completed assignment
Team members	• Give drugs without verbally confirming the order with the team leader • Forget to inform the team leader after giving the drug or performing the procedure

Clear Messages

Clear messages consist of concise communication spoken with distinctive speech in a controlled tone of voice. All healthcare providers should deliver messages and orders in a calm and direct manner without yelling or shouting. Unclear communication can lead to unnecessary delays in treatment or to medication errors.

Yelling or shouting can impair effective high-performance team interaction. Only one person should talk at any time.

Do	
Team leader	• Encourage team members to speak clearly
Team members	• Repeat the medication order • Question an order if the slightest doubt exists

Don't	
Team leader	• Mumble or speak in incomplete sentences • Give unclear messages and drug/medication orders • Yell, scream, or shout
Team members	• Feel patronized by distinct and concise messages

Mutual Respect

The best high-performance teams are composed of members who share a mutual respect for each other and work together in a collegial, supportive manner. To have a high-performance team, everyone must abandon ego and respect each other during the resuscitation attempt, regardless of any additional training or experience that the team leader or specific team members may have.

Do	
Team leader and team members	• Speak in a friendly, controlled tone of voice • Avoid shouting or displaying aggression if you are not understood initially
Team leader	• Acknowledge correctly completed assignments by saying, "Thanks—good job!"

Don't	
Team leader and team members	• Shout or yell at team members—when one person raises his voice, others will respond similarly • Behave aggressively or confuse directive behavior with aggression • Be uninterested in others

Part 6

Recognition of Respiratory Distress and Failure

Overview

Respiratory distress is a condition of abnormal respiratory rate or effort. It encompasses a spectrum of signs from tachypnea with retractions to agonal gasps. Respiratory distress includes increased work of breathing, inadequate respiratory effort (eg, hypoventilation) or rate (bradypnea), and irregular breathing.

PALS providers must identify respiratory conditions that are treatable with simple measures, such as clearing of airway secretions or administration of O_2. Yet it may be even more important to identify those respiratory conditions that are subtly but rapidly progressing toward respiratory failure. These conditions require timely interventions with more advanced airway techniques (eg, assisted bag-mask ventilation).

In infants and children, respiratory distress can quickly progress to respiratory failure and finally to cardiac arrest. Good outcome (ie, neurologically intact survival to hospital discharge) is more likely after respiratory arrest than after cardiac arrest. Once the child with a respiratory problem develops cardiac arrest, outcome is often poor. You can greatly improve outcome by early identification and management of respiratory distress and respiratory failure before the child deteriorates to cardiac arrest.

Identify and Intervene	**Respiratory Distress and Failure**
	The earlier you detect respiratory distress or respiratory failure and start appropriate therapy, the better the chance for a good outcome.

Learning Objective

After completing this section, you should be able to

- Differentiate between respiratory distress and failure

Preparation for the Course

You need to understand the concepts in this Part to be able to quickly identify signs of respiratory distress and respiratory failure. You also must be able to recognize respiratory problems by type so that you can choose appropriate interventions.

Fundamental Issues Associated With Respiratory Problems

Children with respiratory problems have impairment of oxygenation, ventilation, or both. This section discusses

- Impairment of oxygenation and ventilation
- Physiology of respiratory disease

Impairment of Oxygenation and Ventilation in Respiratory Problems

Physiology of the Respiratory System

The main function of the respiratory system is gas exchange. Air is taken into the lungs with inspiration. O_2 diffuses from the alveoli into the blood, where some O_2 dissolves in plasma. Most O_2 that enters the blood is attached (ie, saturated or bound) to hemoglobin. The percent of hemoglobin that is fully saturated with O_2 is called *oxygen saturation*. When blood passes through the lungs, CO_2 diffuses from the blood into the alveoli and is exhaled. Acute respiratory problems can result from alterations in any part of this system, from the airway to the alveoli (lung parenchyma). Central nervous system disease, such as seizures or head trauma, can impair control of respiration, leading to decreased respiratory rate. Muscle weakness, either primary (eg, muscular dystrophy) or secondary (eg, fatigue), may also impair oxygenation or ventilation.

Children have a high metabolic rate, so O_2 demand per kilogram of body weight is high. O_2 consumption in infants is 6 to 8 mL/kg per minute, compared with 3 to 4 mL/kg per minute in adults. Therefore, hypoxemia and tissue hypoxia can develop more rapidly in a child than in an adult if apnea or inadequate alveolar ventilation occurs.

Respiratory problems can result in

- Hypoxemia
- Hypercarbia
- A combination of both hypoxemia and hypercarbia

Hypoxemia (Low Oxygen Saturation)

Hypoxemia is defined as a decreased arterial oxygen saturation detected by pulse oximetry or direct measurement of oxygen saturation in an arterial blood gas sample. Hypoxemia is generally defined as arterial oxygen saturation below 94% in a normal child breathing room air. There are a variety of conditions that may lower the threshold, such as altitude or the presence of cyanotic heart disease. **Permissive hypoxemia** is a pulse oximetry percentage of less than 94%, which may be appropriate in certain circumstances (eg, some cases of congenital heart disease).

It is important to distinguish between *hypoxemia* and *tissue hypoxia*. Hypoxemia is low arterial O_2 saturation (SaO_2 less than 94%). Hypoxia is a pathologic condition in which the body as a whole (*generalized hypoxia*) or a region of the body (*tissue hypoxia*) is deprived of an adequate oxygen supply. Note that hypoxemia does *not* necessarily lead to tissue hypoxia and that tissue hypoxia may occur when arterial oxygen saturation is normal. For example, when hypoxemia is chronic (eg, unrepaired cyanotic heart disease), compensatory increases in blood flow (ie, increased cardiac output) or hemoglobin concentration (polycythemia) increase the O_2-carrying capacity of the blood and help maintain arterial O_2 content at near-normal concentrations despite the fact that hemoglobin saturation is low. This can help maintain oxygen delivery and tissue oxygenation even when hypoxemia is present. Conversely, if tissue perfusion is poor or the patient has severe anemia, tissue hypoxia may occur with normal arterial oxygen saturation.

In response to tissue hypoxia, the child may initially compensate by increasing respiratory rate and depth. This is known as *hyperventilation*. Hyperventilation refers to increased alveolar ventilation resulting in a decrease in $PaCO_2$ to less than 35 mm Hg. This may be caused by an increased respiratory rate, increased tidal volume, or combination of both. To ensure that $PaCO_2$ does not decrease below 30 mm Hg, hyperventilation must be guided by capnography. Tachycardia may also develop in response to hypoxemia as a means of increasing cardiac output. As tissue hypoxia worsens, these signs of cardiopulmonary distress become more severe (Table 29).

Table 29. Signs of Tissue Hypoxia

Early Signs of Tissue Hypoxia	Late Signs of Tissue Hypoxia
Fast respiratory rate (tachypnea)	Slow respiratory rate (bradypnea), inadequate respiratory effort, apnea
Increased respiratory effort: nasal flaring, retractions	Increased respiratory effort: head bobbing, seesaw respirations, grunting
Tachycardia	Bradycardia
Pallor, mottling, cyanosis (can appear as both early and late signs)	
Agitation, anxiety, irritability	Decreased level of consciousness

FYI

Arterial O_2 Content

Arterial O_2 content is the total amount of O_2 carried in the blood (in milliliters O_2 per deciliter of blood). It is the sum of the quantity of O_2 bound to hemoglobin plus the O_2 dissolved in arterial blood. O_2 content is determined largely by the hemoglobin (Hgb) concentration (grams per deciliter) and its saturation with O_2 (SaO_2). Use the following equation to calculate arterial O_2 content:

Arterial O_2 Content = [1.36 × Hgb concentration × SaO_2] + (0.003 × PaO_2)

Under normal conditions, dissolved O_2 (0.003 × PaO_2) is an inconsequential portion of the total arterial O_2 content. But an increase in dissolved O_2 can produce a relatively significant increase in arterial O_2 content for a child with severe anemia.

Hypoxemia can be caused by a number of different mechanisms leading to respiratory distress and failure (Table 30).

Table 30. Mechanisms of Hypoxemia

Factor	Causes	Mechanism	Treatment
Low atmospheric Po_2	High altitude (decreased barometric pressure)	Decreased Pao_2	Supplementary O_2
Alveolar hypoventilation	• Central nervous system infection • Traumatic brain injury • Drug overdose • Neuromuscular weakness • Apnea	Increased arterial CO_2 tension (hypercarbia) displaces alveolar O_2, resulting in decreased alveolar and arterial O_2 tension (low Pao_2 or hypoxemia).	Restore normal ventilation; supplementary O_2
Diffusion defect	• Pulmonary edema • Interstitial pneumonia • Alveolar proteinosis	Impaired movement of O_2 and CO_2 between the alveoli and blood results in decreased Pao_2 (hypoxemia) and, if severe, an increased $Paco_2$ (hypercarbia).	Application of noninvasive ventilation (either continuous positive airway pressure [CPAP] or biphasic/bilevel CPAP)
Ventilation/perfusion (V/Q) imbalance	• Pneumonia • Atelectasis • Acute respiratory distress syndrome • Asthma • Bronchiolitis • Foreign body	Mismatch of ventilation and perfusion: blood flow through areas of the lung that are inadequately ventilated results in incomplete oxygenation of the blood returning to the left side of the heart. The result is a decreased arterial O_2 saturation and Pao_2 and, to a lesser extent, increased $Paco_2$.	Positive end-expiratory pressure to increase mean airway pressure*; supplementary O_2; ventilatory support
Right-to-left shunt	• Cyanotic congenital heart disease • Extracardiac (anatomical) vascular shunt Same causes listed for V/Q imbalance[†]	Shunting of unoxygenated blood from the right side of the heart to the left (or from the pulmonary artery into the aorta) results in a low Pao_2. Effects are similar to right-to-left shunt in the lungs.	Correction of defect (supplementary O_2 alone is insufficient)

*Positive end-expiratory pressure should be used carefully in children with asthma; expert consultation is advised.

[†]With pneumonia, acute respiratory distress syndrome, and other lung tissue diseases, the pathophysiology is often characterized by a mix of mechanisms of hypoxemia. The most extreme form of V/Q mismatch would be a segment of lung with blood flow (Q) but no ventilation (V). In such a situation the blood does not become oxygenated. When it returns to the left side of the heart, it mixes with the oxygenated blood. The result is a lower O_2 saturation. The degree of desaturation depends on the size of the unventilated lung segment.

Hypercarbia (Inadequate Ventilation)

Hypercarbia is an increased CO_2 tension in the arterial blood ($PaCO_2$). When hypercarbia is present, ventilation is inadequate.

CO_2 is a by-product of tissue metabolism. Normally it is eliminated by the lungs to maintain acid-base homeostasis. When ventilation is inadequate, CO_2 elimination is inadequate. The resulting increase in $PaCO_2$ causes the blood to become acidic (respiratory acidosis). Causes of hypercarbia are

- Airway obstruction (upper or lower)
- Lung tissue disease
- Decreased or inadequate respiratory effort (central hypoventilation)

Foundational Facts

Detection of Hypercarbia

Hypercarbia is more difficult to detect than hypoxemia because it produces no obvious clinical sign, such as cyanosis. Precise measurement of PCO_2 requires a blood sample (arterial, capillary, or venous). Exhaled CO_2 detectors are now available for use in children with or without advanced airways. The end-tidal CO_2 (or exhaled CO_2 measured at the end of exhalation) measured by capnography may not be identical to the arterial CO_2. However, if the airway is open/patent, there is no increased dead space from air trapping (eg, asthma), and cardiac output is adequate, the end-tidal CO_2 will increase in the presence of hypercarbia.

Most children with hypercarbia present with respiratory distress and tachypnea. Children may become tachypneic in an attempt to eliminate excess CO_2. However, the child with hypercarbia may also present with poor respiratory effort, including decreased respiratory rate. In this case, hypercarbia results from inadequate ventilation secondary to impaired respiratory drive. This inadequate ventilation may result from drugs, such as a narcotic overdose. It may also result from a central nervous system disorder with respiratory muscle weakness preventing the development of compensatory tachypnea. Detection of an inadequate respiratory drive requires careful observation and assessment. Consequences of inadequate ventilation become more severe as the $PaCO_2$ increases and respiratory acidosis worsens.

When to Suspect Inadequate Ventilation (Hypercarbia)

Decreased level of consciousness is a critical symptom of both inadequate ventilation and hypoxia. If a child's clinical condition deteriorates from agitation and anxiety to decreased responsiveness despite supplementary O_2, this may indicate that the $PaCO_2$ is rising. Note that even if the pulse oximeter indicates adequate O_2 saturation, ventilation may be impaired and hypercarbia may be present. If a child with respiratory distress has a decreased level of consciousness despite adequate oxygenation, suspect that ventilation is inadequate and that hypercarbia and respiratory acidosis may be present.

Signs of inadequate ventilation are nonspecific and include one or more of the following:

- Tachypnea or inadequate respiratory rate for age and clinical condition
- Nasal flaring, retractions
- Change in level of consciousness: initial anxiety, agitation, and then decreased level of consciousness

Physiology of Respiratory Disease

Normal spontaneous breathing is accomplished with minimal work. Breathing is quiet with unlabored, smooth inspiration and passive expiration. In children with respiratory disease, "work of breathing" becomes more apparent. Important factors associated with increased work of breathing include

- Increased airway resistance (upper and lower)
- Decreased lung compliance
- Use of accessory muscles of respiration
- Disordered central nervous system control of breathing

Airway Resistance

Airway resistance is the impedance to airflow within the airways. Resistance is primarily increased by a reduction in the size of the conducting airways (either by airway constriction or inflammation). Turbulent airflow also causes increased airway resistance. Airflow may become turbulent when the flow rate is increased, even if the size of the airway is unchanged. When airway resistance increases, work of breathing increases in an attempt to maintain airflow despite the increase in airway resistance.

Larger airways provide lower resistance to airflow than smaller airways. Airway resistance decreases as lung volume increases (inflation) because airway dilation accompanies lung inflation. Conditions such as edema, bronchoconstriction, secretions, mucus, or a mediastinal mass impinging on large or small airways can decrease airway size, thereby increasing airway resistance. Resistance in the upper airway, particularly in the nasal or nasopharyngeal passages, can represent a significant portion of total airway resistance, especially in infants.

FYI

Airway Resistance

Airway Resistance in Laminar Airflow

During normal breathing, airflow is laminar (ie, quiet, smooth, and orderly) and airway resistance is relatively low. Specifically, only a small driving pressure (ie, difference in pressure between the pleural space and the atmosphere) is needed to produce adequate airflow. When airflow is laminar (quiet), resistance to airflow is inversely proportional to the *fourth* power of the airway radius, so even a small reduction in airway diameter results in a significant increase in airway resistance and work of breathing (Figure 23).

Airway Resistance in Turbulent Airflow

When airflow is turbulent (ie, irregular), resistance is inversely proportional to the *fifth* power of the radius of the airway lumen, a 10-fold increase over the resistance to airflow that occurs during reduction in the airway radius when airflow is normal and laminar. In this state, a much larger driving pressure is required to produce the same rate of airflow. Therefore, patient agitation (causing rapid, turbulent airflow) results in a much greater increase in airway resistance and work of breathing than with quiet, laminar flow. To prevent generation of turbulent airflow (eg, during crying), try to keep a child with airway obstruction as calm as possible.

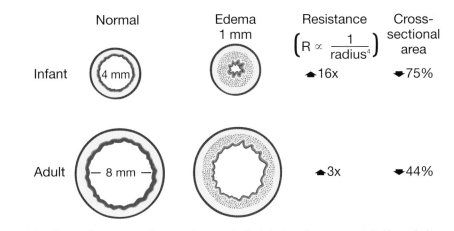

Figure 23. Effects of edema on airway resistance in the infant vs the young adult. Normal airways are shown on the left; edematous airways (with 1 mm of circumferential edema) are on the right. Resistance to flow is inversely proportional to the fourth power of the radius of the airway lumen for laminar flow and to the fifth power of the radius when air flow is turbulent. The net result is a 75% decrease in cross-sectional area and a 16-fold increase in airway resistance in the infant vs a 44% decrease in cross-sectional area and a 3-fold increase in airway resistance in the adult during quiet breathing. Turbulent flow in the infant (eg, crying) increases airway resistance and thus the work of breathing from 16- to 32-fold. Modified from Coté CJ, Todres ID. The pediatric airway. In: Coté CJ, Ryan JF, Todres ID, Goudsouzian NG, eds. *A Practice of Anesthesia for Infants and Children.* 2nd ed. Philadelphia, PA: WB Saunders Co; 1993:55-83, copyright Elsevier.

Lung Compliance

Compliance refers to the distensibility of the lung, chest wall, or both. *Lung compliance* is defined as the change in lung volume produced by a change in driving pressure across the lung. When lung compliance is high, the lungs are easily inflated (there is a large change in volume produced by a slight change in driving pressure). In a child with low lung compliance, the lungs are stiffer; more effort is needed to inflate them. To create a significant pressure gradient to produce air flow into the stiff lung, the diaphragm contracts more forcefully. This increases intrathoracic volume and reduces intrathoracic pressure to create air flow. It also increases work of breathing and, in the younger child, produces retractions. During mechanical ventilation, increased positive airway pressure is needed to achieve adequate ventilation when lung compliance is decreased.

Compliance varies within the lung according to the degree of lung inflation. Extrapulmonary conditions that cause decreased compliance are pneumothorax and pleural effusion. Pneumonia and inflammatory lung tissue disease (eg, ARDS, fibrosis, pulmonary edema) cause decreased compliance. These conditions are associated with an increase in the water content in the interstitial space and alveoli. The impact of this increase in water content on lung compliance is similar to the expansion that occurs when a sponge becomes saturated with water. A normal sponge re-expands quickly when it is compressed. A wet sponge is harder to compress and re-expands more slowly because its normal elasticity is opposed by the extra weight of the fluid in the sponge.

FYI

Disordered Breathing and the Chest Wall

The chest wall in infants and young children is compliant. Therefore, relatively small pressure changes can move the chest wall. During normal breathing, diaphragm contraction in infants pulls the lower ribs slightly inward but does not result in significant chest retraction. However, forceful contraction of the diaphragm results in a large drop in pressure within the chest, pulling the chest inward (ie, retracting it) during inspiration. When lung compliance is reduced, maximum inspiratory effort may not produce adequate tidal volume because marked retractions of the chest wall limit lung expansion during inspiration.

Children with neuromuscular disorders have a weak chest wall and weak respiratory muscles that can make breathing and coughing ineffective. Muscle weakness can result in characteristic seesaw breathing (simultaneous retraction of the chest wall and expansion of the abdomen).

Inspiratory and Expiratory Flow

The inspiratory muscles of respiration include the diaphragm, intercostal muscles, and accessory muscles (primarily of the abdomen and neck). During spontaneous breathing, inspiratory muscles (chiefly the diaphragm) increase intrathoracic volume, resulting in a decrease in intrathoracic pressure. When intrathoracic pressure is less than atmospheric pressure, air flows into the lungs (*inspiration*). The intercostal muscles normally stiffen the chest wall as the diaphragm contracts. Accessory muscles of respiration are not typically needed during normal ventilation. In respiratory disorders that increase airway resistance or reduce lung compliance, accessory muscles help create a decrease in intrathoracic pressure and maintain adequate chest wall stiffness needed to produce inspiratory flow.

Expiratory flow results from relaxation of the inspiratory muscles and elastic recoil of the lung and chest wall. These changes increase intrathoracic pressure to a level that is higher than the atmospheric pressure. During spontaneous breathing, expiratory flow is primarily a passive process. Expiration may become an active process in the presence of increased lower airway resistance and may require involvement of muscles of the abdominal wall and the intercostal muscles.

FYI

The Role of the Diaphragm in Breathing

The normal diaphragm is dome-shaped and contracts most forcefully in this shape. When the diaphragm is flattened, as occurs with lung hyperinflation (eg, acute asthma), contraction is less forceful and ventilation is less efficient. Respiration is compromised if movement of the diaphragm is impeded by abdominal distention and high intra-abdominal pressure (eg, gastric inflation) or by air trapping caused by airway obstruction. During infancy and early childhood, the intercostal muscles serve primarily to stabilize the chest wall. They cannot effectively lift the chest wall to increase intrathoracic volume and compensate for loss of diaphragm motion.

Central Nervous System Control of Breathing

Breathing is controlled by complex mechanisms involving

- Brainstem respiratory centers
- Central and peripheral chemoreceptors
- Voluntary control

Spontaneous breathing is controlled by a group of respiratory centers located in the brainstem. Breathing also can be overridden by voluntary control from the cerebral cortex. Examples of voluntary control include breath holding, panting, and sighing. Conditions such as infection of the central nervous system, traumatic brain injury, and drug overdose can impair respiratory drive, resulting in hypoventilation or even apnea.

FYI

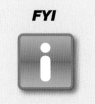

Central Chemoreceptors

Central chemoreceptors respond to changes in the hydrogen ion concentration of cerebrospinal fluid, which is largely determined by the arterial CO_2 tension ($Paco_2$). Peripheral chemoreceptors (eg, in the carotid body) respond primarily to a decrease in arterial O_2 (Pao_2); some receptors also respond to an increase in $Paco_2$.

Identification of Respiratory Problems by Severity

Identifying the severity of a respiratory problem will help you decide the most appropriate interventions. Be alert for signs of

- Respiratory distress
- Respiratory failure

Respiratory Distress

Respiratory distress is a clinical state characterized by increased respiratory rate, effort, and work of breathing. Children can have respiratory distress, which spans a spectrum from mild tachypnea with increased effort to severe distress with impending respiratory failure. A description of the severity of respiratory distress typically includes a description of the respiratory rate and effort, quality of breath sounds, and mental status (Table 31). Note that signs of severe respiratory distress can indicate respiratory failure.

Table 31. Signs of Respiratory Distress*

Mild Respiratory Distress	Severe Respiratory Distress or Possible Respiratory Failure
• Mild tachypnea • Mild increase in respiratory effort (eg, nasal flaring, retractions) • Abnormal airway sounds (eg, stridor, wheezing, grunting) • Mottling	• Marked tachypnea and apnea • Significant or inadequate respiratory effort (eg, hypoventilation or bradypnea) • Abnormal airway sounds • Low oxygen saturation (hypoxemia) despite high-flow supplementary oxygen • Pale, cool skin; cyanosis • Decreased level of consciousness (eg, less responsive or unresponsive)

*These indicators may vary in severity.

Respiratory distress is apparent when a child tries to maintain adequate gas exchange despite airway obstruction, reduced lung compliance, or lung tissue disease. As the child tires or as respiratory function or effort or both deteriorate, adequate gas exchange cannot be maintained. When this happens, clinical signs of respiratory failure develop.

Respiratory Failure

Respiratory failure is a clinical state of inadequate oxygenation, ventilation, or both. Respiratory failure is recognized typically by abnormal appearance (particularly an altered level of consciousness, which may be characterized by agitation or a depressed level of consciousness), poor color, and reduced responsiveness. Although respiratory failure is often the result of progression of respiratory distress, it may occur with little or no respiratory effort. At times, recognition of respiratory failure requires laboratory data (eg, blood gas) to confirm the diagnosis. In other patients, the clinical examination is sufficient to identify respiratory failure.

Suspect *probable respiratory failure* if some of the signs listed in Table 32 are present.

Table 32. Signs of Severe Respiratory Distress and Probable Respiratory Failure

Signs of Severe Respiratory Distress	Signs of Probable Respiratory Failure
• Marked tachypnea • Increased or decreased respiratory effort • Poor distal air movement • Tachycardia • Low oxygen saturation (hypoxemia) despite high-flow oxygen administration • Cyanosis	• Very rapid or inadequate respiratory rate or possible apnea • Significant, inadequate, or absent respiratory effort • Absent distal air movement • Extreme tachycardia; bradycardia often indicates life-threatening deterioration • Low oxygen saturation (hypoxemia) despite high-flow supplementary oxygen • Decreased level of consciousness • Cyanosis

Respiratory failure can result from upper or lower airway obstruction, lung tissue disease, and disordered control of breathing (eg, apnea or shallow, slow respirations). *When respiratory effort is inadequate, respiratory failure can occur without typical signs of respiratory distress.* Respiratory failure is a clinical state that *requires intervention* to prevent deterioration to cardiac arrest.

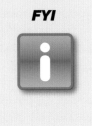

Respiratory Failure and Baseline Physiology

It is difficult to define strict criteria for respiratory failure because the baseline respiratory function of an infant or child may be abnormal. For example, an infant with cyanotic congenital heart disease and a baseline arterial O_2 saturation (SaO_2) of 75% is not in respiratory failure on the basis of low O_2 saturation. But the same degree of hypoxemia would be one sign of respiratory failure in a child with normal baseline cardiopulmonary physiology.

Auscultation With a Stethoscope

Use a stethoscope to auscultate the following points during a respiratory physical exam:

- Anterior (on either side of the breastbone)
- Posterior
- Lateral (under the axillae)

For more information, see "Chest Expansion and Air Movement" in Part 3.

Identification of Respiratory Problems by Type

Respiratory distress or failure can be classified into one or more of the following types:

- Upper airway obstruction
- Lower airway obstruction
- Lung tissue disease
- Disordered control of breathing

Respiratory problems do not always occur in isolation. A child may have more than a single cause of respiratory distress or failure. For example, a child may have disordered control of breathing caused by a head injury and then develop pneumonia (lung tissue disease). A patient may also exhibit symptoms consistent with more than one class of respiratory abnormality.

Upper Airway Obstruction

Obstruction of the upper airways (ie, the airways outside the thorax) can occur in the nose, pharynx, or larynx. Obstruction can range from mild to severe.

Causes of Upper Airway Obstruction

Common causes of upper airway obstruction are foreign-body aspiration (eg, food or a small object), infection, and swelling of the airway (eg, anaphylaxis, tonsillar hypertrophy, croup, or epiglottitis). Other causes of upper airway obstruction are a mass that compromises the airway lumen (eg, pharyngeal or peritonsillar abscess, retropharyngeal abscess, or tumor), thick secretions obstructing the nasal passages, or any congenital airway abnormality (eg, congenital subglottic stenosis) resulting in narrowing of the airway, or poor control of the upper airway due to a decreased level of consciousness. Upper airway obstruction also may be hospital acquired. For example, subglottic stenosis may develop secondary to trauma induced by endotracheal intubation.

Due to their small airway, infants and small children are especially prone to upper airway obstruction. An infant's tongue is large in proportion to the oropharyngeal cavity. If the infant has a decreased level of consciousness, the muscles may relax, allowing the tongue to fall back and obstruct the oropharynx. Infants also have a prominent occiput. If the infant with a decreased level of consciousness is supine, resting on the large occiput can cause flexion of the neck, resulting in upper airway obstruction.

Signs of Upper Airway Obstruction

The major clinical signs typically occur during the inspiratory phase of the respiratory cycle, such as stridor, hoarseness, or a change in voice or cry. Inspiratory retractions, use of accessory muscles, and nasal flaring are often present. The respiratory rate is often only mildly elevated, as upper airway obstruction is worse with faster breathing. Examples include foreign body obstruction, croup, and epiglottitis.

Signs of Upper Airway Obstruction
• Increased respiratory rate and effort
• Increased inspiratory respiratory effort (eg, inspiratory retractions, use of accessory muscles of respiration, nasal flaring)
• Stridor (usually inspiratory but may be expiratory)
• Change in voice (eg, hoarseness), cry, or presence of a barking cough
• Drooling, snoring, or gurgling sounds
• Poor chest rise
• Poor air entry on auscultation

Lower Airway Obstruction

Obstruction of the lower airways (ie, the airways within the thorax) can occur in the lower trachea, the bronchi, or the bronchioles.

Causes of Lower Airway Obstruction

Common causes of lower airway obstruction are

- Asthma
- Bronchiolitis

Signs of Lower Airway Obstruction

The major clinical signs typically occur during the expiratory phase of the respiratory cycle. The child often has wheezing and a prolonged expiratory phase requiring increased expiratory effort. The respiratory rate is usually elevated, particularly in infants. Inspiratory retractions become prominent when the lower airway obstruction impairs inspiration and exhalation, requiring increased respiratory effort. Examples include asthma and bronchiolitis.

Signs of Lower Airway Obstruction
• Increased respiratory rate
• Increased respiratory effort (retractions, nasal flaring, and prolonged expiration)
• Possible decreased air movement on auscultation
• Prolonged expiratory phase associated with increased expiratory effort (ie, expiration becomes an active rather than a passive process)
• Wheezing (most commonly expiratory but may be inspiratory or biphasic)
• Cough

FYI

Airway Obstruction and Respiratory Rate

In children with acute lower airway obstruction (eg, status asthmaticus), the increase in intrapleural pressure produced by forced expiration compresses airways proximal to the alveoli. This airway compression leads to further expiratory obstruction with no increase in expiratory flow. If this small airway collapse is severe, it leads to air trapping and lung hyperinflation. In acute severe asthma, the respiratory rate may slow and the child may attempt to increase tidal volume. These responses minimize frictional forces and the work of breathing.

An infant with lower airway obstruction, by comparison, typically has a rapid respiratory rate. The infant has a compliant chest wall. If the infant attempts to breathe more deeply, the resulting decrease in intrapleural pressure may result in greater chest wall retractions. When there is significant lower airway obstruction, it is more efficient for the infant to breathe at a fast rate with small tidal volumes to maintain minute ventilation, keeping a relatively larger volume of gas in the lungs.

Lung Tissue Disease

This condition is used to describe disease involving the substance (ie, parenchyma or tissue) of the lung. In this state, the child's lungs become stiff because of fluid accumulation in the alveoli, interstitium, or both requiring increased respiratory effort during inspiration and exhalation. Therefore, retractions and accessory muscle use are common. Hypoxemia is often marked due to alveolar collapse or reduced oxygen diffusion caused by pulmonary edema fluid and inflammatory debris in alveoli. Tachypnea is common and often quite marked. The patient frequently attempts to counteract alveolar and small airway collapse by increasing efforts to maintain an elevated end-expiratory pressure. This is often manifested by grunting respirations.

Causes of Lung Tissue Disease

Lung tissue disease has many causes. Pneumonia from any cause (eg, bacterial, viral, chemical, aspiration) and cardiogenic and noncardiogenic pulmonary edema (from congestive heart failure and ARDS) can cause lung tissue disease. Other potential causes are pulmonary contusion (trauma), allergic reaction, toxins, vasculitis, and infiltrative disease. Lung tissue disease can also result from allergic, vascular, widespread inflammatory, environmental, and other factors.

Signs of Lung Tissue Disease

Signs of lung tissue disease are shown below.

Signs of Lung Tissue Disease
• Tachypnea (often marked)
• Increased respiratory effort
• Grunting
• Crackles (rales) and decreased air movement
• Diminished breath sounds
• Tachycardia
• Hypoxemia (despite administration of supplementary O_2)

FYI

Hypercarbia and Grunting in Lung Tissue Disease

Children with lung tissue disease can often maintain ventilation (ie, CO_2 elimination) with a relatively small number of functional alveoli, but they cannot maintain oxygenation as effectively. As a result, hypoxemia is an earlier sign of lung tissue disease than hypercarbia. Compromised ventilation, indicated by hypercarbia, is typically a late manifestation of the disease process.

Grunting produces early glottic closure during expiration. Grunting is a compensatory mechanism to maintain positive airway pressure and prevent collapse of the alveoli and small airways.

Disordered Control of Breathing

In this state, there is inadequate respiratory effort. Often the parent will state that the child is "breathing funny." There may be periods of increased respiratory rate, effort, or both followed by decreased rate, effort, or both, or the child's respiratory rate or effort may be continuously inadequate. Often the net effect is hypoventilation leading to hypoxemia and hypercarbia.

Causes of Disordered Control of Breathing

Disordered control of breathing may result from a host of conditions, including neurologic disorders (eg, seizures, central nervous system infections, head injury, brain tumor, hydrocephalus, neuromuscular disease), metabolic abnormalities, and drug overdose. Because disordered control of breathing is typically associated with conditions that impair neurologic function, these children often have a decreased level of consciousness.

Signs of Disordered Control of Breathing

Signs of disordered control of breathing include the following:

Signs of Disordered Control of Breathing
• Variable or irregular respiratory rate and pattern (tachypnea alternating with bradypnea)
• Variable respiratory effort
• Shallow breathing with inadequate effort (frequently resulting in hypoxemia and hypercarbia)
• Central apnea (ie, apnea without any respiratory effort)
• Normal or decreased air movement

Summary: Recognition of Respiratory Problems Flowchart

Figure 24 summarizes recognition and identification of respiratory problems. Note that this chart does not include all respiratory emergencies; it provides key characteristics for a limited number of diseases.

Pediatric Advanced Life Support
Signs of Respiratory Problems

	Clinical Signs	Upper Airway Obstruction	Lower Airway Obstruction	Lung Tissue Disease	Disordered Control of Breathing
A	Patency	Airway open and maintainable/not maintainable			
B	Respiratory Rate/Effort	Increased			Variable
	Breath Sounds	Stridor (typically inspiratory) Barking cough Hoarseness	Wheezing (typically expiratory) Prolonged expiratory phase	Grunting Crackles Decreased breath sounds	Normal
	Air Movement	Decreased			Variable
C	Heart Rate	Tachycardia (early) Bradycardia (late)			
	Skin	Pallor, cool skin (early) Cyanosis (late)			
D	Level of Consciousness	Anxiety, agitation (early) Lethargy, unresponsiveness (late)			
E	Temperature	Variable			

Pediatric Advanced Life Support
Identification of Respiratory Problems by Severity

Respiratory Distress ➡ Respiratory Failure

A	Open and maintainable ➡ **Not maintainable**
B	Tachypnea ➡ **Bradypnea to apnea**
	Work of breathing (nasal flaring/retractions) **Increased effort** ➡ **Decreased effort** ➡ **Apnea**
	Good air movement ➡ **Poor to absent air movement**
C	Tachycardia ➡ **Bradycardia**
	Pallor ➡ **Cyanosis**
D	Anxiety, agitation ➡ **Lethargy to unresponsiveness**
E	Variable temperature

Figure 24. Recognition of Respiratory Problems Flowchart.

Part 7

Management of Respiratory Distress and Failure

Overview

Respiratory problems are a major cause of cardiac arrest in children. In fact, many infants and children who require CPR (both in and out of hospital) have respiratory problems that progress to cardiopulmonary failure. It may not be possible to differentiate between respiratory distress and respiratory failure on the basis of clinical examination alone. Respiratory failure can develop even without significant signs of distress. In children, clinical deterioration in respiratory function may progress rapidly, so there is little time to waste. Prompt recognition and effective management of respiratory problems are fundamental to PALS.

Critical Concepts

Intervene Quickly to Restore Respiratory Function

PALS providers must intervene quickly to restore adequate respiratory function. You can greatly improve outcome by early identification and prompt management of respiratory distress and failure. Once respiratory failure progresses to cardiac arrest, outcome is often poor.

Learning Objective

After completing this Part, you should be able to

- Perform early interventions for respiratory distress and failure

Preparation for the Course

During the course you will participate in the Airway Management Skills Station. You will have an opportunity to practice and demonstrate your proficiency in performing basic airway management skills, such as insertion of airway adjuncts, effective bag-mask ventilation, and suctioning. See the Appendix for a checklist of required competencies. See the "Resources for Management of Respiratory Emergencies" at the end of this Part for details on bag-mask ventilation, respiratory function monitoring devices (eg, monitoring of O_2 saturation by pulse oximetry, monitoring of exhaled CO_2), and O_2 delivery systems.

Rescue Breathing

Respiratory Arrest

Respiratory arrest is the absence of respirations (ie, apnea) with detectable cardiac activity. The provider must provide rescue breathing to prevent cardiac arrest.

Rescue Breathing

Guidelines for rescue breathing are as follows:

Rescue Breathing for Infants and Children
• Give 12 to 20 breaths per minute (about 1 breath every 3 to 5 seconds). • Give each breath in 1 second. • Each breath should result in visible chest rise. • Check the pulse about every 2 minutes; if the child becomes pulseless, shout for help and provide compressions as well as ventilation (CPR). • Use oxygen as soon as it is available.

Identify and Intervene

Life-Threatening Problems

If at any time you identify a life-threatening problem, immediately begin appropriate interventions. Activate the emergency response system as indicated in your practice setting.

Initial Management of Respiratory Distress and Failure

The first priority in the management of a seriously ill or injured child who is not in cardiac arrest is evaluation of airway and breathing. If there are signs of respiratory distress or failure, initial interventions must support or restore adequate oxygenation and ventilation.

Respiratory conditions are a major cause of cardiac arrest in infants and children. As a result, when respiratory distress or failure is detected, it is important to begin appropriate interventions quickly.

Initial interventions include a rapid, focused evaluation of respiratory function to identify the type and severity, rather than the precise etiology, of the respiratory problem. Once oxygenation and ventilation are stabilized, identify the cause of the problem to facilitate targeted interventions. Use the evaluate-identify-intervene sequence to monitor progression of symptoms or response to therapy and to prioritize further interventions.

Initial stabilization and management of a child in respiratory distress or respiratory failure may include the interventions listed in Table 33.

Table 33. Initial Management of Respiratory Distress or Failure

Evaluate	Interventions (as Indicated)

Airway	• Support an open airway (allow child to assume position of comfort) or, if necessary, open the airway with
	  – Head tilt–chin lift
	  – Jaw thrust without head tilt if cervical spine injury is suspected. If this maneuver does not open the airway, use the head tilt–chin lift or jaw thrust with gentle head extension
	• Clear the airway if indicated (eg, suction nose and mouth, remove visualized foreign body).
	• Consider an oropharyngeal airway or nasopharyngeal airway to improve airway openness/patency.

Breathing	• Monitor O_2 saturation by pulse oximetry. • Provide O_2 (humidified if available). Use a high-concentration delivery device such as a nonrebreathing mask for treatment of severe respiratory distress or possible respiratory failure. • Administer inhaled medication (eg, albuterol, epinephrine) as needed. • Assist ventilation with bag-mask device and supplementary O_2 if needed. • Prepare for insertion of an advanced airway if indicated.
Circulation	• Monitor heart rate, heart rhythm, and blood pressure. • Establish vascular access (for fluid therapy and medications) as indicated.

Principles of Targeted Management

Once oxygenation and ventilation are stabilized, identify the type of respiratory problem to help prioritize the next interventions. This Part reviews principles of targeted management for the following 4 types of respiratory problems:

- Upper airway obstruction
- Lower airway obstruction
- Lung tissue disease
- Disordered control of breathing

Management of Upper Airway Obstruction

Upper airway obstruction is an obstruction of the large airways outside the thorax (ie, in the nose, pharynx, or larynx). The obstruction can range from mild to severe. Causes of upper airway obstruction are airway swelling, foreign body, or infection. Other causes of obstruction are edema or swelling of the soft tissue of the upper airway (large tonsils or adenoids), a mass in the airway, thick secretions, congenital narrowing of the upper airway, or poor control of the upper airway due to a decreased level of consciousness.

Infants and small children are especially prone to upper airway obstruction. If the infant has a decreased level of consciousness, the muscles may relax, allowing the tongue to fall back and obstruct the oropharynx. Also, if the infant with a decreased level of consciousness is supine, resting on their large occiput can cause flexion of the neck, resulting in upper airway obstruction. In young infants, nasal obstruction can impair ventilation. Secretions, blood, and debris in the nose, pharynx, and larynx from infection, inflammation, or trauma also can obstruct the airway. It is important to remember that the smaller the airway is, the more easily it can become obstructed.

General Management of Upper Airway Obstruction

General management of upper airway obstruction includes initial interventions listed in Table 33. Additional measures focus on relieving the obstruction. These measures may include opening the airway by

- Allowing the child to assume a position of comfort
- Performing manual airway maneuvers, such as a jaw thrust or head tilt–chin lift
- Removing a foreign body
- Suctioning the nose or mouth
- Reducing airway swelling with medications
- Minimizing agitation (agitation often worsens upper airway obstruction)
- Deciding whether an airway adjunct or advanced airway is needed
- Deciding early if a surgical airway (tracheostomy or needle cricothyroidotomy) is needed

Suctioning is helpful in removing secretions, blood, or debris; *however, if the upper airway obstruction is caused by edema from infection (eg, croup) or allergic reaction, carefully weigh potential benefits vs risks of suctioning.* Suctioning may increase the child's agitation and may increase respiratory distress. Instead, consider allowing the child to assume a position of comfort. Give nebulized epinephrine, particularly if the swelling is beyond the tongue. Corticosteroids (inhaled, IV, oral, or intramuscular [IM]) also may be helpful in this situation.

When upper airway obstruction is severe, *call early* for advanced help. The provider with the greatest skill and experience in airway management is the most likely person to safely establish an airway. Failure to aggressively treat an acute partial upper airway obstruction may lead to complete airway obstruction and, ultimately, to cardiac arrest.

In less severe cases of upper airway obstruction, infants and children may benefit from specific airway adjuncts. For example, in a child with a decreased level of consciousness, an oropharyngeal airway or nasopharyngeal airway may be helpful in relieving obstruction caused by the tongue. Use an oropharyngeal airway only if the child is deeply unconscious with no gag reflex. A child with a gag reflex may tolerate a nasopharyngeal airway. Insert a nasopharyngeal airway carefully to avoid nasopharyngeal trauma and bleeding. Avoid using a nasopharyngeal airway in children with increased bleeding risk or severe trauma to the head or face.

An infant or child with upper airway obstruction from redundant tissues or tissue edema may benefit from the application of noninvasive ventilation with positive airway pressure.

Specific Management of Upper Airway Obstruction by Etiology

Specific causes of upper airway obstruction require specific interventions. This section reviews management of upper airway obstruction due to

- Croup
- Anaphylaxis
- Foreign-body airway obstruction (FBAO)

Management of Croup Based on Severity

Croup is managed according to your assessment of clinical severity. The following characteristics of croup are listed by degree of severity:

- **Mild croup:** Occasional barking cough, little or no stridor at rest, absent or mild retractions
- **Moderate croup:** Frequent barking cough, easily audible stridor at rest, retractions at rest, little or no agitation, good air entry by auscultation of the peripheral lung fields
- **Severe croup:** Frequent barking cough, prominent inspiratory and occasional expiratory stridor, marked retractions, significant agitation, decreased air entry by auscultation of the lungs
- **Impending respiratory failure:** Barking cough (may not be prominent if the child's respiratory effort is growing weaker with the development of severe hypoxemia and hypercarbia), audible stridor at rest (can be difficult to hear with failing respiratory effort), retractions (may not be severe if respiratory effort is failing), poor air movement on auscultation, lethargy or decreased level of consciousness, and, sometimes, pallor or cyanosis despite administration of supplementary O_2

O_2 saturation may be slightly low in mild and moderate croup and is commonly well below normal in severe croup.

General management for upper airway obstruction includes the initial interventions listed in Table 33 and may include the *specific interventions for management of croup* listed in Table 34.

Table 34. Management of Croup

Severity of Croup	Interventions
Mild	• Consider dexamethasone.
Moderate to severe	• Administer humidified O_2. • Give nothing by mouth. • Administer nebulized epinephrine. • Observe for at least 2 hours after giving nebulized epinephrine to ensure continued improvement (no recurrence of stridor). • Administer dexamethasone. • Consider use of heliox (helium-oxygen mixture) for severe disease if the child requires no higher than 40% inspired oxygen concentration.
Impending respiratory failure	• Administer a high concentration of O_2; use a nonrebreathing mask if available. • Provide assisted ventilation (ie, bag-mask ventilation timed to support child's own inspiration) for persistent, severe hypoxemia (<90% O_2 saturation) despite O_2 administration, inadequate ventilation, or changes in level of consciousness. • Administer dexamethasone IV/IM. • Perform endotracheal (ET) intubation if indicated; to avoid injury to the subglottic area, use a smaller ET tube size (a half size smaller than predicted for the child's age). • Prepare for surgical airway if needed.

Critical Concepts

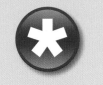

Endotracheal Intubation

Endotracheal intubation of the child with upper airway obstruction is a high-risk procedure and should be performed by a team with significant pediatric airway expertise. Use neuromuscular blockade only if you are confident the child's oxygenation and ventilation can be supported with bag-mask ventilation.

Management of Anaphylaxis

In addition to the initial interventions listed in Table 33, specific interventions that may be used for the *management of anaphylaxis* are listed in Table 35. Campbell et al. *Ann Allergy Asthma Immunol.* 2014;113:599-608 in the Suggested Reading List on the Student Website for more information.

Table 35. Management of Anaphylaxis

Severity of Allergic Reaction	Interventions
Mild	• Remove the offending agent (eg, stop the IV antibiotic). • Get help. • Ask the child or caregiver about any history of allergy or anaphylaxis; look for a medical alert bracelet or necklace. • Consider an oral dose of antihistamine.

Moderate to Severe	• Administer IM epinephrine by autoinjector or regular syringe every 10 to 15 minutes as needed; repeated doses may be needed.
	• Administer methylprednisolone or equivalent corticosteroid IV.
	• Treat bronchospasm (wheezing) with albuterol administered by metered-dose inhaler or nebulizer solution.
	• Give continuous nebulization if indicated (ie, severe bronchospasm).
	• For severe respiratory distress, anticipate further airway swelling and prepare for ET intubation.
	• To treat hypotension:
	  – Place the child in the supine position as tolerated
	  – Administer isotonic crystalloid (eg, normal saline or lactated Ringer's) 20 mL/kg bolus IV (repeat as needed)
	  – For hypotension unresponsive to fluids and IM epinephrine, administer an epinephrine infusion titrated to achieve adequate blood pressure for age
	• Administer diphenhydramine and H_2 blocker (eg, ranitidine) IV.

Management of Foreign-Body Airway Obstruction

If you suspect an FBAO that is mild (the child is able to make sounds and cough forcefully), do not intervene. Call for help and allow the child to try to clear the obstruction by coughing. If you suspect that the FBAO is severe (child makes no sound, is unable to speak or cough, has poor or no air exchange, makes a high-pitched noise while inhaling or no noise at all, has increased respiratory difficulty), perform the following maneuvers:

Interventions for a Responsive Infant or Child With FBAO	
Infant **(Younger Than 1 Year of Age)**	**Child** **(1 Year to Adolescent [Puberty])**
1. Confirm severe airway obstruction. 2. Give up to 5 back slaps and up to 5 chest thrusts. 3. Repeat Step 2 until object is expelled or victim becomes unresponsive.	1. Ask, "Are you choking?" If the child nods or otherwise indicates "yes," say you're going to help. 2. Stand or kneel behind the child. Give abdominal thrusts/ Heimlich maneuver. 3. Repeat abdominal thrusts until object is expelled or victim becomes unresponsive.
Victim Becomes Unresponsive	
1. Shout for help. Send someone to activate the emergency response system. 2. Lower the child to the floor. If the child is unresponsive with no breathing or only gasping, begin CPR (no pulse check). 3. Each time you open the airway to deliver breaths, look into the mouth. If you see an object that can be easily removed, remove it. If you do not see an object, continue CPR. *Note:* Do not perform a *blind finger sweep* in an effort to dislodge a foreign body. This may push the foreign body farther into the airway. It also may cause trauma and bleeding. 4. Continue CPR for 5 cycles or about 2 minutes.* If you are alone, leave the child to activate the emergency response system. Continue CPR until more skilled providers arrive.	

*Providing effective ventilation by using a bag-mask device during CPR to a child with an FBAO may be difficult. Consider using the 2-person bag-mask ventilation technique.

Management of Lower Airway Obstruction

Lower airway obstruction involves the smaller bronchi and bronchioles inside the thorax. Common causes are bronchiolitis and asthma.

General Management of Lower Airway Obstruction

General management of lower airway obstruction includes the initial interventions listed in Table 33.

In a child with severe respiratory distress or respiratory failure, your first priority is to restore adequate oxygenation; immediate correction of hypercarbia to the child's baseline level is not required because most children can tolerate hypercarbia without adverse effects.

If bag-mask ventilation is needed for a child with lower airway obstruction, provide effective ventilation at a relatively slow rate. Providing ventilation at a slow rate allows more time for expiration. This reduces the risk that air will remain inside the chest at the end of expiration. Providing too many breaths or breaths with too much volume may result in complications (Table 36).

Table 36. Complications of Hyperventilation

Complication	Result
Air enters the stomach (gastric distention)	• Increased risk of vomiting and aspiration • Can prevent adequate movement of the diaphragm, limiting effective ventilation
Risk of pneumothorax (air leak into space surrounding the lungs)	• Decreased blood return to the heart • Risk of lung collapse and resultant complications (severe hypoxemia, obstructive shock)
Severe air trapping	• Severe decrease in oxygenation • Decreased venous return to the heart and cardiac output

Specific Management of Lower Airway Obstruction by Etiology

Specific causes of lower airway obstruction require specific interventions. This section reviews management of lower airway obstruction due to the following:

- Bronchiolitis
- Acute asthma

Distinguishing between bronchiolitis and asthma in a wheezing infant can be difficult. A history of previous wheezing episodes suggests that the infant has reversible bronchospasm (ie, asthma). Consider a trial of bronchodilators if the diagnosis is unclear.

Management of Bronchiolitis

In addition to initial management in Table 33, specific measures that may be used for the *management of bronchiolitis* are listed in Table 37.

Table 37. Management of Bronchiolitis

Interventions
• Perform oral or nasal suctioning as needed. • Consider laboratory and other tests, which may include viral studies, chest x-ray, and arterial blood gas.

Randomized controlled trials of bronchodilator or corticosteroid therapy for bronchiolitis have shown mixed results. Some infants improve when treated with nebulized epinephrine or albuterol. In some infants, however, respiratory symptoms are aggravated by nebulizer therapy. Consider a trial of nebulized epinephrine or albuterol treatment. Discontinue it if there is no improvement. Administer supplementary O_2 if O_2 saturation is less than 94%.

Management of Acute Asthma

Manage asthma according to your assessment of clinical severity (Table 38). In addition to initial interventions listed in Table 33, there are specific interventions for the management of acute asthma (Table 39).

Table 38. Severity Score: Classification of Mild, Moderate, and Severe Asthma

Parameter*	Mild	Moderate	Severe	Respiratory Arrest Imminent
Breathless	Walking Can lie down	Talking (Infant will have softer, shorter cry; difficulty feeding) Prefers sitting	At rest (Infant will stop feeding) Hunched forward	
Talks in	Sentences	Phrases	Words	
Alertness	May be agitated	Usually agitated	Usually agitated	Drowsy or confused
Respiratory rate	Increased	Increased	Often >30/min	
	Age <2 months 2-12 months 1-5 years 6-8 years	**Normal rate** <60/min <50/min <40/min <30/min		
Accessory muscles and suprasternal retractions	Usually not	Usually	Usually	Paradoxical thoraco-abdominal movement
Wheeze	Moderate, often only end-expiration	Loud	Usually loud	Absence of wheeze
Pulse/min	<100	100-120	>120	Bradycardia
	Guide to limits of normal pulse rate in children: **Age** Infants (2-12 months) Toddler (1-2 years) Preschool/school age (2-8 years)	**Normal rate** <160/min <120/min <110/min		
Pulsus paradoxus	Absent <10 mm Hg	May be present 10-25 mm Hg	Often present >25 mm Hg (adult) 25-40 mm Hg (child)	Absence suggests respiratory muscle fatigue
PEF after initial bronchodilator % predicted or % personal best	>80%	Approximately 60%-80%	<60% predicted or personal best (<100 L/min adults) or response lasts <2 hours	
Pao_2 (on air) and/or $Paco_2$	Normal, test usually not necessary <45 mm Hg	>60 mm Hg <45 mm Hg	<60 mm Hg Possible cyanosis >45 mm Hg; possible respiratory failure	
Sao_2 %	>95%	91%-95%	<90%	

*The presence of several parameters, but not necessarily all, indicates the general classification of the attack.
Reproduced from National Heart, Lung, and Blood Institute and World Health Organization. *Global Strategy for Asthma Management and Prevention NHLBI/WHO Workshop Report.* Bethesda, MD: US Department of Health and Human Services; 1997. Publication 97-4051.

Table 39. Management of Acute Asthma

Asthma Severity	Interventions
Mild to moderate	• Administer humidified O_2 in high concentration via nasal cannula or O_2 mask; titrate according to pulse oximetry. Keep O_2 saturation ≥94%. • Administer albuterol by metered-dose inhaler or nebulizer solution. • Administer oral corticosteroids.
Moderate to severe	• Administer humidified O_2 in high concentrations to keep O_2 saturation 95%; use a nonrebreathing mask if needed. If this is unsuccessful, further support such as noninvasive positive-pressure ventilation or ET intubation may be indicated. • Administer albuterol by metered-dose inhaler (with spacer) or nebulizer solution. If wheezing and aeration are not alleviated, continuous albuterol administration may be required. • Administer ipratropium bromide by nebulizer solution. Albuterol and ipratropium may be mixed for nebulization. Consider establishing vascular access for administration of fluids and medications. • Administer corticosteroids PO/IV. • Consider administering magnesium sulfate by slow (15-30 minutes) IV bolus infusion while monitoring heart rate and blood pressure. • Perform diagnostic assessments (eg, arterial blood gas, chest x-ray) as indicated.
Impending respiratory failure	All of the above therapies are indicated in addition to the following: • Administer O_2 in high concentrations; use a nonrebreathing mask if available. • Administer albuterol by continuous nebulizer. • Administer corticosteroid IV if not already given. • Consider giving terbutaline subcutaneously or by continuous IV infusion; titrate to response while monitoring for toxicity. You may administer subcutaneous or IM epinephrine as an alternative. • Consider bilevel positive airway pressure (noninvasive positive-pressure ventilation), especially in alert, cooperative children. • Consider ET intubation for children with refractory hypoxemia (low O_2 saturation), worsening clinical condition (eg, decreasing level of consciousness, irregular breathing), or both despite the aggressive medical management described above. Intubation in an asthmatic child carries significant risk for respiratory and circulatory complications. Consider using a cuffed ET tube.

Management of Lung Tissue Disease

Lung tissue disease (also called *parenchymal lung disease*) refers to a variety of clinical conditions. Common causes of lung tissue disease are pneumonia (eg, infectious, chemical, aspiration) and cardiogenic pulmonary edema. ARDS and traumatic pulmonary contusion are other causes. Lung tissue disease can also result from allergic, vascular, widespread inflammatory, environmental, and other factors.

General Management of Lung Tissue Disease

General management of lung tissue disease includes the initial interventions listed in Table 33. In children with hypoxemia refractory to high inspired O_2 concentrations, positive expiratory pressure (CPAP, noninvasive ventilation, or mechanical ventilation with positive end-expiratory pressure [PEEP]) is usually helpful in the management of lung tissue disease.

Specific Management of Lung Tissue Disease by Etiology

Specific causes of lung tissue disease require specific interventions. This section reviews the management of lung tissue disease from the following causes:

- Infectious pneumonia
- Chemical pneumonitis
- Aspiration pneumonitis
- Cardiogenic pulmonary edema
- Noncardiogenic pulmonary edema (ARDS)

Management of Infectious Pneumonia

Infectious pneumonia results from viral, bacterial, or fungal inflammation of the alveoli. The common causes of acute community-acquired pneumonia in children include viruses, bacteria (*Streptococcus pneumoniae*), and atypical bacteria (*Mycoplasma pneumoniae* and *Chlamydia pneumoniae*). Methicillin-resistant *Staphylococcus aureus* is increasingly common and may cause empyema (ie, a collection of pus and fluid in the pleural cavity).

In addition to initial interventions listed in Table 33, there are also specific interventions for the *management of acute infectious pneumonia* (Table 40).

Table 40. Management of Acute Infectious Pneumonia

Interventions
Perform diagnostic assessments (eg, arterial blood gas, chest x-ray, viral studies, complete blood count, blood culture, sputum gram stain and culture) as indicated.
Administer antibiotic therapy* (goal is to administer within first hour of medical contact).
Treat wheezing with albuterol by metered-dose inhaler or nebulizer solution.
Consider using CPAP or noninvasive positive-pressure ventilation. In severe cases, endotracheal intubation and mechanical ventilation may be required.
Reduce metabolic demand by normalizing temperature (ie, treating fever) and reducing the work of breathing.

*It may not be necessary to draw blood cultures before antibiotics are given. Follow facility protocol.

Management of Chemical Pneumonitis

Chemical pneumonitis is an inflammation of the lung tissue caused by inhalation or aspiration of toxic liquids, gases, or particulate matter such as dust or fumes. Aspiration of hydrocarbons or inhalation of irritant gases (eg, chlorine) can result in noncardiogenic pulmonary edema with increased capillary permeability.

In addition to initial interventions listed in Table 33, the *management of chemical pneumonitis* may include the specific interventions listed in Table 41.

Table 41. Management of Chemical Pneumonitis

Interventions
Treat wheezing with nebulized bronchodilator.
Consider using CPAP or noninvasive ventilation. Intubation and mechanical ventilation may be required. Consider early intubation particularly if the child requires transport to a tertiary care facility, is not tolerating secretions, or demonstrates evidence of upper airway edema and obstruction.
In a child with rapidly progressive symptoms, obtain early consultation. Consider referral to a specialized center for advanced technologies (eg, high-frequency oscillation or pediatric extracorporeal membrane oxygenation).

Management of Aspiration Pneumonitis

Aspiration pneumonitis is a form of chemical pneumonitis that results from the toxic effects of aspirated oral secretions or stomach acid and enzymes and the subsequent inflammatory response.

General management of lung tissue disease includes the initial interventions listed in Table 33. Specific interventions for the *management of aspiration pneumonitis* are listed in Table 42.

Table 42. Management of Aspiration Pneumonitis

Interventions
Consider using CPAP or noninvasive ventilation. Intubation and mechanical ventilation may be required in severe cases.
Consider administration of antibiotics if the child has a fever and an infiltrate is present on chest x-ray. Prophylactic antimicrobial therapy is not indicated.

Management of Cardiogenic Pulmonary Edema

In cardiogenic pulmonary edema, high pressure in the pulmonary capillaries causes fluid to leak into the lung interstitium and alveoli. The most common cause of acute cardiogenic pulmonary edema in children is left ventricular myocardial dysfunction. This can be caused by congenital heart disease, myocarditis, cardiomyopathy, inflammatory processes, hypoxia, and cardiac-depressant drugs (eg, β-adrenergic blockers, tricyclic antidepressants, calcium channel blockers).

In addition to initial interventions listed in Table 33, specific interventions for the *management of cardiogenic pulmonary edema* are listed in Table 43.

Table 43. Management of Cardiogenic Pulmonary Edema

Interventions
Provide ventilator support (ie, noninvasive ventilation or mechanical ventilation with PEEP) as needed.
Consider diuretics to reduce left atrial pressure, inotropic infusions, and afterload-reducing agents to improve ventricular function. Obtain expert consultation.
Reduce metabolic demand by normalizing temperature (treat fever) and reducing the work of breathing.

Indications for ventilator support (noninvasive ventilation or ET intubation with mechanical ventilation) in children with cardiogenic pulmonary edema include

- Persistent hypoxemia despite oxygen administration and noninvasive ventilation
- Impending respiratory failure
- Hemodynamic compromise (eg, hypotension, severe tachycardia, signs of shock)

PEEP is added during mechanical ventilation to help reduce the need for high O_2 concentrations. It is usually started at about 5 cm H_2O and adjusted upward until O_2 saturation and oxygen delivery improve. Too much PEEP may create pulmonary hyperinflation that impedes both systemic and venous return to the heart, thus reducing cardiac output and O_2 delivery.

Management of Noncardiogenic Pulmonary Edema

ARDS usually follows a pulmonary (eg, pneumonia or aspiration) or systemic (eg, sepsis, pancreatitis, trauma) disease process that injures the interface between the alveoli and pulmonary capillaries and triggers release of inflammatory mediators. As a result, oxygen diffusion into the blood and, to a lesser degree, CO_2 diffusion from the blood to the alveoli is compromised. Early recognition and treatment of bacteremia, shock, and respiratory failure may help prevent the progression to ARDS.

The following are characteristics of ARDS:

- Acute onset (within 7 days of insult)
- PaO_2/FIO_2 300 or less (with full face-mask bilevel ventilation or CPAP 5 cm H_2O or greater)
- Oxygenation Index (OI: $[FIO_2 \times$ mean airway pressure $\times 100]/PaO_2$) 4 or greater
- New infiltrate on chest x-ray consistent with acute pulmonary parenchymal disease
- No evidence for a cardiogenic or fluid overload cause of pulmonary edema

For more details, see Khemani et al. *Pediatr Crit Care Med.* 2015;16(5 suppl 1):S23-S40 in the Suggested Reading List on the Student Website.

In addition to initial interventions listed in Table 33, specific interventions for the *management of ARDS* may include those listed in Table 44.

Table 44. Management of ARDS

Interventions
Monitor heart rate and rhythm, blood pressure, respiratory rate, pulse oximetry, and end-tidal CO_2.
Obtain laboratory studies, including arterial blood gas, central venous blood gas, and complete blood count.
Provide ventilatory support (ie, noninvasive ventilation or mechanical ventilation with PEEP) as needed.

Indications for ventilatory support (noninvasive ventilation or ET intubation with mechanical ventilation) in children with ARDS are

- Worsening clinical and radiographic lung disease
- Hypoxemia refractory to high concentrations of inspired O_2

Correction of hypoxemia is the most important intervention. This is accomplished by increasing PEEP until O_2 saturation is adequate. "Permissive" hypercarbia is a treatment approach that recognizes that correction of increased $Paco_2$ is less important than correction of hypoxemia. Maintaining low tidal volumes (5-8 mL/kg; lower for children with decreased lung compliance) and keeping peak inspiratory pressure less than 30 to 35 cm H_2O is more important than correcting the $Paco_2$.

FYI

ET Intubation in Children With Lung Tissue Disease

When ET intubation is anticipated in children with lung tissue disease, providers should anticipate the need to use PEEP and airway pressures as high as 29 to 32 cm H_2O. To ensure that both can be provided effectively, a cuffed ET tube is helpful to prevent glottic air leak. When using a cuffed tube, carefully monitor cuff inflation pressure and maintain it according to manufacturer's recommendations (typically less than 20 to 25 cm H_2O).

Management of Disordered Control of Breathing

Disordered control of breathing results in an abnormal respiratory pattern that produces inadequate minute ventilation. Common causes of disordered control of breathing are neurologic disorders, including increased intracranial pressure (ICP), neuromuscular disease (weakness), central nervous system infections, head injury, brain tumor, and hydrocephalus. Conditions that depress the level of consciousness (eg, deep sedation, central nervous system infection, seizures, metabolic disorders such as hyperammonemia, poisoning, or drug overdose) also cause disordered control of breathing.

General Management of Disordered Control of Breathing

General management for treatment of disordered control of breathing includes the initial interventions listed in Table 33.

Specific Management of Disordered Control of Breathing by Etiology

Specific causes of *disordered control of breathing* require specific interventions. This section reviews the management of disordered control of breathing caused by the following:

- Increased ICP
- Neuromuscular disease
- Poisoning or drug overdose

Management of Respiratory Distress/ Failure With Increased ICP

Increased ICP can be a complication of meningitis, encephalitis, intracranial abscess, subarachnoid hemorrhage, subdural or epidural hematoma, traumatic brain injury, hypoxic/ischemic insult, hydrocephalus, and central nervous system tumor. An irregular respiratory pattern is one sign of increased ICP. A combination of irregular breathing or apnea, an increase in mean arterial pressure, and bradycardia is called *Cushing's triad*. This triad suggests a marked increase in ICP and impending brain herniation. However, children with increased ICP also can present with irregular breathing, hypertension, and tachycardia rather than with bradycardia.

If increased ICP is suspected, obtain neurosurgical consult. In addition to initial interventions listed in Table 33, specific interventions for *disordered control of breathing due to increased ICP* may include those listed in Table 45.

Table 45. Management of Disordered Control of Breathing Due to Increased ICP

Interventions
If trauma is suspected and you need to open the airway, ensure the head is midline, manually stabilize the cervical spine, and use a jaw-thrust maneuver.
Verify open/patent airway, adequate oxygenation, and adequate ventilation. A brief period of mild hyperventilation may occasionally be used as temporizing rescue therapy in response to signs of impending brain herniation (eg, irregular respirations or apnea, bradycardia, hypertension, unequal or dilated pupil[s] not responsive to light, decerebrate or decorticate posturing) in the initial 48 hours after injury. If hyperventilation is used, advanced neuromonitoring for evaluation of cerebral ischemia may be considered.
If the child has poor perfusion or other evidence of poor end-organ function, administer 20 mL/kg IV isotonic crystalloid (normal saline or lactated Ringer's).
Administer pharmacologic therapy for management of increased ICP (eg, osmotic agents, hypertonic saline).
Treat agitation and pain aggressively once the airway is established and ventilation is adequate.
Avoid or aggressively treat fever.
Severe prophylactic hyperventilation (to $PaCO_2$ less than 30 mm Hg) should be avoided because hyperventilation can depress cardiac output by impairing venous return. Hyperventilation must be used cautiously—if at all—in the child with traumatic brain injury, as excessive hyperventilation may cause cerebral vasoconstriction, leading to brain ischemia and a worse outcome. In patients with severe traumatic brain injury, hyperventilation may be considered in the initial 48 hours after injury only when there are acute signs of cerebral herniation and must be guided by neuromonitoring for evaluation of cerebral ischemia.

Respiratory Management in Neuromuscular Disease

Chronic progressive neuromuscular diseases can affect the muscles of respiration. Affected children can develop an ineffective cough and difficulty managing secretions. Complications include atelectasis, restrictive lung disease, pneumonia (including aspiration pneumonitis and pneumonia), chronic respiratory insufficiency, and respiratory failure. Consider the initial interventions listed in Table 33 for disordered control of breathing due to neuromuscular disease. For children with advanced restrictive lung disease, long-term noninvasive ventilation may be used.

Management of Respiratory Distress/ Failure in Poisoning or Drug Overdose

One of the most common causes of respiratory distress or failure after a poisoning or drug overdose is depression of central respiratory drive; less common causes are weakness or paralysis of respiratory muscles, loss of consciousness, and upper airway obstruction by the tongue.

Complications of disordered breathing in this setting include upper airway obstruction, poor respiratory effort and rate, hypoxemia, aspiration, and respiratory failure. Complications from a decreased level of consciousness (eg, aspiration pneumonitis and noncardiogenic pulmonary edema) may also result in respiratory failure. If you suspect poisoning, contact your local poison control center.

Support of airway and ventilation is the main therapeutic intervention for management of respiratory distress or failure caused by poisoning or drug overdose. In addition to initial interventions listed in Table 33, specific interventions for *disordered control of breathing due to poisoning or drug overdose* may include those listed in Table 46.

Table 46. Management of Disordered Control of Breathing Due to Poisoning or Drug Overdose

Interventions
Contact a poison control center (1-800-222-1222).
Be prepared to suction the airway in case of vomiting.
Administer antidote as indicated. Administer naloxone for opioid overdose (IM and intranasal preparations available) in addition to standard BLS support for patients with known or suspected opioid overdose who have respiratory arrest but with a definite pulse).
Perform diagnostic assessments as indicated (eg, arterial blood gas, ECG, chest x-ray, electrolytes, glucose, serum osmolality, drug screen).
Potentially prepare for transfer when in a rural or nonchildren's hospital.

FYI

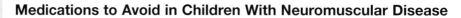

Medications to Avoid in Children With Neuromuscular Disease

Recall that the use of succinylcholine for intubation of children with neuromuscular diseases may trigger life-threatening conditions, such as hyperkalemia or malignant hyperthermia. Several commonly used pediatric acute care drugs, such as aminoglycosides, have intrinsic neuromuscular blocking activity that can worsen respiratory muscle weakness.

Summary: Management of Respiratory Emergencies Flowchart

The Management of Respiratory Emergencies Flowchart summarizes general management of respiratory emergencies and specific management by etiology (Figure 25). Note that this chart does not include all respiratory emergencies; it provides key management strategies for a limited number of diseases.

Management of Respiratory Emergencies Flowchart

- Airway positioning
- Suction as needed
- Oxygen
- Pulse oximetry
- ECG monitor (as indicated)
- BLS as indicated

Upper Airway Obstruction
Specific Management for Selected Conditions

Croup	Anaphylaxis	Aspiration Foreign Body
• Nebulized epinephrine • Corticosteroids	• IM epinephrine (or autoinjector) • Albuterol • Antihistamines • Corticosteroids	• Allow position of comfort • Specialty consultation

Lower Airway Obstruction
Specific Management for Selected Conditions

Bronchiolitis	Asthma
• Nasal suctioning • Bronchodilator trial	• Albuterol ± ipratropium • Corticosteroids • Subcutaneous epinephrine • Magnesium sulfate • Terbutaline

Lung Tissue Disease
Specific Management for Selected Conditions

Pneumonia/Pneumonitis Infectious Chemical Aspiration	Pulmonary Edema Cardiogenic or Noncardiogenic (ARDS)
• Albuterol • Antibiotics (as indicated) • Consider CPAP	• Consider noninvasive or invasive ventilatory support with PEEP • Consider vasoactive support • Consider diuretic

Disordered Control of Breathing
Specific Management for Selected Conditions

Increased ICP	Poisoning/Overdose	Neuromuscular Disease
• Avoid hypoxemia • Avoid hypercarbia • Avoid hyperthermia	• Antidote (if available) • Contact poison control	• Consider noninvasive or invasive ventilatory support

Figure 25. Management of Respiratory Emergencies Flowchart.

Resources

Resources for Management of Respiratory Emergencies

Bag-Mask Ventilation

Overview

Bag-mask ventilation can provide adequate oxygenation and ventilation for a child with no breathing or inadequate breathing despite an open/patent airway. Signs of inadequate breathing are apnea, abnormal respiratory rate, inadequate breath sounds, and hypoxemia despite supplementary O_2. When properly performed, bag-mask ventilation is as effective as ventilation through an endotracheal (ET) tube for short periods and may be safer. In the out-of-hospital setting, bag-mask ventilation is especially useful if the transport time is short or providers are inexperienced in insertion of advanced airways or have insufficient opportunities to maintain competence in this skill.

Preparation for the Course

All healthcare providers who care for infants and children should be able to provide ventilation effectively with a bag and mask. In the PALS Provider Course you will be required to demonstrate effective bag-mask ventilation during BLS testing, in the Airway Management Skills Station, and in some case simulations.

How to Select and Prepare the Equipment

For ventilation to be effective with a bag-mask device, you must know how to select the face mask, prepare the ventilation bag, and provide supplementary O_2 if needed.

Face Mask

Select a face mask that extends from the bridge of the child's nose to the cleft of the chin, covering the nose and mouth but not compressing the eyes (Figure 26). The mask should have a soft rim (eg, flexible cuff) that molds easily to create a tight seal against the face. If the face-mask seal is not tight, O_2 intended for ventilation will escape under the mask, and ventilation will not be effective.

Select a transparent mask if available. A transparent mask allows you to see the color of the child's lips and condensation on the mask (which indicates exhalation). You will also be able to observe for regurgitation.

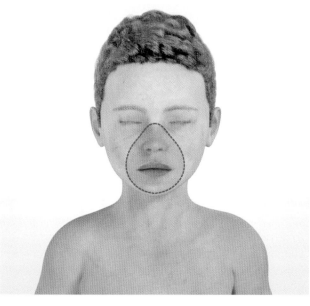

Figure 26. Proper area of the face for face-mask application. Note that no pressure is applied to the eyes.

Ventilation Bag

There are 2 basic types of ventilation bags:

- Self-inflating bag
- Flow-inflating bag

Self-Inflating Bag

A self-inflating bag is typically used for initial resuscitation. A self-inflating bag consists of a bag with an intake valve and a nonrebreathing outlet valve. The intake valve allows the bag to fill with either O_2 (Figures 27A and B) or room air (Figures 27C and D). When you compress the bag, the intake valve closes and the nonrebreathing outlet valve opens, allowing either room air or an air-O_2 gas mixture to flow to the child. When the child exhales, the nonrebreathing outlet valve closes and exhaled gases are vented. The nonrebreathing outlet valve is designed to prevent the child from rebreathing CO_2.

Even when supplementary O_2 is attached, the concentration of delivered O_2 varies from 30% to 80%. The amount of delivered O_2 is affected by tidal volume and peak inspiratory flow rate. To deliver a high O_2 concentration (60% to 95%), attach an O_2 reservoir to the intake valve (Figures 27A and B). Maintain an O_2 flow of 10 to 15 L/min into a reservoir attached to a pediatric bag and a flow of at least 15 L/min into an adult bag.

Critical Concepts

Use O₂ During Resuscitation

Attach an O_2 reservoir to the self-inflating bag as soon as possible during a resuscitation attempt. Frequently verify that O_2 is attached and flowing to the bag. Remember to

- Listen for O_2 flow
- Check O_2 tank pressure or verify connection to a wall O_2 source

Once circulation is adequate and when appropriate equipment is available, titrate O_2 administration to maintain an O_2 saturation of 94% to 99%.

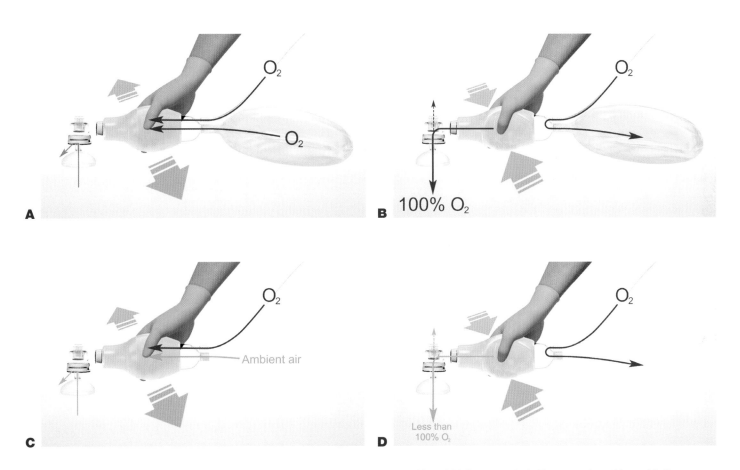

Figure 27. Self-inflating ventilation bag with face mask, with (**A** and **B**) and without (**C** and **D**) O_2 reservoir. **A,** Re-expansion of bag with O_2 reservoir. When the provider's hand releases the bag, O_2 flows into the bag from the O_2 source and from the reservoir, so the concentration of O_2 in the bag remains 100%. **B,** Compression of bag with O_2 reservoir delivers 100% O_2 to the patient (purple arrow). O_2 continuously flows into the reservoir. **C,** Re-expansion of the bag without an O_2 reservoir. When the provider's hand releases the bag, O_2 flows into the bag from the O_2 source, but ambient air is also entrained into the bag, so the bag becomes filled with a mixture of O_2 and ambient air. **D,** Compression of the bag without O_2 reservoir delivers O_2 mixed with room air (aqua arrow). Note that with both setups, exhaled patient air flows into the atmosphere near the connection of the mask and bag (see gray arrows from mask in **A** and **C**).

Check to see if the bag has a pop-off valve. Many self-inflating bags have a pressure-limited pop-off valve set at 35 to 45 cm H_2O to prevent development of excessive airway pressures. If the child's lung compliance is poor or airway resistance is high or CPR is needed, an automatic pop-off valve may prevent delivery of sufficient tidal volume, resulting in inadequate ventilation and chest expansion. Ventilation bags used during CPR should have *no pop-off valve* or the valve should be twisted into the closed position.

Critical Concepts

Caution: Continuous O₂ Flow Not Possible With Some Self-Inflating Bags

Self-inflating bag-mask devices with a fish-mouth or leaf-flap–operated nonrebreathing outlet valve do not provide a continuous flow of O_2 to the mask. Such valves open *only* if the bag is squeezed *or* the mask is sealed tightly to the face and the child generates significant inspiratory force to open the valve. Many infants cannot generate the inspiratory pressure required to open the outlet valve. *Do not use this type of bag to provide supplementary O_2 to a spontaneously breathing infant or child.*

FYI

Providing Positive End-Expiratory Pressure (PEEP) During Bag-Mask Ventilation

Use of PEEP may improve oxygenation in children with lung tissue disease or low lung volumes. Provide PEEP during ventilation with a bag by adding a compatible spring-loaded ball or disk or a magnetic-disc PEEP valve to the bag-mask or bag-tube system. Do *not* use self-inflating bag-mask devices equipped with PEEP valves to provide CPAP *during spontaneous breathing* because the outlet valve in the bag will not open (and provide gas flow) unless the child generates significant negative inspiratory pressure.

Flow-Inflating Bag

A flow-inflating bag (Figure 28), also called an *anesthesia bag*, may be used in the intensive care unit, delivery room, and operating room. It requires O_2 flow to operate. Safe and effective ventilation with a flow-inflating bag requires more experience than is needed to use a self-inflating bag. To provide effective ventilation with a flow-inflating bag, the provider must be able to adjust the flow of O_2, adjust the outlet control valve, ensure a proper seal with the face mask, and deliver the appropriate tidal volume at the correct rate. For these reasons, flow-inflating bags should be used only by trained and experienced providers.

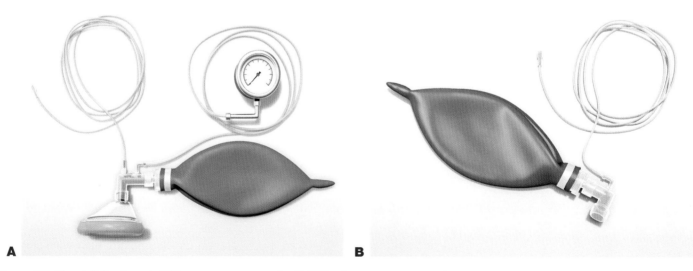

A **B**

Figure 28. Flow-inflating bag. **A,** With a pressure manometer. **B,** Without a pressure manometer.

Bag Size

Use a self-inflating bag with a volume of at least 450 to 500 mL or larger for infants and young children. Smaller bags may not deliver an effective tidal volume over the longer inspiratory times required by full-term neonates and infants. In older children or adolescents, you may need to use an adult self-inflating bag (1000 mL or larger) to achieve chest rise and minute ventilation.

How to Test the Bag-Mask Device

Check all components of any bag and mask system before use to ensure proper function. To test the device

- Check the bag for leaks by occluding the patient outlet valve with your hand and squeezing the bag
- Check the gas flow control valves (including any CPAP valve) to verify proper function
- Check the pop-off valve (if present) to ensure that it can be closed
- Check that the O_2 tubing is securely connected to the device and the O_2 source
- Listen for the sound of O_2 flowing into the bag
- Ensure that the cuff of the mask (if present) is adequately inflated

How to Position the Child

Properly position the child to maintain an open airway. During bag-mask ventilation it may be necessary to move the child's head and neck gently through a range of positions to optimize ventilation. A "sniffing" position without hyperextension of the neck is usually best for infants and toddlers.

To achieve a "sniffing" position, place the child supine. Flex the child's neck forward at the level of the shoulders while extending the head. Position the opening of the external ear canal at the level of or in front of the anterior aspect of the shoulder while the head is extended (Figure 29). Avoid hyperextending the neck because this may obstruct the airway.

Children older than 2 years may require padding under the occiput. Younger children and infants may need padding under the shoulders or upper torso to prevent excessive flexion of the neck that can occur when the prominent occiput rests on a flat surface.

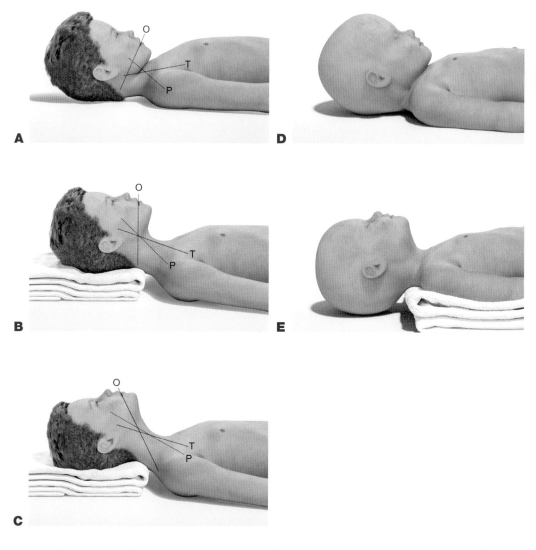

Figure 29. Correct positioning of the child older than 2 years for ventilation and ET intubation. **A,** With the child on a flat surface (eg, bed or table), the oral (O), pharyngeal (P), and tracheal (T) axes pass through 3 divergent planes. **B,** A folded sheet or towel placed under the occiput aligns the pharyngeal and tracheal axes. **C,** Extension of the atlanto-occipital joint results in the alignment of the oral, pharyngeal, and tracheal axes when the head is extended and the chin is lifted. Note that proper positioning places the external ear canal anterior to the shoulder. **D,** Incorrect position with neck flexion. **E,** Correct position for ventilation and ET intubation for infant. Note that the external ear canal is anterior to the shoulder. Modified from Coté CJ, Todres ID. The pediatric airway. In: Coté CJ, Ryan JF, Todres ID, Goudsouzian NG, eds. *A Practice of Anesthesia for Infants and Children.* 2nd ed. Philadelphia, PA: WB Saunders Co; 1993:55-83, copyright Elsevier.

How to Perform Bag-Mask Ventilation

Bag-mask ventilation can be performed by 1 or 2 providers. Because effective bag-mask ventilation requires complex steps, bag-mask ventilation is not recommended for a lone rescuer during CPR. During CPR, the lone rescuer should use the mouth-to–barrier device technique for ventilation. Bag-mask ventilation can be provided effectively during 2-rescuer CPR.

1-Person Bag-Mask Ventilation Technique

If 1 healthcare provider is performing bag-mask ventilation, the provider must open the airway and keep the mask sealed to the child's face with one hand (Figure 30) and squeeze the bag with the other hand. Effective bag-mask ventilation requires a tight seal between the mask and the child's face. Use the E-C clamp technique described below to open the airway and achieve a tight seal (Table 47).

Table 47. E-C Clamp Technique

Step	Action
1	To open the airway and make a seal between the mask and the face *in the absence of suspected cervical spine injury*, tilt the head back. Use the E-C clamp technique to lift the jaw against the mask, pressing and sealing the mask on the face. This technique moves the tongue away from the posterior pharynx, moves the jaw forward, and opens the mouth. Lifting the jaw toward the mask helps seal the mask against the face. If possible, the mouth should be open under the mask, as a result of either lifting the jaw or insertion of an oropharyngeal airway.
2	With the other hand, squeeze the ventilation bag until the chest rises. Deliver each breath over 1 second. Avoid excessive ventilation (see "How to Deliver Effective Ventilation" in this Part).

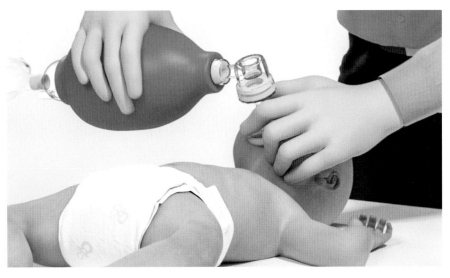

Figure 30. One-handed E-C clamp face-mask application technique. Three fingers of one hand lift the jaw (forming the "E") while the thumb and index finger hold the mask to the face (making a "C").

Critical Concepts

E-C Clamp Technique

The technique of opening the airway and making a seal between the mask and the face is called the *E-C clamp technique*. The third, fourth, and fifth fingers of one hand (forming an "E") are positioned along the jaw to lift it forward; then the thumb and index finger of the same hand (forming a "C") make a seal to hold the mask to the face. Avoid pressure on the soft tissues underneath the chin (the submental area) because this can push the tongue into the posterior pharynx, resulting in airway compression and obstruction.

2-Person Bag-Mask Ventilation Technique

If 2 healthcare providers are available to perform bag-mask ventilation, one provider uses both hands to open the airway and keep the mask sealed to the child's face and the other provider squeezes the bag (Figure 31). Both providers should observe the child's chest to ensure that chest rise is visible. Be careful to avoid delivering too large a tidal volume, which may result in excessive ventilation.

The 2-person technique may provide more effective bag-mask ventilation than a 1-person technique. Also, 2-person bag-mask ventilation may be necessary when

- There is difficulty making a seal between the face and the mask
- The provider's hands are too small to reach from the front of the mask to behind the jaw or to open the airway and create a seal between the face and mask
- There is significant airway resistance (ie, asthma) or poor lung compliance (ie, pneumonia or pulmonary edema)
- Spinal motion restriction is necessary

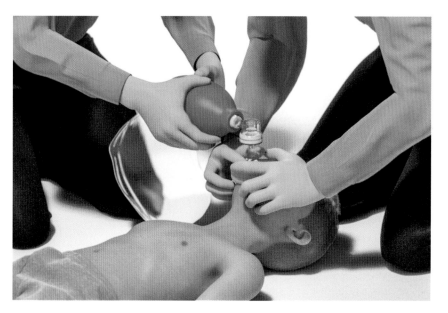

Figure 31. Two-person bag-mask ventilation technique. This technique may provide more effective ventilation than 1-person ventilation when there is significant airway obstruction or poor lung compliance. One provider uses both hands to open the airway and maintain a tight mask-to-face seal, while the other provider squeezes the ventilation bag.

How to Deliver Effective Ventilation

Avoid excessive ventilation; use only the force and tidal volume necessary to just make the chest rise.

Critical Concepts

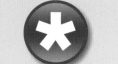

Effective Ventilation With a Bag-Mask

Give each breath slowly over about 1 second. Watch for chest rise. If the chest does not rise, reopen the airway. Verify that there is a tight seal between the mask and the face. Reattempt ventilation.

Precaution

Healthcare providers often deliver excessive ventilation during CPR. Excessive ventilation is harmful because it

- Increases intrathoracic pressure and impedes venous return, which decreases filling of the heart between compressions and reduces blood flow generated by the next compression, reducing coronary perfusion and cerebral blood flow
- Causes air trapping and barotrauma in children with small airway obstruction
- Increases the risk of regurgitation and aspiration in children without an advanced airway

Clinical Parameters of Oxygenation and Ventilation

Frequently monitor the following parameters to assess the effectiveness of oxygenation and ventilation:

- Visible chest rise with each breath
- O_2 saturation
- Exhaled CO_2
- Heart rate
- Blood pressure
- Distal air entry
- Signs of improvement or deterioration (eg, appearance, color, agitation)

Troubleshooting Ineffective Ventilation

If effective ventilation is not achieved (ie, the chest does not rise), do the following:

- Reposition/reopen the airway: attempt to further lift the jaw and ensure that the child is placed in a sniffing position
- Verify mask size and ensure a tight face-mask seal
- Suction the airway if needed
- Check the O_2 source
- Check the ventilation bag and mask
- Treat gastric inflation
- Consider 2-person bag-mask ventilation and insertion of an oropharyngeal airway (OPA)

Spontaneously Breathing Child

In a spontaneously breathing child, give gentle positive-pressure breaths with a bag-mask device. Time these breaths carefully to supplement the child's inspiratory efforts. If you do not coordinate the delivered breaths with the child's efforts, bag-mask ventilation may be ineffective. Poorly timed breaths may stimulate coughing, vomiting, laryngospasm, and gastric inflation, which prevent effective ventilation.

FYI

Detecting for Changes in Lung Compliance

When performing bag-mask ventilation, be aware of the child's lung compliance. A poorly compliant lung is "stiff" or difficult to inflate. A sudden increase in lung stiffness during ventilation with a bag may indicate airway obstruction, decreased lung compliance, or development of a pneumothorax. Lung distention from excessive inflating pressures, PEEP, or rapid assisted respiratory rates with short exhalation time may also cause the feel of "stiff lungs" during ventilation.

Gastric Inflation and Cricoid Pressure

Inflation or distention of the stomach frequently develops during bag-mask ventilation. Gastric inflation is more likely to develop during assisted ventilation if

- A partial airway obstruction is present
- High airway pressures are needed, such as in a child with poor lung compliance
- The bag-mask ventilation rate is too fast
- The volume delivered is too high
- The pressure created is too high
- The child is unconscious or is in cardiac arrest (because the gastro-esophageal sphincter opens at a lower than normal pressure)

Gastric inflation can impair a child's ventilation by limiting lung volumes.

Ways to Minimize Gastric Inflation

Gastric inflation may interfere with effective ventilation and cause regurgitation. To minimize gastric inflation

- Ventilate at a rate of 1 breath every 3 to 5 seconds (about 12 to 20 breaths per minute)
- Avoid creation of excessive peak inspiratory pressures by delivering each breath over about 1 second
- Deliver enough volume and pressure to produce visible chest rise
- Because there is insufficient evidence to recommend routine cricoid pressure application to prevent aspiration during ET intubation in children, consider application of cricoid pressure—but only in an unresponsive victim and only if there is an additional provider able to perform it separate from other duties
- Avoid excessive cricoid pressure so as not to obstruct the trachea and interfere with delivering positive-pressure breaths

Advanced providers may perform gastric decompression by inserting a nasogastric or orogastric tube.

Suctioning

Suction Devices

Suction devices can be either portable or wall-mounted units.

- Portable suction devices are easy to transport. However, they may not have adequate suction power. A suction force of –80 to –120 mm Hg is generally needed to remove airway secretions.
- Bulb or syringe suction devices are simple to use and require no outside vacuum source. These devices may be inadequate in larger patients or when secretions are thick or copious.
- Wall-mounted suction units can provide high suction force of more than –300 mm Hg.

Suction devices used in children should have adjustable suction regulators so that you can use sufficient suction force and minimize tissue trauma. Large-bore, noncollapsible suction tubing should always be joined to the suction unit. Semirigid pharyngeal tips (tonsil suction tips) and appropriate sizes of catheters should be available.

Indications

Suctioning of secretions, blood, or vomit from the oropharynx, nasopharynx, or trachea may be needed to achieve or maintain an open/patent airway.

Complications

Complications of suctioning can include

- Hypoxia
- Vagal stimulation resulting in bradycardia
- Gagging and vomiting
- Soft tissue injury
- Agitation

Soft vs Rigid Catheters

Both soft, flexible and rigid suctioning catheters are available.

Use	For
A soft, flexible plastic suction catheter	- Aspiration of thin secretions from the oropharynx and nasopharynx - Suctioning an advanced airway (eg, ET tube)
A rigid wide-bore suction cannula ("tonsil tip")	- Suctioning of the oropharynx, particularly if thick secretions, vomit, or blood are present

Catheter Sizes

For a guide to selecting the appropriate-sized suction catheter, use a color-coded length-based resuscitation tape or other reference.

Oropharyngeal Suctioning Procedure

Follow the steps in Table 48 to suction the oropharynx.

Table 48. Oropharynx Suctioning Technique

Step	Interventions
1	Gently insert the distal end of the suction catheter or device into the oropharynx over the tongue. Guide it into the posterior pharynx (back of the throat).
2	Apply suction by covering the catheter side opening. At the same time, withdraw the catheter with a rotating or twisting motion.
3	Try to limit suction attempts to 10 seconds or less. This will help reduce the risk of hypoxemia (low oxygen saturation). You may give short periods of 100% oxygen immediately before and after each suctioning attempt. *Note:* Suction attempts may need to be longer than 10 seconds if the airway is obstructed (eg, by blood). You cannot provide adequate oxygenation or ventilation unless the airway is open and clear.

Monitoring During Suctioning

Monitor the child's heart rate, oxygen saturation, and clinical appearance during suctioning. In general, if bradycardia develops or clinical appearance deteriorates, interrupt suctioning. Give high-flow oxygen and bag-mask ventilation, if needed, until the heart rate and clinical appearance return to normal.

Oropharyngeal Airway

Description

The OPA consists of a flange, a short bite-block segment, and a curved body. The curved body is usually made of plastic. It is shaped to provide an air channel and a passage for a suction catheter to the pharynx. The OPA fits over the tongue to prevent it and other soft structures of the throat from obstructing the airway. An OPA is not intended to be used long-term as a bite-block device in agitated patients.

Indications

An OPA may relieve upper airway obstruction caused by the tongue. If an OPA of correct size is used (see below), it will not damage laryngeal structures. An OPA may be used in the *unconscious* child with no gag reflex if procedures to open the airway (eg, head tilt–chin lift or jaw thrust) fail to provide and maintain a clear, unobstructed airway. An OPA should not be used in a *conscious* or *semiconscious* child because it may stimulate gagging and vomiting. Before using an OPA, check to see if the child has a gag reflex. If so, do not use an OPA.

Complications

It is important to choose the correct-sized OPA. If the OPA is *too large*, it can block the airway or cause trauma to the laryngeal structures (Figure 32B).

If the OPA is *too small* or is inserted improperly, it can push the tongue into the back of the throat and contribute to airway obstruction (Figure 32C).

Airway Selection and Insertion Procedure

OPA sizes range from 4 to 10 cm in length (Guedel sizes 000 to 4). Follow the steps in Table 49 to choose the correct-sized OPA and insert it into the airway.

Table 49. Choosing and Inserting an OPA

Step	Interventions
1	Place the OPA against the side of the child's face. The tip of the OPA should extend from the corner of the mouth to the angle of the jaw (Figure 32A).
2	Gently insert the OPA directly into the oropharynx. The use of a tongue blade to depress the tongue may be helpful.
3	After insertion of an OPA, monitor the child. Keep the head and jaw positioned properly to maintain an open/patent airway. Suction the airway as needed.

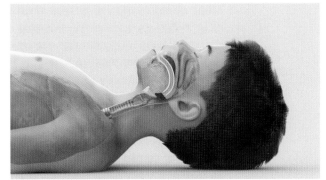

A

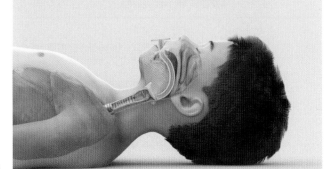

B

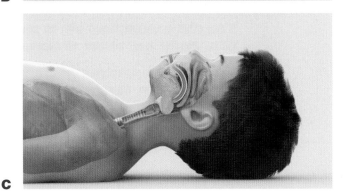

C

Figure 32. Selection of an OPA. A properly sized OPA relieves airway obstruction caused by the tongue without damaging the larynx. **A,** The tip of the OPA should end just at the angle of the jaw, so that once inserted, it will align with the glottis opening. **B,** If the OPA is too large, it will obstruct the airway by pushing the epiglottis down. **C,** If the OPA is too small, it will worsen airway obstruction by pushing the tongue into the back of the throat. Modified from Coté CJ, Todres ID. The pediatric airway. In: Coté CJ, Ryan JF, Todres ID, Goudsouzian NG, eds. *A Practice of Anesthesia for Infants and Children*. 2nd ed. Philadelphia, PA: WB Saunders Co; 1993:55-83, copyright Elsevier.

Oxygen Delivery Systems

Indications for Oxygen

For children with respiratory distress or shock, oxygen uptake by the lungs and oxygen delivery to the tissues are typically reduced. At the same time, tissue demand for oxygen may be increased. Give high-flow oxygen to all seriously ill or injured children with severe respiratory distress, shock, or changes in mental status. As soon as possible, add humidification to the oxygen delivery system. This may help prevent airway dryness.

Giving Oxygen to a Conscious Child

When giving oxygen to an alert child in respiratory distress, balance the need to improve oxygen delivery against the possible agitation that may result from applying an oxygen delivery device. Agitation can increase oxygen demand and respiratory distress. If a child is agitated by one method of oxygen delivery, try an alternative technique. For example, if the child is upset by an oxygen mask, try directing a "blow-by" stream of humidified oxygen toward the child's mouth and nose. It may be helpful to have a person familiar to the child, such as a parent, introduce the oxygen delivery equipment.

When giving oxygen to an alert child in respiratory distress, allow the child to remain in a position of comfort. This will minimize respiratory effort and help keep the airway as open as possible. For infants and young children, the best position might be in the arms of the parent or caregiver.

Giving Oxygen to a Child With a Decreased Level of Consciousness

If a child has a decreased level of consciousness, the airway may become obstructed by a combination of the following:

- Flexion of the neck
- Relaxation of the jaw
- Displacement of the tongue against the back of the throat
- Accumulation of secretions

If the child is unconscious with no cough or gag reflex, open the airway and insert an OPA. Use the head tilt–chin lift maneuver or a jaw thrust to open the airway.

If no trauma is suspected and the child is breathing normally, roll the child onto her side in a neutral position. Place the child on her side only if no other interventions are needed.

Suction the oropharynx and nasopharynx to clear secretions, mucus, or blood if needed. Once the airway is open and clear, you can give oxygen by a variety of oxygen delivery systems.

Critical Concepts

Jaw Thrust

A properly performed jaw thrust is the most effective means to open the pediatric airway. Providers, however, are often inexperienced with this technique because it is difficult to practice the skill with some CPR manikins.

Types of Oxygen Delivery Systems

For a spontaneously breathing child who needs supplementary oxygen, you need to know which oxygen delivery system to use. Oxygen delivery systems are either low flow or high flow (Table 50). Consider the child's clinical status and the desired concentration of inspired oxygen when choosing the appropriate system.

Table 50. Types of Oxygen Delivery Systems

Oxygen Delivery System	Device
Low-flow oxygen	• Nasal cannula • Simple oxygen mask
High-flow oxygen	• Nonrebreathing mask with reservoir • High-flow nasal cannula

The concentration of inspired oxygen delivered is determined by several factors. These include oxygen flow into the device, the child's inspiratory flow, and how tightly the device fits against the child's face.

Low-Flow Oxygen Delivery Systems

A low-flow oxygen delivery system delivers air through a nasal cannula or a simple mask that does not fit tightly against the child's face. The oxygen flow into the delivery device is less than the child's inspiratory flow rate. When the child inhales, the child inspires some room air in addition to the oxygen provided by the device. As a result, the oxygen from the device mixes with room air, so a variable concentration of oxygen is delivered to the child. The higher the oxygen flow provided, the higher the inspired oxygen concentration.

Low-flow systems generally provide an inspired oxygen concentration of about 22% to 60%. Low-flow oxygen systems are used when the child requires a relatively low inspired oxygen concentration and is relatively stable, such as when the child is not in severe respiratory distress or shock.

The nasal cannula and simple oxygen mask are examples of low-flow oxygen delivery systems.

Nasal Cannula

The nasal cannula is typically a low-flow oxygen delivery device. It delivers an inspired oxygen concentration of 22% to 60%. The appropriate oxygen flow rate for the nasal cannula is 0.25 to 4 L/min.

The nasal cannula is suitable for infants and children who require only low concentrations of supplementary oxygen. Note that in small infants, a nasal cannula may deliver a high inspired oxygen concentration (see, also, "High-Flow Nasal Cannula" later in this Part). The inspired oxygen concentration delivered via nasal cannula cannot be reliably determined from the oxygen flow rate alone. It is also influenced by other factors, such as

- The child's size
- Inspiratory flow rate
- Volume of inspired air
- Nasopharyngeal and oropharyngeal volume
- Nasal resistance (eg, oxygen delivery is compromised if nares are obstructed)
- Oropharyngeal resistance

Simple Oxygen Mask

The simple oxygen mask is a low-flow device. It delivers an inspired oxygen concentration of 35% to 60%. The appropriate flow rate for the simple oxygen mask is 6 to 10 L/min.

The simple oxygen mask cannot deliver an inspired oxygen concentration greater than 60%. This is because room air enters the mask between the mask and the face and through ports in the side of the mask during inspiration. The oxygen concentration delivered to the child is reduced if

- The child's inspiratory flow is high
- The mask does not fit tightly against the face
- The oxygen flow into the mask is low

A minimum oxygen flow rate of 6 L/min is needed to maintain an increased inspired oxygen concentration and prevent rebreathing of exhaled CO_2.

There are several types of oxygen masks that can deliver humidified oxygen in a wide range of concentrations. The soft vinyl pediatric mask may cause infants and toddlers to become agitated and upset. This increases oxygen demand and could result in increased respiratory distress. This mask may be used effectively in older children.

High-Flow Oxygen Delivery Systems

High-flow oxygen systems reliably deliver an oxygen concentration of greater than 60%. In a high-flow oxygen delivery system, the oxygen flow rate is high, at least 10 L/min. A nonrebreathing mask is the most common example of a high-flow system. Another example of a high-flow oxygen delivery system is high-flow nasal cannula.

High-flow systems should be used in emergency settings whenever the child has respiratory distress or shock.

Nonrebreathing Mask

The nonrebreathing mask (Figure 33) is a high-flow delivery device. An inspired oxygen concentration of 95% can be achieved with an oxygen flow rate of 10 to 15 L/min and the use of a well-sealed face mask.

A nonrebreathing mask consists of a face mask and reservoir bag with the addition of 2 one-way valves:

- A valve in 1 or both exhalation port(s) to prevent room air from entering the mask during inspiration
- A valve placed between the reservoir bag and the mask to prevent the flow of exhaled gas into the reservoir

Adjust the oxygen flow rate into the mask to prevent collapse of the bag (usually greater than 10 L/min). The bag is filled with oxygen to meet the child's total maximum inspired flow requirements. During inspiration, the child draws 100% oxygen from the reservoir bag and the oxygen inflow. Room air does not enter the mask if the mask is tight-fitting and the delivery system is closed.

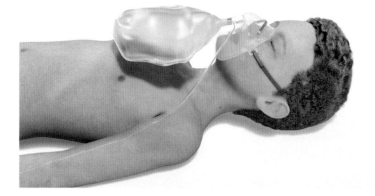

Figure 33. Nonrebreathing mask with reservoir.

High-Flow Nasal Cannula

The nasal cannula can also be used as a high-flow delivery device. The oxygen flow rate can be adjusted from 4 L in infants to up to 40 L or more in adolescents. The flow can be titrated to provide additional inspiratory and expiratory pressure to improve the patient's work of breathing.

High-flow nasal cannula systems deliver a combination of both room air and oxygen. With these systems, the oxygen concentration is titrated based on the patient's needs and oxyhemoglobin saturations.

Nebulizer

Components

A nebulizer has the following components:

- Nebulizer reservoir
- Nebulizer cap
- T-piece
- Spacer
- Handheld mouthpiece or face mask
- Plastic oxygen tubing
- Oxygen source or compressed air

Older children may use the handheld mouthpiece instead of the face mask.

Steps for Using a Nebulizer With a Handheld Mouthpiece

General steps for using a nebulizer with a handheld mouthpiece (Figure 34) are listed in Table 51.

Table 51. Using a Nebulizer With a Handheld Mouthpiece

Step	Action
1	Unscrew the cap of the nebulizer reservoir, add medication (eg, albuterol) to the nebulizer reservoir, and reattach the cap.
2	Connect the bottom of the T-piece to the top of the nebulizer reservoir, and then connect the spacer to one end of the T-piece and the mouthpiece to the other end.
3	Connect plastic tubing between the bottom of the nebulizer bottle and the pressurized oxygen/gas source.
4	Set the gas flow at 5 to 6 L/min.
5	Hold the nebulizer reservoir upright during delivery of the medication through the mouthpiece. Place the mouthpiece in the child's mouth and show him how to hold it. Tell the child, "Take long, slow, deep breaths through your mouth." Continue the treatment (about 8-10 minutes) until the nebulizer reservoir is empty and no mist flows from the T-piece.

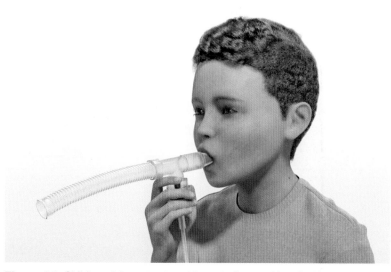

Figure 34. Child receiving a treatment by nebulizer and handheld mouthpiece.

Steps for Using a Nebulizer With a Face Mask

Follow these steps to use a nebulizer with a face mask (Table 52).

Table 52. Using a Nebulizer With a Face Mask

Step	Action
1	Unscrew the cap of the nebulizer reservoir, add medication (eg, albuterol) to the nebulizer reservoir, and reattach the cap.
2	Attach the face mask to the top of the nebulizer reservoir.
3	Connect plastic tubing between the bottom of the nebulizer reservoir and the pressurized oxygen/gas source.
4	Set the gas flow at 5 to 6 L/min.
5	Hold the nebulizer reservoir upright during delivery of the medication through a face mask. • Place the face mask over the child's face so that it covers both the nose and mouth; press the mask to the face to ensure a light seal. • Tell the child, "Take long, slow, deep breaths through your mouth." Continue the treatment (about 8 to 10 minutes) until the nebulizer bottle is empty and no mist flows from the mask.

Metered-Dose Inhaler

Using a Metered-Dose Inhaler With a Spacer Device

Follow the steps in Table 53 to use a metered-dose inhaler (MDI) with a spacer device (with and without a face mask).

Table 53. Using a Metered-Dose Inhaler With a Spacer Device

Step	Action
1	Remove the cap from the spacer, and insert the mouthpiece of the MDI into the rubber-sealed end of the spacer (Figure 35). Once assembled, shake the MDI and the spacer vigorously. Place the mouthpiece of the spacer device into the child's mouth. *or* If you are using a spacer device with a face mask, place the mask over the child's face so that it covers both the nose and the mouth (Figure 36). Press the mask to the face to ensure a tight seal. 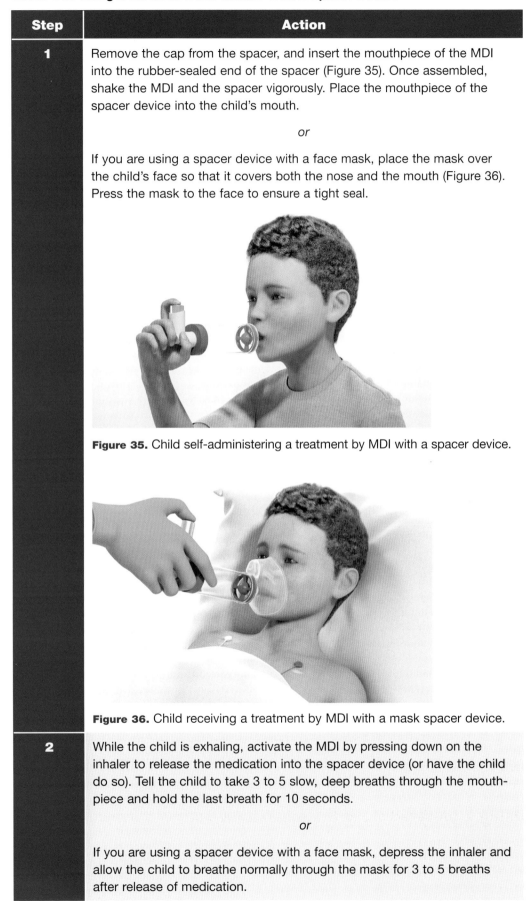 **Figure 35.** Child self-administering a treatment by MDI with a spacer device. **Figure 36.** Child receiving a treatment by MDI with a mask spacer device.
2	While the child is exhaling, activate the MDI by pressing down on the inhaler to release the medication into the spacer device (or have the child do so). Tell the child to take 3 to 5 slow, deep breaths through the mouthpiece and hold the last breath for 10 seconds. *or* If you are using a spacer device with a face mask, depress the inhaler and allow the child to breathe normally through the mask for 3 to 5 breaths after release of medication.

Pulse Oximetry

When to Use Pulse Oximetry

When caring for a seriously ill or injured child, use pulse oximetry to monitor

- Oxygen saturation
- Trends in oxygen saturation

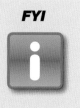

FYI

Oxygen Saturation

The pulse oximeter measures the percent of hemoglobin that is fully saturated or bound with oxygen. Hemoglobin is usually bound with oxygen, but it is important to note that it may be bound with any agent that binds to hemoglobin (eg, carbon monoxide). It is also important to note that oxygen saturation does not equate to oxygen delivery to the tissues, and the pulse oximeter does not provide information about effectiveness of ventilation (carbon dioxide elimination).

Confirm the Validity of Oximeter Data

The pulse oximeter requires pulsatile blood flow to determine oxygen saturation. Different brands of pulse oximeters vary in how quickly they reflect the development of hypoxemia and in their accuracy when the child has decreased blood flow; all pulse oximetry devices are inaccurate unless the pulse rate displayed by the oximeter is consistent with the heart rate displayed by the cardiac monitor. Note that skin pigment does not affect the accuracy or function of the pulse oximeter.

Critical Concepts

Validity of Oximeter Data

Confirm validity of oximeter data by evaluating the child's appearance. Also compare the heart rate displayed by the pulse oximeter with the heart rate displayed by the bedside cardiorespiratory monitor or counted during physical examination.

You should immediately evaluate the child if the oximeter

- Fails to detect a signal
- Displays an inaccurate pulse rate
- Indicates a weak signal
- Indicates a fall in oxygen saturation

If the oximeter fails to detect a signal or indicates a fall in oxygen saturation, you should immediately evaluate the child. Do not assume that the pulse oximeter is malfunctioning.

The pulse oximeter may not be functioning correctly if

- The displayed heart rate does not correlate with the child's heart rate
- The child's appearance does not correspond with the reported concentration of oxygen saturation

Accuracy of Values in Clinical Settings

Pulse oximetry can accurately estimate oxygen saturation but does not provide evidence of oxygen delivery. It also does not directly evaluate the effectiveness of ventilation (carbon dioxide concentration).

Pulse oximetry may be inaccurate in some settings (Table 54).

Table 54. Settings Where a Pulse Oximeter May Be Inaccurate

Setting	Cause/Solution
Cardiac arrest	Cause: Absence of blood flow Solution: None. Many devices will not be useful during cardiac arrest.
Shock or hypothermia	Cause: Decreased blood flow Solution: Improve blood flow (treat the shock). You may be able to find an alternative site (particularly one that is closer to the heart) where the device can detect pulsatile blood flow.
Motion, shivering, or bright overhead lighting	Cause: False signals and inaccurate oxygen saturation values Solution: Move the sensor unit closer to the heart. Lightly cover the device in position (ie, if it is placed on a finger, lightly cover the finger to reduce ambient light).
Problem with the skin probe interface	Cause: Low or absent pulse signals Solution: Try an alternate site or alternate skin probe
Misalignment of sensor with light source	Cause: Low or absent pulse signals Solution: Reposition the device so that the light source is located directly across the tissue bed from the sensor.
Cardiac arrhythmias with low cardiac output	Cause: Arrhythmias interfere with detection of a pulse and calculation of pulse rate Solution: Get help to treat the arrhythmia.

Correct Use of Oximetry Equipment

Correct probe positioning is critical for accurate oxygen saturation values. The probe is typically applied to a finger or toe. Falsely low values can occur when the probe is not positioned correctly. Repositioning of the probe can result in immediate improvement in the detection of oxygen saturation by the device.

In addition to applying the probe to a finger or toe, the following locations can be used to solve placement problems:

If	Then
Infant probes are unavailable	Use an adult probe around the hand or foot of an infant
Blood flow is significantly reduced, and no signal is detected in the extremities	Assess and support systemic perfusion Apply an infant probe to the earlobe

Endotracheal Intubation

Potential Indications

Consider ET intubation if the child is unable to maintain effective airway, oxygenation, or ventilation despite initial intervention.

Preparation of Endotracheal Intubation

In the Airway Management Skills Station, you will need to know the equipment needed for ET intubation (Table 55).

Critical Concepts

Sudden Deterioration in an Intubated Patient (DOPE Mnemonic)

Sudden deterioration in an intubated patient may be caused by one of several complications. Use the mnemonic **DOPE** to help remember these:

Displacement of the tube	The tube may be displaced out of the trachea or advanced into the right or left main bronchus.
Obstruction of the tube	Obstruction may be caused by • Secretions, blood, pus, or a foreign body • Kinking of the tube
Pneumothorax	• Simple pneumothorax usually results in a sudden deterioration in oxygenation (reflected by a sudden decrease in SpO_2) and decreased chest expansion and breath sounds on the involved side. • Tension pneumothorax may result in the above plus evidence of hypotension and a decrease in cardiac output. The trachea is usually shifted away from the involved side.
Equipment failure	Equipment may fail for a number of reasons, such as • Disconnection of the O_2 supply from the ventilation system • Leak in the ventilator circuit • Failure of power supply to the ventilator • Malfunction of valves in the bag or circuit

Evaluating the Patient's Status

If the condition of an intubated patient deteriorates, the first priority is to support oxygenation and ventilation. While attempting this support, rapidly assess the child and attempt to determine and correct the cause of deterioration. If the child is being mechanically ventilated, hand ventilate with a bag while you assess the patient's airway, ventilation, and oxygenation as follows:

• Observe for chest rise and symmetry of chest movement.
• Auscultate over both sides of the anterior chest and at the midaxillary line and over the stomach. Listen carefully over the lateral lung fields for asymmetry in breath sounds or abnormal sounds such as wheezing.
• Check monitors (eg, pulse oximetry and, if available, capnography).
• Check heart rate.
• Suction the ET tube if you suspect obstruction with secretions.
• Use sedatives or analgesics, with or without neuromuscular blockers, if needed to reduce the child's agitation and control ventilation. Administer these agents only *after* you rule out a correctable cause of the acute distress and are sure that you can provide positive-pressure ventilation.

Your initial assessment will determine the urgency of the required response. If you cannot verify that the ET tube is in the airway, direct visualization of the tube passing through the glottis is advised. If the child's condition is deteriorating and you strongly suspect that the tube is no longer in the trachea, you may need to remove it and ventilate with a bag-mask device.

Patient Agitation

Once the ET tube position and openness/patency are confirmed and failure of ventilation equipment and pneumothorax are ruled out, evaluate oxygenation and perfusion. If oxygenation and perfusion are adequate or unchanged, it is possible that agitation, pain, or excessive movement is interfering with adequate ventilation.

If so, try one or more of the following:

- Analgesia (eg, fentanyl or morphine) to control pain
- Sedation (eg, lorazepam, midazolam) for anxiety or agitation
- Neuromuscular blocking agents and analgesia or sedation to optimize ventilation and minimize the risk of barotrauma and unintentional tube displacement

Continuous capnography is the gold standard during mechanical ventilation as an adjunct to clinical assessment. A sudden decrease in exhaled CO_2 can indicate ET tube displacement or cardiac arrest, while a gradual decrease in exhaled CO_2 may indicate development of ET tube obstruction or decreasing cardiac output. In addition, capnography may help to detect hypoventilation or hyperventilation, and so is particularly useful during transport and diagnostic procedures. A colorimetric detector or capnography should be used during intrahospital and interhospital transport.

Table 55. Pre-event Equipment Checklist for Endotracheal Intubation

☐	Universal precautions (gloves, masks, eye protection)
☐	Cardiac monitor, pulse oximeter, and blood pressure monitoring device
☐	End-tidal CO_2 detector or exhaled CO_2 capnography (or esophageal detector device, if appropriate)
☐	Intravenous and intraosseous infusion equipment
☐	Oxygen supply, bag mask (appropriate size)
☐	Oral/tracheal suction equipment (appropriate size); confirm that it is working
☐	Oral and nasopharyngeal airways (appropriate size)
☐	Endotracheal tubes with stylets (all sizes, with and without cuffs) and sizes 0.5 mm (i.d.) above and below anticipated size for patient
☐	Laryngoscope (curved and straight blades) and/or video laryngoscope; backup laryngoscope available
☐	Cuff pressure monitor (if using cuffed tubes)
☐	3-, 5-, and 10-mL syringes to test inflate endotracheal tube balloon
☐	Adhesive/cloth tape or commercial endotracheal tube holder to secure tube
☐	Towel or pad to align airway by placing under head or torso
☐	Specialty equipment as needed for difficult airway management or anticipated complications (supraglottic, transtracheal, and/or cricothyrotomy)

Part 8

Recognition of Shock

Overview

When shock is present, rapid identification and prompt intervention are critical to improving outcomes. If left untreated, shock can quickly progress to cardiopulmonary failure followed by cardiac arrest. Once an infant or child develops cardiac arrest secondary to inadequately treated shock, the outcome is poor.

This Part discusses the following:

- Pathophysiology of shock
- Effect of different types of shock on blood pressure
- Systolic blood pressure as a method of categorizing the severity of shock (ie, compensated or hypotensive)
- Etiology and signs of the 4 most common types of shock
- Systematic approach to evaluation of the cardiovascular system

Your evaluation will help you identify the child's shock based on type and severity. These clinical findings will direct your interventions, as discussed in "Part 9: Management of Shock."

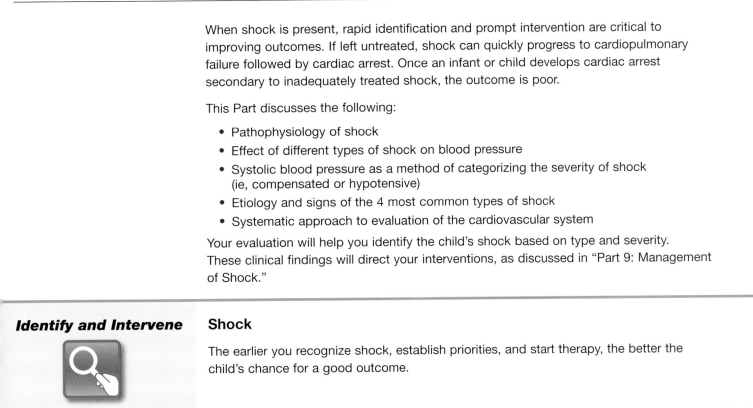

Identify and Intervene

Shock

The earlier you recognize shock, establish priorities, and start therapy, the better the child's chance for a good outcome.

Learning Objective

After completing this Part, you should be able to

- Differentiate between compensated and hypotensive shock

Preparation for the Course

During the PALS Provider Course you will need to identify different types and severities of shock. Your evaluation of patient information will help determine effective interventions.

Definition of Shock

Shock is defined as a physiologic state characterized by inadequate tissue perfusion to meet metabolic demand and tissue oxygenation. Shock is often, but not always, characterized by inadequate peripheral and end-organ perfusion. In children, most shock is characterized by low cardiac output; however, in some types of shock (eg, caused by sepsis or anaphylaxis), cardiac output may be high. All types of shock can result in impaired function of vital organs, such as the brain (decreased level of consciousness) and kidneys (low urine output, ineffective filtering).

Critical Concepts 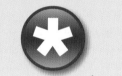	**Shock and Blood Pressure** The definition of shock does not require the presence of hypotension. Shock can be present with a normal, increased, or decreased systolic blood pressure.

Shock can result from

- Inadequate blood volume or oxygen-carrying capacity (hypovolemic shock, including hemorrhagic shock)
- Inappropriate distribution of blood volume and flow (distributive shock)
- Impaired cardiac contractility (cardiogenic shock)
- Obstructed blood flow (obstructive shock)

Conditions such as fever, infection, injury, respiratory distress, and pain may contribute to shock by increasing tissue demand for O_2 and nutrients. Whether due to inadequate supply, increased demand, or a combination of both, *O_2 and nutrient delivery to the tissues is inadequate relative to metabolic needs*. Inadequate tissue perfusion can lead to tissue hypoxia, anaerobic metabolism, accumulation of lactic acid and CO_2, irreversible cell damage, and, ultimately, organ damage. Death may then result rapidly from cardiovascular collapse or more slowly from multiorgan failure.

Critical Concepts	**Goal for Treating Shock** In the treatment of shock, the goal is to improve systemic perfusion and O_2 delivery. This will help prevent end-organ injury and stop the progression to cardiopulmonary failure and cardiac arrest.

Pathophysiology of Shock

The major function of the cardiopulmonary system is to deliver O_2 to body tissues and remove metabolic by-products of cellular metabolism (primarily CO_2). When O_2 delivery is inadequate to meet tissue demand, cells use anaerobic metabolism to produce energy, but this generates lactic acid as a by-product. Anaerobic metabolism can only maintain limited cell function. Unless O_2 delivery is restored, organ dysfunction or failure will result.

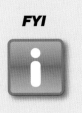

FYI

Central Venous O_2 Saturation ($Scvo_2$) and Cardiac Output

In healthy children with normal metabolic demand, the arterial blood contains more O_2 than the tissues need. If demand increases and/or O_2 delivery decreases, the tissues will extract a greater percent of the O_2 delivered. This results in reduced O_2 saturation in the venous blood returning to the heart. The $Scvo_2$, therefore, can be used to assess the balance between O_2 delivery and demand. If metabolic demand and O_2 content are unchanged, a decreased $Scvo_2$ indicates a fall in cardiac output and, therefore, a fall in O_2 delivered to the tissues. In addition, greater extraction of O_2 has occurred as the result of reduced delivery.

Components of Tissue Oxygen Delivery

Adequate tissue O_2 delivery (Figure 37) depends on

- Sufficient O_2 content in the blood
- Adequate blood flow to the tissues (cardiac output)
- Appropriate distribution of blood flow to the tissues

O_2 content of the blood is determined primarily by the hemoglobin concentration and percent of the hemoglobin that is saturated with O_2 (ie, the arterial oxygen saturation or Sao_2). A small amount of oxygen is carried dissolved in plasma.

FYI

Compensatory Mechanisms for Hypoxemia

Tissue hypoxia is present when a region of the body or an organ is deprived of adequate O_2 supply. Low O_2 saturation (hypoxemia) alone does not necessarily result in tissue hypoxia. Oxygen delivery to the tissues is the product of the arterial O_2 content (determined by the oxygen bound to hemoglobin plus dissolved O_2) and the volume of blood pumped per minute (cardiac output). O_2 delivery may be normal despite hypoxemia if cardiac output increases commensurate with the decrease in O_2 content.

When hypoxemia is chronic (eg, unrepaired cyanotic heart disease), hemoglobin concentration increases (polycythemia). The increased hemoglobin concentration will increase the O_2-carrying capacity of the blood and help maintain arterial O_2 content at near-normal concentrations, despite the fact that hemoglobin oxygen saturation is low.

If cardiac output decreases or hypoxemia worsens, these compensatory mechanisms may not be sufficient to maintain tissue O_2 delivery, and tissue hypoxia will likely develop.

Adequate blood flow to the tissues is determined by the cardiac output and vascular resistance. Cardiac output (the volume of blood pumped by the heart per minute) is the product of stroke volume (the volume of blood pumped by the ventricles with each contraction) and heart rate (number of times the ventricles contract per minute):

Cardiac Output = Stroke Volume · Heart Rate

According to this formula, if the heart rate decreases, stroke volume must increase commensurately to maintain the cardiac output. Cardiac output can increase either by an increase in heart rate, in stroke volume, or both. However, the increase in cardiac output produced by increasing heart rate does have its limit. If the heart rate is too fast, as can happen with extreme tachyarrhythmias (eg, supraventricular tachycardia), stroke volume can fall because there is inadequate time to fill the heart (ie, the diastolic phase is too short). Some arrhythmias, such as complete heart block or junctional tachycardia can be associated with a decrease in ventricular filling because atrial contraction (which normally contributes about 25% of ventricular filling) does not precede ventricular contraction.

Critical Concepts

Infant Cardiac Output Dependent on Heart Rate

Infants have a very small stroke volume with limited ability to increase. Infants are therefore very dependent on an adequate heart rate to maintain or increase cardiac output. The adolescent and adult have greater ability to increase stroke volume, and cardiac output is less dependent on the heart rate.

Appropriate distribution of blood flow is determined by the size of the blood vessels supplying a specific organ. This property is known as *vascular resistance*. If the vessel is large, vascular resistance is low; if the vessel is small, vascular resistance is high. Vascular resistance is adjusted by tissues to locally regulate blood flow to meet metabolic demands. Abnormally increased resistance (vasoconstriction) or decreased resistance (vasodilation) can interfere with blood flow distribution, even if cardiac output is adequate.

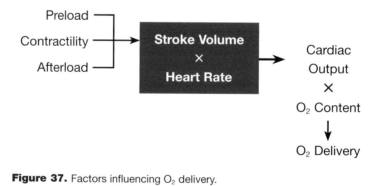

Figure 37. Factors influencing O_2 delivery.

Stroke Volume

Stroke volume is the amount of blood ejected by the ventricles with each contraction. Stroke volume is determined by 3 factors (Table 56).

Table 56. Factors Used to Determine Stroke Volume

Factor	Clinical Definition
Preload	Volume of blood present in the ventricle before contraction
Contractility	Strength of contraction
Afterload	Resistance against which the ventricle is ejecting

Inadequate *preload* is the most common cause of low stroke volume and, therefore, low cardiac output. A number of conditions (eg, hemorrhage, severe dehydration, vasodilation) can cause inadequate preload. Inadequate preload results in hypovolemic shock.

FYI

Preload

Preload is often assessed indirectly by measuring the central venous pressure, but the relationship between central venous pressure and preload is complex. Preload to the ventricles is the *volume* of blood in the ventricles that stretches the ventricular fibers before a contraction (ie, the end-diastolic volume). However, the measurements used clinically are measurements of *pressure*. The relationship between changes in ventricular volume and changes in ventricular end-diastolic pressure is affected by ventricular compliance (or, conversely, ventricular stiffness).

In general, assessment of the right ventricle preload is made through measurement of the central venous pressure, measured in the superior vena cava or right atrium. In general, an increase in the central venous pressure corresponds to an increase in right ventricular end-diastolic volume and preload. However, if there is increased pressure around the right atrium and ventricle from a tension pneumothorax or pericardial tamponade, or if the right ventricle is stiff (ie, not compliant) as the result of a congenital heart defect or pulmonary hypertension, ventricular end-diastolic pressure may be increased despite no increase (or even a decrease) in right ventricular end-diastolic volume and preload.

Preload is not the same as total blood volume. At steady state, most of the blood (about 70%) is in the veins. If the veins are dilated, the total blood volume may be normal or increased, but an inadequate amount of blood may be returning to the heart, so right ventricular preload may be inadequate. This is part of the problem with sepsis: there is often severe venodilation, so preload to the heart may be inadequate. In addition, the maldistribution of blood flow results in some tissue hypoxia.

Poor contractility (also referred to as *myocardial dysfunction*) impairs stroke volume and cardiac output. It can lead to cardiogenic shock. Poor contractility can be due to an intrinsic problem with pump function or an acquired abnormality, such as an inflamed heart muscle (ie, myocarditis). Poor contractility also can occur from metabolic problems, such as hypoglycemia, or from toxic ingestions (eg, calcium channel blockers).

Increased afterload is an uncommon primary cause of low stroke volume and impaired cardiac output in children. Certain conditions, such as severe pulmonary or systemic hypertension or congenital abnormalities of the aorta, can increase afterload so significantly that cardiogenic shock results.

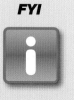

Negative Effects of High Afterload in Cardiogenic Shock

High afterload in children with poor myocardial function can further impair stroke volume and cardiac output. When cardiac output is reduced, the body responds with vasoconstriction in an attempt to maintain blood pressure and blood flow to vital organs. Paradoxically, vasoconstriction increases impedance to ventricular ejection and further decreases stroke volume and cardiac output. An essential component of the advanced treatment of cardiogenic shock is afterload reduction.

Compensatory Mechanisms

As shock develops, compensatory mechanisms attempt to maintain O_2 delivery to vital organs. Compensatory mechanisms include

- Tachycardia
- Increase in systemic vascular resistance (SVR) (vasoconstriction)
- Increase in strength of cardiac contraction (contractility)
- Increase in venous smooth muscle tone

The body's first action to maintain cardiac output is to increase heart rate (tachycardia). *Tachycardia* can increase cardiac output to a limited degree.

When O_2 delivery to the tissues is compromised, blood flow is redirected or shunted from nonvital organs and tissues (eg, skin, skeletal muscles, gut, kidneys) to vital organs (eg, brain, heart). This redirection occurs by a selective *increase in SVR (vasoconstriction)*. Clinically, this results in reduced peripheral perfusion (ie, delayed capillary refill, cool extremities, less easily palpable peripheral pulses), and reduced perfusion to the gut and kidneys (decreased urine volume).

Another compensatory mechanism to maintain stroke volume and cardiac output is an *increase in strength of cardiac contractions (contractility)* with more complete emptying of the ventricles. Stroke volume may also be supported by an *increase in venous smooth muscle tone,* improving venous return to the heart and preload.

Effect on Blood Pressure

Blood pressure is determined by cardiac output and SVR. As cardiac output decreases, blood pressure can be maintained by an increase in SVR. In children with shock, this compensatory mechanism can be so effective that systolic blood pressure may initially remain normal or even slightly elevated. Pulse pressure, the difference between the systolic and diastolic blood pressure, is often narrowed because an increase in SVR raises the diastolic pressure. In contrast, if SVR is low (as in sepsis), diastolic blood pressure decreases and pulse pressure widens.

If cardiac output is inadequate, tissue perfusion is compromised, even if blood pressure is normal. Signs of poor tissue perfusion, including lactic acidosis and end-organ dysfunction, will be present even if blood pressure is normal.

When SVR cannot increase further, blood pressure begins to decline. At that point, delivery of O_2 to vital organs is severely compromised. Clinical signs include metabolic acidosis and evidence of end-organ dysfunction (eg, impaired mental status and decreased urine output). Ultimately O_2 delivery to the myocardium becomes inadequate, causing myocardial dysfunction, decreased stroke volume, and hypotension. These may rapidly lead to cardiovascular collapse, cardiac arrest, and irreversible end-organ injury.

Identification of Shock by Severity (Effect on Blood Pressure)

The severity of shock is frequently characterized by its effect on systolic blood pressure. Shock is described as *compensated* if compensatory mechanisms are able to maintain a systolic blood pressure within a normal range (ie, above the fifth percentile systolic blood pressure for age). When compensatory mechanisms fail and systolic blood pressure declines, shock is classified as *hypotensive* (previously referred to as *decompensated*). It's important to remember that shock may be present even if the child's blood pressure is normal.

You can easily identify hypotensive shock by measuring blood pressure; compensated shock is more difficult to diagnose. Shock can range from mild to severe. Its manifestations are affected by the type of shock and the child's compensatory responses. Blood pressure is used to determine severity of shock; however, children with both compensated and hypotensive shock are at high risk for deterioration. The child with low cardiac output (ie, hypovolemic shock) but normal blood pressure associated with severe vasoconstriction may have more end-organ compromise than the child with normal or increased cardiac output (ie, septic shock) and low systolic blood pressure.

Because blood pressure is one method of categorizing the severity of shock, it is important to recognize that automated blood pressure devices are accurate only when there is adequate distal perfusion. If you cannot palpate distal pulses, and the extremities are cool and poorly perfused, automated blood pressure values may not be reliable. Treat the child based on your entire clinical evaluation. If measurement of blood pressure is not feasible, use clinical evaluation of tissue perfusion to guide treatment.

Compensated Shock

Compensated shock refers to a clinical state in which there are clinical signs of inadequate tissue perfusion, but the patient's blood pressure is in the normal range. In this stage of shock, the body is able to maintain blood pressure despite impaired delivery of O_2 and nutrients to the vital organs. Clinical findings include tachycardia, delayed capillary refill, and decreased urine output.

Critical Concepts

Systolic Blood Pressure in Identification of Shock

Note that the term *compensated shock* refers to the child with signs of poor perfusion but a normal systolic blood pressure (ie, with blood pressure compensation). Systolic blood pressure is used by convention and consensus to determine the presence or absence of hypotension with shock. Infants and children with compensated shock may be critically ill despite an adequate systolic blood pressure.

When O_2 delivery is limited, compensatory mechanisms try to maintain normal blood flow to the brain and heart. These compensatory mechanisms are clues to the presence of shock and vary according to the type of shock. Table 57 lists common compensatory mechanisms in shock and the cardiovascular signs associated with these mechanisms.

Signs specific to shock type are discussed in "Identification of Shock by Type" later in this Part.

Table 57. Common Signs of Shock Resulting From Cardiovascular Compensatory Mechanisms

Compensatory Mechanism	Area	Sign
Increased heart rate	Heart	Tachycardia
Increased SVR	Skin	Cold, pale, mottled, diaphoretic
	Peripheral circulation	Delayed capillary refill
	Pulses	Weak peripheral pulses; narrow pulse pressure (increased diastolic blood pressure)
Increased renal and splanchnic vascular resistance (redistribution of blood flow away from these areas)	Kidney	Oliguria (decreased urine output)
	Intestine	Vomiting, ileus
Cerebral autoregulation	Brain	Altered mental status, anxiety/restlessness, disorientation or decreased level of consciousness or even coma

Hypotensive Shock

Hypotensive (decompensated) shock can result from many causes and is characterized by evidence of impaired perfusion that will rapidly progress to cardiac arrest if not corrected. Signs include abnormal clinical appearance and evidence of severely impaired perfusion (ie, absent distal pulses and weak central pulses, cool extremities, mottled skin, or altered level of consciousness). Shock represents a continuum of severity, and the presence of signs and symptoms of shock should prompt immediate action rather than waiting for direct measurement of blood pressure to document hypotension.

Hypotension is a late finding in most types of shock and may signal impending cardiac arrest. Hypotension can occur early in septic shock because mediators of sepsis produce vasodilation and reduce SVR. In this setting the child may initially appear to have warm extremities, brisk capillary refill, and full peripheral pulses despite hypotension.

Critical Concepts

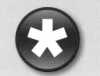

Hypotension in Septic Shock

SVR may be increased or decreased in septic shock. When SVR is decreased, hypotension will be an early rather than a late sign of shock.

Hypotension Formula

In children 1 to 10 years of age, hypotension is present if the systolic blood pressure is less than

70 mm Hg + [child's age in years · 2] mm Hg

For more information, see Table 11: Definition of Hypotension by Systolic Blood Pressure and Age in Part 3.

Physiologic Continuum

Be alert to the progression of clinical signs that may signal a worsening of the child's condition. These signs will develop along a continuum from compensated shock to hypotensive shock and ultimately to cardiac arrest. Decreased peripheral pulses and prolonged capillary refill time occur early in shock progression. Progressive tachypnea and tachycardia are indicators of worsening status. Later, warning signs include loss of peripheral pulses and decreasing level of consciousness. Bradycardia and weak central pulses in a child with signs of shock are ominous signs of impending cardiac arrest.

Accelerating Process

Shock progression is unpredictable. It may take hours for compensated shock to progress to hypotensive shock, but only minutes for hypotensive shock to progress to cardiopulmonary failure and cardiac arrest. This progression is typically an *accelerating process* (Figure 38).

Compensated Shock

↓ Possibly hours

Hypotensive Shock

↓ Potentially minutes

Cardiac Arrest

Figure 38. Accelerating process of shock.

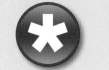

Critical Concepts

Halting the Progression

Early recognition and rapid intervention are critical to halting the progression from compensated shock to hypotensive shock to cardiopulmonary failure and cardiac arrest.

These and other clinical manifestations are discussed in greater detail later in this Part.

Identification of Shock by Type

Shock can be categorized into 4 basic types (see Table 58 and Figure 39 later in this Part).

Table 58. Basic Types of Shock

Type	Etiology
Hypovolemic	Gastroenteritis, burns, hemorrhage, inadequate fluid intake, increased body fluid losses, osmotic diuresis
Cardiogenic	Congenital heart disease, myocarditis, cardiomyopathy, arrhythmia
Distributive	Sepsis, anaphylaxis, spinal cord injury
Obstructive	Tension pneumothorax, cardiac tamponade, pulmonary embolism, constriction of the ductus arteriosus in infants with ductal-dependent congenital heart lesions (eg, coarctation, hypoplastic left ventricle)

Hypovolemic Shock

Hypovolemic shock refers to a clinical state of reduced intravascular volume. It is the most common type of shock in pediatric patients. It can be caused by extravascular fluid loss (eg, diarrhea, dehydration) or intravascular volume loss (eg, hemorrhage) and results in decreased preload and cardiac output. Volume loss that can lead to hypovolemic shock can result from

- Diarrhea
- Vomiting
- Hemorrhage (internal and external)
- Inadequate fluid intake
- Osmotic diuresis (eg, DKA)
- Third-space losses (fluid leak into tissues)
- Large burns

Hypovolemic shock is the result of an absolute deficiency of intravascular blood volume, but, in fact, it typically represents depletion of both intravascular and extravascular fluid volume. As a result, adequate fluid resuscitation often requires administration of fluid boluses that exceed the volume of the estimated intravascular deficit.

Tachypnea, a respiratory compensation to maintain acid-base balance, is often present in hypovolemic shock. The respiratory alkalosis that results from hyperventilation partially compensates for the metabolic acidosis (lactic acidosis) that accompanies shock.

Physiology of Hypovolemic Shock

Hypovolemic shock is characterized by decreased preload leading to reduced stroke volume and low cardiac output. Tachycardia, increased SVR, and increased cardiac contractility are the main compensatory mechanisms.

Hypovolemic Shock		
Preload	**Contractility**	**Afterload**
Decreased	Initially normal or increased	Increased

Signs of Hypovolemic Shock

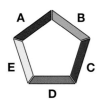

Table 59 outlines typical signs of hypovolemic shock found during the initial impression and primary assessment. The **bold** text denotes type-specific signs that distinguish hypovolemic shock from other forms of shock.

Although septic, anaphylactic, neurogenic, and other distributive forms of shock are not classified as hypovolemic, they are characterized by *relative* hypovolemia. The relative hypovolemia results from arterial and venous vasodilation, increased capillary permeability, and plasma loss into the interstitium ("third spacing" or capillary leak).

Table 59. Findings Consistent With Hypovolemic Shock

Primary Assessment	Finding
A	Typically, open/patent unless level of consciousness is significantly impaired
B	Tachypnea without increased effort (quiet tachypnea)
C	<ul><li>Tachycardia</li><li>**Adequate systolic blood pressure, narrow pulse pressure, or systolic hypotension with a narrow pulse pressure**</li><li>Weak or absent peripheral pulses</li><li>Normal or weak central pulses</li><li>Delayed capillary refill</li><li>Cool to cold, pale, mottled, diaphoretic skin</li><li>Dusky/pale distal extremities</li><li>Changes in level of consciousness</li><li>Oliguria</li></ul>
D	Decreasing level of consciousness as shock progresses
E	Extremities often cooler than trunk

Distributive Shock

Distributive shock refers to a clinical state characterized by reduced SVR leading to maldistribution of blood volume and blood flow. This group includes

- Septic shock
- Anaphylactic shock
- Neurogenic shock (eg, spinal injury)

In septic and anaphylactic shock, there may also be increased capillary permeability, leading to loss of volume from the intravascular space (ie, decreased preload). In neurogenic shock, there is loss of sympathetic tone leading to vasodilation and lack of compensatory mechanisms (ie, tachycardia and peripheral vasoconstriction).

Distributive shock caused by sepsis is characterized by reduced or increased SVR result-ing in maldistribution of blood flow. The vasodilation and venodilation causes pooling of blood in the venous system and a relative hypovolemia. Septic shock also causes increased capillary permeability, so there is loss of plasma from the vascular space. This increases the severity of the hypovolemia. Myocardial contractility may also be depressed in septic shock.

In anaphylactic shock, venodilation, arterial dilation, and increased capillary permeability combined with pulmonary vasoconstriction result in reduced cardiac output. The low cardiac output is caused by relative hypovolemia and increased right ventricular afterload.

Neurogenic shock is characterized by generalized loss of vascular tone, most often after a high cervical spine injury. The loss of vascular tone leads to severe vasodilation and hypotension. Normally, the sympathetic nervous system increases heart rate in response to hypotension. Children with neurogenic shock may be unable to generate a faster heart rate in response to hypotension. As a result, cardiac output and blood flow to tissues decrease dramatically.

Pathophysiology of Distributive Shock

In distributive shock, cardiac output may be increased, normal, or decreased. Although myocardial dysfunction may be present, stroke volume can be adequate, particularly if there is aggressive volume resuscitation and decreased SVR. Tachycardia and an increase in ventricular end-diastolic volume (from volume resuscitation) help maintain cardiac output. Tissue perfusion is compromised by maldistribution of blood flow. Some tissue beds (eg, splanchnic circulation) may be inadequately perfused; in other tissues (eg, some skeletal muscle and skin) perfusion may exceed metabolic needs. Hypoxic tissues generate lactic acid, leading to metabolic acidosis. Early in the clinical course, a child with distributive shock may present with decreased SVR and increased blood flow to the skin. This produces warm extremities and bounding peripheral pulses ("warm shock").

The high cardiac output and low SVR often observed in distributive shock differ from the low cardiac output and high SVR seen in hypovolemic, cardiogenic, and obstructive shock. As distributive shock progresses, concomitant hypovolemia and/or myocardial dysfunction produce a decrease in cardiac output. SVR can then increase, resulting in inadequate blood flow to the skin, cold extremities, and weak pulses ("cold shock"). The late phase of distributive shock, therefore, can be similar to the clinical picture of hypovolemic and cardiogenic shock.

FYI

Central ScvO$_2$ in Septic Shock

In contrast to hypovolemic and cardiogenic shock, ScvO$_2$ may be normal, increased, or decreased in septic shock. There are 2 mechanisms to explain a normal, or even increased, ScvO$_2$, despite the presence of inadequate cardiac output/index.

- Children with low SVR and increased cardiac output will extract less O$_2$ from the blood because some tissues are receiving more blood flow than they need. Other tissues don't receive enough blood flow so they don't have the opportunity to extract the O$_2$.
- Children with sepsis may be unable to utilize O$_2$ at the cellular level

Toxins and inflammatory mediators circulating in sepsis can prevent aerobic metabolism even in the setting of adequate O$_2$ delivery. As a result, lactic acidosis and end-organ dysfunction can occur even in the setting of normal or increased ScvO$_2$.

Distributive Shock		
Preload	**Contractility**	**Afterload**
Normal or decreased	Normal or decreased	Variable

Distributive shock is most often characterized by many changes in cardiovascular function, including

- Low SVR, which causes the wide pulse pressure characteristic of distributive shock and contributes to early hypotension; late in the clinical course, SVR may increase
- Increased blood flow to some peripheral tissue beds
- Inadequate perfusion of the splanchnic (gut and kidney) vascular beds
- Release of inflammatory and other mediators and vasoactive substances
- Volume depletion caused by capillary leak
- Accumulation of lactic acid in poorly perfused tissue beds

Critical Concepts

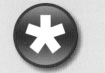

Relative Hypovolemia

Although most types of distributive shock are not typically classified as hypovolemic shock, all are characterized by relative hypovolemia unless adequate fluid resuscitation is provided.

Signs of Distributive Shock

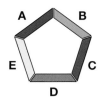

Table 60 outlines typical signs of distributive shock seen during the initial impression and primary assessment. The **bold** text denotes type-specific signs that distinguish distributive shock from other forms of shock.

Table 60. Findings Consistent With Distributive Shock

Primary Assessment	Finding
A	Usually open/patent unless level of consciousness is significantly impaired
B	Tachypnea, usually without increased work of breathing ("quiet tachypnea") unless the child has pneumonia or is developing ARDS or cardiogenic pulmonary edema
C	• Tachycardia or, less commonly, bradycardia • **Bounding or decreased peripheral pulses** • **Flash or delayed capillary refill** • **Warm, flushed skin peripherally (warm extremities)** *or* **Pale, mottled skin with vasoconstriction (cold extremities)** • **Hypotension with a wide pulse pressure (when warm extremities are present)** *or* **Hypotension with a narrow pulse pressure (when cold extremities are present)** *or* **Normotension may be present** • Changes in level of consciousness • Oliguria
D	Changes in level of consciousness
E	• Fever or hypothermia • Extremities may be warm or cool • **Petechial or purpuric rash (septic shock)**

Septic Shock

Sepsis represents an important cause of shock in infants and children. *Sepsis* and *septic shock* are terms used to characterize shock caused by an infectious agent or inflammatory stimulus.

Septic shock is the most common form of distributive shock. It is caused by infectious organisms or their by-products (eg, endotoxin) that cause the small blood vessels to dilate and to leak fluid into the tissues.

Infection is a pathologic process caused by invasion of normally sterile tissue, fluid, or a body cavity by pathogenic or potentially pathogenic microorganisms. Infection may be suspected or proven by positive result of a culture, tissue stain, or polymerase chain reaction test. In the absence of these tests, evidence of infection includes positive findings on clinical examination, imaging, or laboratory tests consistent with tissue invasion by a pathogenic organism leading to a host response (eg, white blood cells in normally sterile body fluid, perforated viscus, chest radiograph consistent with pneumonia, petechial or purpuric rash, purpura fulminans).

Pathophysiology of Septic Shock

Septic shock in children typically evolves along a continuum from a systemic inflammatory response in the early stages to septic shock in the late stages. This continuum may evolve over days or just a few hours; there is wide variability in clinical presentation and progression.

FYI

Inflammatory Cascade Response to Sepsis

The pathophysiology of the septic cascade includes the following, often referred to as the *systemic inflammatory response*:

- The infectious organism or its by-products (eg, endotoxin) activates the immune system, including neutrophils, monocytes, and macrophages.
- These cells, or their interaction with the infecting organism, stimulate release or activation of inflammatory mediators (cytokines) that perpetuate the inflammatory response.
- Cytokines produce vasodilation and damage to the lining of the blood vessels (endothelium), causing increased capillary permeability.
- Cytokines activate the coagulation cascade and may result in microvascular thrombosis and disseminated intravascular coagulation (DIC).
- Specific inflammatory mediators can impair cardiac contractility and cause myocardial dysfunction.

FYI

The Challenge of Treating Septic Shock

In septic shock, the combination of inadequate perfusion and possible microvascular thrombosis leads to ischemia, which is diffuse and patchy so that individual organs have varying levels of hypoxia and ischemia. The variability of perfusion throughout the body is what makes treatment of sepsis so difficult.

Septic Shock		
Preload	**Contractility**	**Afterload**
Decreased	Normal to decreased	Variable

FYI

Adrenal Insufficiency in Septic Shock

The adrenal glands are especially prone to microvascular thrombosis and hemorrhage in septic shock. Because adrenal glands produce cortisol, an important hormone in the body's stress response, children with sepsis may develop absolute or relative adrenal insufficiency. Adrenal insufficiency contributes to low SVR and myocardial dysfunction in septic shock.

Signs of Septic Shock

In the early stages, signs of septic shock are often subtle and may be difficult to recognize because peripheral perfusion may initially appear to be adequate. Because septic shock is triggered by an infection or its by-products, the child may have fever or hypothermia, and the white blood cell (WBC) count may be decreased, normal, or increased.

In addition to the findings listed in Table 58, the child with septic shock may have other abnormalities identified by diagnostic assessments. Examples include metabolic acidosis, respiratory alkalosis, leukocytosis (high WBC count), leukopenia (low WBC count), or left shift (increased percent of bands or immature white blood cells). With some types of infections, the child may develop a petechial or purpuric rash.

Identify and Intervene

Septic Shock

Early recognition and treatment of septic shock are critically important determinants of outcome. You should evaluate temperature, heart rate, systemic perfusion, blood pressure, and clinical signs of end-organ function to identify sepsis and septic shock before severe organ dysfunction develops. If you suspect sepsis, and especially if shock develops, provide appropriate volume resuscitation and hemodynamic support (see "Part 9: Management of Shock" for details). Search for and treat the underlying cause.

Anaphylactic Shock

Anaphylactic shock is an acute multisystem response caused by a severe reaction to a drug, vaccine, food, toxin, plant, venom, or other antigen. The reaction is characterized by venodilation, arterial vasodilation, increased capillary permeability, and pulmonary vasoconstriction. It can occur within seconds to minutes after exposure.

Physiology of Anaphylactic Shock

Pulmonary vasoconstriction acutely increases right heart afterload. It may reduce pulmonary blood flow, pulmonary venous return, and preload to the left ventricle, and decrease cardiac output. Death may occur immediately or the child may develop acute-phase symptoms, which typically begin 5 to 10 minutes after exposure.

Anaphylactic Shock		
Preload	**Contractility**	**Afterload**
Decreased	Variable	Left ventricle: Decreased
		Right ventricle: Increased

Signs of Anaphylactic Shock

Signs and symptoms may include those listed in Table 61. The **bold** text denotes type-specific signs that distinguish anaphylactic shock from other forms of shock.

Table 61. Findings Consistent With Anaphylactic Shock

Primary Assessment	Finding	Resulting From
A	**Angioedema (swelling of the face, lips, and tongue)**	Swelling of the tongue and tissues related to fluid leak from blood vessels
B	**Respiratory distress with stridor, wheezing, or both**	Constriction of airways by inflammatory response
C	Hypotension	Vasodilation, hypovolemia, and diminished cardiac output
C	Tachycardia	Inadequate blood flow to the tissues
D	Anxiety and agitation	Low oxygen concentration
E	**Urticaria (hives)**	Histamine release
	Nausea and vomiting	Histamine and other mediator release

Angioedema may cause partial or complete upper airway obstruction. Hypotension results from vasodilation, hypovolemia, and diminished cardiac output. Relative hypovolemia is caused by the vasodilation, and absolute volume loss is caused by capillary leak.

Neurogenic Shock

Neurogenic shock, also known as *spinal shock*, results from a cervical (neck) or upper thoracic (above T6) injury that disrupts the sympathetic nervous system innervation of blood vessels and of the heart.

Physiology of Neurogenic Shock

The sudden loss of sympathetic nervous system signals to the smooth muscle in the vessel walls results in uncontrolled vasodilation. The same disruption prevents development of tachycardia as a compensatory mechanism.

Neurogenic Shock		
Preload	**Contractility**	**Afterload**
Decreased	Normal	Decreased

Signs of Neurogenic Shock

Primary signs of neurogenic shock are

- Hypotension with a wide pulse pressure
- Normal heart rate or bradycardia
- Hypothermia

Other signs may include increased respiratory rate, diaphragmatic breathing (use of muscles in the diaphragm rather than the chest wall), and other evidence of a high thoracic or cervical spine injury (ie, motor or sensory deficits).

Neurogenic shock must be differentiated from hypovolemic shock. Hypovolemic shock is typically associated with hypotension, a narrow pulse pressure from compensatory vasoconstriction, and compensatory tachycardia. In neurogenic shock, these compensatory mechanisms are not apparent because sympathetic innervation of the heart and blood vessels is interrupted.

Cardiogenic Shock

Cardiogenic shock refers to reduced cardiac output secondary to abnormal cardiac function or pump failure. This results in decreased systolic function and cardiac output. Common causes of cardiogenic shock include

- Congenital heart disease
- Myocarditis (inflammation of the heart muscle)
- Cardiomyopathy (an inherited or acquired abnormality of pumping function)
- Arrhythmias
- Sepsis
- Poisoning or drug toxicity
- Myocardial injury (eg, trauma)

Physiology of Cardiogenic Shock

Cardiogenic shock is characterized by marked tachycardia, high SVR, and decreased cardiac output. End-diastolic volume within the left and right ventricles is increased, resulting in congestion within the pulmonary and systemic venous systems. Pulmonary venous congestion leads to pulmonary edema and increased work of breathing. Typically, intravascular volume is normal or increased unless a concurrent illness causes hypovolemia (eg, in a child who has viral myocarditis with recent vomiting and fever).

Cardiogenic Shock		
Preload	**Contractility**	**Afterload**
Variable	Decreased	Increased

Cardiogenic shock is often characterized by sequential compensatory and pathologic mechanisms, including

- Increase in heart rate and left ventricular afterload, which increases left ventricular work and myocardial O_2 consumption
- Compensatory increase in SVR to redirect blood from peripheral and splanchnic tissues to the heart and brain
- Decrease in stroke volume due to decreased myocardial contractility and increased afterload
- Increased venous tone, which increases central venous (right atrial) and pulmonary capillary (left atrial) pressures
- Diminished renal blood flow resulting in fluid retention
- Pulmonary edema resulting from myocardial failure and high left ventricular end-diastolic, left atrial, and pulmonary venous pressures, and from increased venous tone and fluid retention

The same compensatory mechanisms that maintain perfusion to the brain and heart in hypovolemic shock are often detrimental during cardiogenic shock. For example, compensatory peripheral vasoconstriction can maintain blood pressure in hypovolemic shock. However, because it increases left ventricular afterload (commonly thought of as increased resistance to left ventricular ejection), compensatory vasoconstriction has detrimental effects in cardiogenic shock.

Because the heart muscle also needs O_2, almost all children with severe or sustained shock may eventually have inadequate myocardial O_2 delivery relative to myocardial O_2 demand. Therefore, severe or sustained shock of any type eventually causes impaired myocardial function (ie, these children develop cardiogenic shock in addition to the primary cause of shock). Once myocardial function declines, the child's clinical status usually deteriorates rapidly.

Signs of Cardiogenic Shock

Table 62 outlines signs of cardiogenic shock typically found during the initial impression and primary assessment of the child. The **bold** text denotes type-specific signs that distinguish cardiogenic shock from other forms of shock.

Table 62. Findings Consistent With Cardiogenic Shock

Primary Assessment	Finding
A	Usually open/patent unless level of consciousness is significantly impaired
B	<ul><li>Tachypnea</li><li>**Increased respiratory effort (retractions, nasal flaring, grunting) resulting from pulmonary edema**</li></ul>
C	<ul><li>Tachycardia</li><li>Normal or low blood pressure with a narrow pulse pressure</li><li>Weak or absent peripheral pulses</li><li>Normal and then weak central pulses</li><li>Delayed capillary refill with cool extremities</li><li>**Signs of congestive heart failure (eg, pulmonary edema, hepatomegaly, jugular venous distention)**</li><li>**Cyanosis (caused by cyanotic congenital heart disease or pulmonary edema)**</li><li>Cold, pale, mottled, diaphoretic skin</li><li>Changes in level of consciousness</li><li>Oliguria</li></ul>
D	Changes in level of consciousness
E	Extremities often cooler than trunk

Critical Concepts

Distinguishing Signs of Cardiogenic Shock

Increased respiratory effort often distinguishes cardiogenic shock from hypovolemic shock. Hypovolemic shock is characterized by "quiet tachypnea," while children with cardiogenic shock may demonstrate retractions, grunting, and use of accessory muscles.

In cardiogenic shock, there may be decreased arterial O_2 saturation secondary to pulmonary edema.

Rapid volume resuscitation of *cardiogenic* shock in the setting of poor myocardial function can aggravate pulmonary edema and further impair myocardial function. This can further compromise oxygenation, ventilation, and cardiac output. Volume resuscitation for cardiogenic shock should be gradual; give smaller (5-10 mL/kg) boluses of isotonic crystalloid and deliver over a longer period of time (ie, over 10 to 20 minutes). Carefully monitor hemodynamic parameters during fluid infusion, and repeat infusion as needed.

Infants and children with cardiogenic shock often require medications to increase and redistribute cardiac output, improve myocardial function, and reduce SVR. Additional treatment includes reducing metabolic demand, such as decreasing work of breathing and controlling fever. This will allow a limited cardiac output to better meet tissue metabolic demands. For more details, see "Part 9: Management of Shock."

Obstructive Shock

Obstructive shock refers to conditions that physically impair blood flow by limiting venous return to the heart or limit the pumping of blood from the heart. The end result is decreased cardiac output. Causes of obstructive shock include

- Pericardial tamponade
- Tension pneumothorax
- Ductal-dependent congenital heart defects (eg, coarctation of the aorta, hypoplastic left ventricle)
- Massive pulmonary embolism

The physical obstruction to blood flow results in low cardiac output, inadequate tissue perfusion, and a compensatory increase in SVR. The early clinical presentation of obstructive shock can be indistinguishable from hypovolemic shock. However, careful clinical examination may reveal signs of systemic or pulmonary venous congestion that are not consistent with hypovolemia. As the condition progresses, increased respiratory effort, cyanosis, and signs of vascular congestion become more apparent.

Obstructive Shock		
Preload	**Contractility**	**Afterload**
Variable	Normal	Increased

Pathophysiology and Clinical Signs of Obstructive Shock

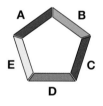

Pathophysiology and clinical signs vary according to the cause of the obstructive shock.

Cardiac Tamponade

Cardiac tamponade is caused by an accumulation of fluid, blood, or air in the pericardial space. Increased intrapericardial pressure and compression of the heart impede systemic venous and pulmonary venous return. This reduces ventricular filling and causes a decrease in stroke volume and cardiac output. If untreated, cardiac tamponade results in cardiac arrest with pulseless electrical activity.

In children, cardiac tamponade most often occurs after penetrating trauma or cardiac surgery. It also may develop as a result of pericardial effusion complicating an inflammatory disorder, an infection of the pericardium, a tumor, or an extremely high white blood cell count. Table 63 outlines signs of cardiac tamponade typically found during the initial impression and primary assessment. The signs unique to pericardial tamponade are in **bold** type.

Table 63. Findings Consistent With Cardiac Tamponade

Primary Assessment	Finding
A	Usually open/patent unless level of consciousness is significantly impaired
B	Respiratory distress with increased respiratory rate and effort

(continued)

(continued)

C	• Tachycardia • Poor peripheral perfusion (weak distal pulses, cool extremities, delayed capillary refill) • **Muffled or diminished heart sounds** • Narrowed pulse pressure • **Pulsus paradoxus** (decrease in systolic blood pressure by >10 mm Hg during spontaneous inspiration) • Distended neck veins (may be difficult to see in infants, especially with severe hypotension)
D	Changes in level of consciousness
E	Extremities often cooler than trunk

Note that after cardiovascular surgery in children, signs of tamponade may be indistinguishable from those of cardiogenic shock. Favorable outcome depends on urgent diagnosis and immediate treatment. In children with a large pericardial effusion, the electrocardiogram typically shows small QRS complexes (low voltage), but echocardiography provides a definitive diagnosis.

FYI

Pulsus Paradoxus

Pulsus paradoxus is an exaggerated manifestation of a normal variation in stroke volume that occurs during the phases of spontaneous respiration. Stroke volume decreases slightly during inspiration and increases slightly during expiration. In pulsus paradoxus, the systolic blood pressure declines by greater than 10 mm Hg on inspiration, compared with expiration. True assessment for pulsus paradoxus requires measurement of blood pressure with a manual pressure cuff. Inflate the cuff until no sounds are heard (as usual). Slowly decrease the cuff pressure and note the point at which the first Korotkoff sounds are initially heard, which will be when the child is exhaling. Continue to slowly deflate the cuff and note the point at which the Korotkoff sounds are heard consistently throughout the respiratory cycle. If the difference between these 2 points is greater than 10 mm Hg, the child has a clinically significant pulsus paradoxus.

You may be able to detect a significant pulsus paradoxus by palpation of the pulse, noting a distinct variation in pulse amplitude as the child inhales and exhales. Pulsus paradoxus may also be apparent on arterial and pulse oximetry waveforms but is not as easily quantified unless the waveform can be saved on the monitor screen or printed for review.

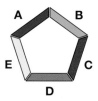

Tension Pneumothorax

Tension pneumothorax is caused by the entry of air into the pleural space and accumulation under pressure. This air can enter from lung tissue injured by an internal tear or from a penetrating chest injury. An air leak that enters the pleural space but then stops spontaneously is called a *simple pneumothorax*. An ongoing leak can result from positive-pressure ventilation or chest trauma that forces air out of the injured lung and into the pleural space. If air continues to leak into the pleural space, it accumulates under pressure, creating a tension pneumothorax. As this pressure increases, it compresses the underlying lung and pushes the mediastinum to the opposite side of the chest. Compression of the lung rapidly causes respiratory failure. The high intrathoracic pressure and direct pressure on mediastinal structures (heart and great vessels) impede venous return, resulting in a rapid decline in cardiac output and hypotension. Untreated tension pneumothorax leads to cardiac arrest characterized by pulseless electrical activity.

Suspect tension pneumothorax in a victim of chest trauma or in any intubated child who deteriorates suddenly while receiving positive-pressure ventilation (including bag-mask or noninvasive ventilation). Table 64 outlines signs of tension pneumothorax typically found during the initial impression and primary assessment. Signs unique to tension pneumothorax are in **bold** type.

Table 64. Findings Consistent With Tension Pneumothorax

Primary Assessment	Finding
A	• Variable depending on situation and primary cause of respiratory distress • Advanced airway may already be in place • **Tracheal deviation toward contralateral side (the side opposite the side of the pneumothorax). This deviation may be difficult to appreciate in infants.**
B	• Respiratory distress with increased respiratory rate and effort • **Hyperresonance of affected side; hyperexpansion of affected side** • **Diminished breath sounds on affected side**
C	• Distended neck veins (may be difficult to appreciate in infants or in children with severe hypotension) • Pulsus paradoxus (decrease in systolic blood pressure by >10 mm Hg during spontaneous inspiration) • Rapid deterioration in perfusion; commonly, rapid evolution from tachycardia to bradycardia and hypotension as cardiac output decreases
D	Changes in level of consciousness
E	Extremities often cooler than trunk

Favorable outcome depends on immediate diagnosis and treatment.

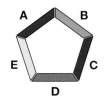

Ductal-Dependent Lesions

Ductal-dependent congenital cardiac abnormalities usually present in the first days to weeks of life. Ductal-dependent lesions include

- Cyanotic congenital heart lesions (ductal dependent for pulmonary blood flow)
- Left ventricular outflow obstructive lesions (ductal dependent for systemic blood flow)

The congenital heart lesions that depend on the ductus for pulmonary blood flow present with cyanosis rather than signs of shock. The left ventricular outflow obstructive lesions often present with signs of obstructive shock in the first few days or weeks of life when the ductus arteriosus closes. These left heart and aortic lesions include coarctation of the aorta, interrupted aortic arch, critical aortic valve stenosis, and hypoplastic left heart syndrome. Restoring and maintaining openness/patency of the ductus arteriosus is critical for survival until surgical intervention is possible, because the ductus serves as a conduit for systemic blood flow that bypasses the obstruction.

Table 65 outlines findings consistent with left ventricular outflow obstructive lesions that may be found during evaluation of the child. Those unique to left ventricular outflow obstructive lesions are in **bold** type.

Table 65. Findings Consistent With Left Ventricular Outflow Obstructive Lesions

Primary Assessment	Finding
A	Usually open/patent unless level of consciousness is significantly impaired
B	Respiratory failure with signs of pulmonary edema or inadequate respiratory effort
C	<ul><li>Rapid progressive deterioration in systemic perfusion</li><li>Congestive heart failure (cardiomegaly, hepatomegaly)</li><li>**Higher preductal vs postductal blood pressure (coarctation or interrupted aortic arch)**</li><li>**Higher (greater than 3% to 4%) preductal vs postductal arterial O$_2$ saturation (coarctation or interrupted aortic arch)**</li><li>Absence of femoral pulses (coarctation or interrupted aortic arch)</li><li>Metabolic acidosis (elevated lactate)</li></ul>
D	Rapid deterioration in level of consciousness
E	Cool skin

Identify and Intervene

Ductal-Dependent Lesions

If the infant is to survive, you must quickly recognize the presence of a ductal-dependent lesion and promptly provide treatment to open and maintain an open/patent ductus arteriosus.

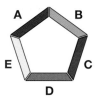

Massive Pulmonary Embolism

Pulmonary embolism is a total or partial obstruction of the pulmonary artery or its branches by a blood clot, fat, air, amniotic fluid, catheter fragment, or injected matter. Most commonly, a pulmonary embolus is a thrombus that migrates to the pulmonary circulation. Pulmonary embolism is rare in children but may develop when an underlying condition predisposes the child to intravascular thrombosis. Examples include central venous catheters, sickle cell disease, malignancy, connective tissue disorders, and inherited disorders of coagulation (eg, antithrombin III, protein S, and protein C deficiencies).

Pulmonary embolism results in ventilation/perfusion mismatch, hypoxemia, increased pulmonary vascular resistance leading to right heart failure, decreased left ventricular filling, and decreased cardiac output. Pulmonary embolism may be difficult to diagnose because signs may be subtle and nonspecific (cyanosis, tachycardia, and hypotension). Providers may not suspect pulmonary embolus, especially in children. However, signs of systemic venous congestion and right heart failure do help distinguish it from hypovolemic shock. Some children with pulmonary embolism will say they have chest pain, reflecting lack of oxygenated blood flow to the lung tissue itself.

Table 66 outlines findings consistent with pulmonary embolism that may be found during evaluation of the child.

Table 66. Findings Consistent With Pulmonary Embolism

Primary Assessment	Finding
A	Usually open/patent unless level of consciousness is significantly impaired
B	Respiratory distress with increased respiratory rate and effort
C Assessment of Cardiovascular Function	• Tachycardia • Cyanosis • Hypotension • Systemic venous congestion and right heart failure • Chest pain
D	Changes in level of consciousness
E	Extremities may be cool and mottled

Summary

Treatment of obstructive shock is cause specific; immediate recognition and correction of the underlying cause of the obstruction can be lifesaving. The most critical tasks for PALS providers are prompt recognition, diagnosis, and treatment of obstructive shock.

Identify and Intervene

Obstructive Shock

Without early recognition and immediate treatment, children with obstructive shock often progress rapidly to cardiopulmonary failure and cardiac arrest.

Recognition of Shock Flowchart

Clinical Signs		Hypovolemic Shock	Distributive Shock	Cardiogenic Shock	Obstructive Shock
A	Patency	Airway open and maintainable/not maintainable			
B	Respiratory rate	Increased			
	Respiratory effort	Normal to increased		Labored	
	Breath sounds	Normal	Normal (± crackles)	Crackles, grunting	
C	Systolic blood pressure	**Compensated Shock ➝ Hypotensive Shock**			
	Pulse pressure	Narrow	Variable	Narrow	
	Heart rate	Increased			
	Peripheral pulse quality	Weak	Bounding or weak	Weak	
	Skin	Pale, cool	Warm or cool	Pale, cool	
	Capillary refill	Delayed	Variable	Delayed	
	Urine output	Decreased			
D	Level of consciousness	Irritable early Lethargic late			
E	Temperature	Variable			

Figure 39. Recognition of Shock Flowchart.

Part 9

Management of Shock

Overview

Once you identify shock in a critically ill or injured child, early intervention can reduce morbidity and mortality. This Part discusses goals and priorities of shock management, fundamentals of treatment, general and advanced management, and specific management according to etiology.

Learning Objective

After completing this Part, you should be able to

- Perform early interventions for the treatment of shock

Preparation for the Course

During the course, you will be asked to manage children in shock. To do this, you will need to know general and specific treatment based on the different types of shock.

Goals of Shock Management

The goals in treatment of shock are to

- Improve O_2 delivery
- Balance tissue perfusion and metabolic demand
- Reverse perfusion abnormalities
- Support organ function
- Prevent progression to cardiac arrest

Speed of intervention is crucial; having the knowledge to identify shock and the skill to respond quickly may be lifesaving. The longer the interval is between the onset of signs of shock and the restoration of adequate O_2 delivery and organ perfusion, the poorer the outcome is. Once a child develops cardiac arrest secondary to shock, prognosis is very poor.

Warning Signs

Be alert to signs that compensatory mechanisms are failing in a seriously ill or injured child. Once you recognize that the child's condition is deteriorating, act decisively with the resuscitation team to provide effective resuscitation therapy. Warning signs that indicate progression from compensated to hypotensive shock include

- Increasing tachycardia
- Diminishing or absent peripheral pulses
- Weakening central pulses
- Narrowing pulse pressure
- Cold distal extremities with prolonged capillary refill
- Decreasing level of consciousness
- Hypotension (late finding)

Once the child is hypotensive, organ perfusion is typically severely compromised, and organ dysfunction may develop even if the child does not progress to cardiac arrest.

Identify and Intervene

Compensated Shock

Early identification of compensated shock is critical to effective treatment and good outcome.

Fundamentals of Shock Management

The acute treatment of shock focuses on restoring O_2 delivery to the tissues and improving the balance between tissue perfusion and metabolic demand. The acute treatment of shock consists of

- Optimizing O_2 content of the blood
- Improving volume and distribution of cardiac output
- Reducing O_2 demand
- Correcting metabolic derangements

Try to identify and reverse the underlying cause of shock while providing prompt interventions.

Optimizing Oxygen Content of the Blood

O_2 content of the blood is determined by the hemoglobin concentration and its saturation with oxygen. To optimize O_2 content

- Administer a high concentration of O_2 (use nonrebreathing mask to deliver 100% O_2)
- Use invasive or noninvasive mechanical ventilation to improve oxygenation by correcting a ventilation/blood flow (V/Q) mismatch or other respiratory disorders
- If hemoglobin concentration is low, consider packed red blood cell (PRBC) transfusion

Improving Volume and Distribution of Cardiac Output

For most forms of shock, bolus fluid administration is used to improve volume and distribution of cardiac output. Noninvasive or invasive positive-pressure ventilation may also be considered to reduce the work of breathing and improve oxygenation. Children in shock may also benefit from vasoactive agents such as vasopressors, vasodilators, inodilators, and/or inotropes.

Reducing Oxygen Demand

For all forms of shock, try to improve the balance between O_2 delivery and supply by using measures to reduce O_2 demand. The most common factors that contribute to increased O_2 demand are

- Increased work of breathing
- Pain and anxiety
- Fever

Support breathing with noninvasive or invasive ventilation and assisted ventilation. To facilitate intubation and mechanical ventilation, you may administer sedatives or analgesics and neuromuscular blockade. Pain and anxiety may also need to be controlled with analgesics and sedatives. Use sedative and analgesic agents with extreme caution; they may suppress the child's endogenous stress response, impair compensatory mechanisms such as tachycardia, and reduce blood pressure. The sedative effects of these agents can also make it more difficult to evaluate the child's level of consciousness and response to treatment. Control fever by administering antipyretics and other cooling measures.

Correcting Metabolic Derangements

Many conditions that lead to shock may result in or be complicated by metabolic derangements, such as

- Hypoglycemia
- Hypocalcemia
- Hyperkalemia
- Metabolic (lactic) acidosis

All of these conditions can adversely affect cardiac contractility. Metabolic acidosis is characteristic of all forms of shock.

Hypoglycemia is low serum glucose concentration. Glucose is vital for proper cardiac and brain function. Glucose stores may be low in infants and chronically ill children. Untreated hypoglycemia can cause seizures and brain injury.

Hypocalcemia is a low serum ionized calcium concentration. Calcium is essential for effective cardiac function and vasomotor tone. Hypocalcemia can result from administration of blood products, colloid, and buffering medications such as sodium bicarbonate. The serum ionized calcium concentration will change in a direction opposite the change in pH (ie, it will rise when acidosis causes a fall in pH and fall when correction of acidosis or development of alkalosis causes a rise in pH).

Hyperkalemia is a high serum potassium concentration, which may result from renal dysfunction, cell death, excess potassium administration, or acidosis. Acidosis causes a shift of potassium from the intracellular to the extracellular—including the intravascular—

space. As a result, acidosis, or a fall in serum pH, typically is associated with a rise in serum potassium. The serum potassium will fall when acidosis is corrected or alkalosis develops.

Metabolic acidosis develops from production of acids, such as lactic acid, when tissue perfusion is inadequate. Renal or gastrointestinal dysfunction can also cause metabolic acidosis. Renal dysfunction can cause retention of organic acids or loss of bicarbonate ions. Gastrointestinal dysfunction, such as diarrhea, can result in loss of bicarbonate ions. Severe metabolic acidosis may depress myocardial contractility and reduce the effect of vasopressors. Unless metabolic acidosis is due solely to bicarbonate losses, it does not respond well to buffer therapy. Treat the acidosis by attempting to restore tissue perfusion with fluid resuscitation and vasoactive agents. If treatment is effective, the metabolic acidosis will resolve.

On occasion, buffers (eg, sodium bicarbonate) may be needed to acutely correct profound metabolic acidosis that is impairing vital organ function. Sodium bicarbonate works by combining with hydrogen ions (acids) to produce carbon dioxide and water; carbon dioxide is then eliminated through increased alveolar ventilation. Support of ventilation is always important in the critically ill child, but it is especially important if metabolic acidosis is treated with sodium bicarbonate.

Correction of metabolic derangements may be essential to optimizing organ function. Measure ionized calcium concentration (the active form of calcium in the body) and glucose concentration. Replenish them as indicated. It is important to measure glucose a few times during resuscitation, particularly if it is borderline or the patient has already received dextrose for a previously low glucose. Consider administration of sodium bicarbonate to treat metabolic acidosis refractory to attempts to increase cardiac output or redistribute blood flow to vital organs.

General Management of Shock

Components of General Management

General management of shock consists of the following (note that several of these interventions may be implemented by the team simultaneously):

- Positioning
- Supporting airway, oxygenation, and ventilation
- Establishing vascular access
- Providing fluid resuscitation
- Monitoring
- Performing frequent reassessment
- Obtaining laboratory studies
- Providing medication therapy
- Consulting appropriate subspecialists

Positioning

Initial management of shock includes positioning the critically ill or injured child. If the child is responsive and hemodynamically stable, allow the child to remain in the most comfortable position (eg, sitting in the arms of a caregiver) to decrease anxiety and activity as you form your initial impression and conduct the primary assessment. If the child is hypotensive and breathing is not compromised, place the child in the supine position.

Supporting Airway, Oxygenation, and Ventilation	Maintain an open/patent airway and support oxygenation and ventilation. Give a high concentration of supplementary O_2 to all children with shock. Usually this is best delivered by a high-flow O_2 delivery system. Sometimes O_2 delivery needs to be combined with ventilatory support if respirations are ineffective, mental status is impaired, or work of breathing is significantly increased. Appropriate interventions may include noninvasive positive airway pressure or mechanical ventilation after endotracheal intubation.
Vascular Access	Once the airway is open/patent and oxygenation and ventilation are supported, obtain vascular access for fluid resuscitation and administration of medications. For compensated shock, initial attempts at peripheral venous cannulation are appropriate. For hypotensive shock, immediate vascular access is critical and is best accomplished by the intraosseous (IO) route if peripheral IV access is not readily achieved. Depending on the provider's experience and expertise and clinical circumstances, central venous access may be useful. However, gaining central venous access takes longer than placement of IO access.

Critical Concepts

✱

IO Access

If peripheral vascular access cannot be readily obtained in a child with compensated or hypotensive shock, be prepared to establish IO access.

For more information on establishment of IO access, see "Intraosseous Access" in "Resources for Management of Circulatory Emergencies" at the end of Part 9.

Fluid Resuscitation	Once vascular access is established, start fluid resuscitation immediately.

Critical Concepts

✱

Fluid Resuscitation

In general, isotonic crystalloid should be given in a 20 mL/kg bolus over 5 to 20 minutes. In children with severe, hypotensive, hypovolemic shock, fluid should be given over 5 to 10 minutes. If you suspect cardiogenic shock, use smaller fluid boluses of 5 to 10 mL/kg given over 10 to 20 minutes. Carefully monitor for signs of pulmonary edema or worsening tissue perfusion. Stop the infusion if such signs occur. Be prepared to support oxygenation and ventilation as necessary.

Reassess* and repeat 20 mL/kg boluses to restore blood pressure and tissue perfusion.

*Repeat fluid boluses based on clinical signs of end-organ perfusion, including heart rate, capillary refill, level of consciousness, and urine output.

Monitoring	No single resuscitation end point has been identified as a consistent marker of adequate tissue perfusion and cellular homeostasis. However, the effectiveness of fluid resuscitation and medication therapy can be assessed by frequent or continuous monitoring (Table 67).

Table 67. Monitoring in Circulatory Emergencies

Frequently or Continuously Monitor	Indication of Positive Response to Shock Therapy
Oxygen saturation with pulse oximetry	94% or higher when breathing room air
Heart rate	Appropriate for age and clinical condition. Typically will fall from a rapid rate toward a normal range (see Table 8: Normal Heart Rates in Part 3)
Peripheral pulses	Weak pulses will become stronger, and bounding pulses will be less bounding but still strong
Capillary refill	Will shorten toward 2 seconds or less
Skin color and temperature	Normal skin color and mucous membranes; warm extremities
Blood pressure	Increase to within normal range for age (Table 10: Normal Blood Pressures in Part 3) with normal pulse pressure
Level of consciousness	Child will respond more appropriately (ie, mental status improves)
Ongoing fluid losses	Bleeding and diarrhea controlled
Urine output	*Infants and young children* approximately 1.5 to 2 mL/kg per hour *Older children and adolescents* approximately 1 mL/kg per hour

As soon as possible, start noninvasive monitoring (SpO_2, heart rate, blood pressure). Assess mental status. Measure temperature and measure urine output with an indwelling bladder catheter. Consider invasive monitoring (eg, arterial and central venous catheterization), depending on the providers' experience and available resources. Signs that indicate clinical improvement toward a normal hemodynamic state are decreased serum lactate, smaller base deficit, and central venous oxygen saturation ($ScvO_2$) greater than 70%.

Foundational Facts

Accurate Assessment of Tissue Perfusion

Although blood pressure is easily measured, it is important to assess other clinical parameters to evaluate tissue perfusion. Remember that blood pressure may be normal in children with severe shock, and noninvasive blood pressure measurement may be inaccurate if perfusion is poor.

Frequent Reassessment Frequently reassess the child's respiratory, cardiovascular, and neurologic status to

- Evaluate trends in the child's condition
- Determine response to therapy
- Plan the next interventions

A child in shock is in a dynamic clinical condition that can deteriorate at any moment and require lifesaving interventions, such as endotracheal intubation. Continue frequent reassessment until the child's condition becomes stable or the child is transferred to advanced care.

Critical Concepts

Monitor to Evaluate Trends

The condition of a child in shock is dynamic. Continuous monitoring and frequent reassessment are essential to evaluate trends in the child's condition and determine response to therapy.

Laboratory Studies Laboratory studies provide important information to help you

- Identify the etiology and severity of shock
- Evaluate organ dysfunction secondary to shock
- Identify metabolic derangements
- Evaluate response to therapy

See "Part 12: Post–Cardiac Arrest Care" for additional information on evaluation of end-organ function. Also consider expert consultation in diagnosis and management of end-organ failure.

Table 68 outlines some laboratory studies that can help identify the etiology and severity of shock and guide therapy.

Table 68. Laboratory Studies to Evaluate Shock and Guide Therapy

Laboratory Study	Finding	Possible Etiology	Possible Interventions
Complete blood cell count	Hemoglobin/hematocrit decreased	• Hemorrhage • Fluid resuscitation (dilution) • Hemolysis	• Administer 100% O₂ • Control bleeding • Transfuse blood • Titrate fluid administration
	White blood cell count increased or decreased	• Sepsis	• Obtain appropriate cultures • Give antibiotics
	Platelets decreased	• Disseminated intravascular coagulation • Decreased platelet production	• Transfuse platelets if child has serious bleeding • Obtain prothrombin time/partial thromboplastin time, fibrinogen, and D-dimers
Glucose	Increased or decreased	• Stress (usually increased but may be decreased in infants) • Sepsis • Decreased production (eg, liver failure) • Adrenal insufficiency	• If hypoglycemia is present, give dextrose bolus and start infusion of dextrose-containing solution if needed • Severe hyperglycemia may require treatment (per institutional protocols or obtain expert consultation)
Potassium	Increased or decreased	• Renal dysfunction • Acidosis (increases serum potassium concentration) • Diuresis (decreased) • Adrenal insufficiency (increased)	• Treat significant or symptomatic hyperkalemia or hypokalemia • Correct acidosis

(continued)

(continued)

Laboratory Study	Finding	Possible Etiology	Possible Interventions
Calcium	Decreased (ionized calcium concentration)	• Sepsis • Transfusion of blood preserved with citrate-phosphate-dextran • Colloid administration • Buffering agents (eg, sodium bicarbonate)	• Give calcium
Lactate	Increased as product of anaerobic metabolism from tissue hypoperfusion	• Tissue hypoxia • Increased glucose production (gluconeogenesis) • Decreased metabolism (eg, liver failure)	• Improve tissue perfusion • Treat acidosis if end-organ function is impaired
Arterial blood gas	pH decreased in acidosis; increased with alkalosis	• Lactic acid accumulation caused by tissue hypoperfusion • Renal failure • Inborn error of metabolism • Diabetic ketoacidosis • Poisoning/overdose • Diarrhea or ileostomy losses • Hyper/hypoventilation (sepsis, poisoning) • Vomiting	• Give fluid • Support ventilation • Correct shock • Consider buffer • Evaluate anion gap* to determine if acidosis is from increased unmeasured ions (increased anion gap) or is more likely from loss of bicarbonate (normal anion gap)
ScvO₂	Variable	• Low central venous O_2 saturation—inadequate O_2 delivery or increased consumption • High central venous O_2 saturation—maldistribution of blood flow or decreased O_2 utilization	• Attempt to maximize O_2 delivery and minimize O_2 demand

*Anion gap = ([serum Na^+] + [serum K^+]) − ([serum Cl^-] + [serum HCO_3^-]); normal = approximately 10 to 12 mEq/L.

Medication Therapy

Medication therapy is used in the management of shock to affect myocardial contractility, heart rate, and vascular resistance. The choice of agent(s) is determined by the child's physiologic state.

Vasoactive agents are indicated when shock persists despite adequate volume resuscitation to optimize preload. For example, a child with septic shock who remains hypotensive with signs of vasodilation despite administration of fluid boluses may benefit from a vasoconstrictor. Administration of vasoactive medications is potentially harmful if the child has not been adequately fluid resuscitated first. However, in children with cardiogenic shock, vasoactive agents should be used early because fluid resuscitation is not key to improving myocardial function and may contribute to pulmonary edema and respiratory failure. Most children with cardiogenic shock benefit from a vasodilator (provided that blood pressure is adequate) to decrease systemic vascular resistance (SVR) and increase cardiac output and tissue perfusion.

Inotropes, phosphodiesterase inhibitors (eg, the inodilator milrinone), vasodilators, and vasopressors are classes of pharmacologic agents commonly used in shock. Table 69 lists vasoactive medications by class and pharmacologic effects.

Table 69. Vasoactive Therapy Used in the Treatment of Shock

Class	Medication	Effect
Inotropes	• Dopamine • Epinephrine • Dobutamine	• Increase cardiac contractility • Increase heart rate • Produce variable effects on SVR *Note:* Includes agents with both α-adrenergic and β-adrenergic effects
Phosphodiesterase inhibitors (inodilators)	• Milrinone	• Decrease SVR • Improve coronary artery blood flow • Improve contractility
Vasodilators	• Nitroglycerin • Nitroprusside	• Decrease SVR and venous tone
Vasopressors (vasoconstrictors)	• Epinephrine (doses >0.3 mcg/kg per minute) • Norepinephrine • Dopamine (doses >10 mcg/kg per minute) • Vasopressin	• Increase SVR • Increase myocardial contractility (except vasopressin)

Critical Concepts

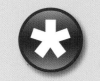

Color-Coded Length-Based Tape

Use a color-coded length-based tape to determine the child's weight (if not known) for calculating drug doses and for selecting the correct sizes of resuscitation equipment. See "Resources for Management of Circulatory Emergencies" at the end of Part 9 for an example.

Subspecialty Consultation

For specific categories of shock, lifesaving diagnostic assessments and therapeutic interventions may be required that are beyond the scope of practice of many PALS providers. For example, a provider may not be trained to interpret an echocardiogram or perform a thoracostomy or pericardiocentesis. Recognize limitations to your own scope of practice and call for help when needed. Early subspecialty consultation (eg, pediatric critical care, pediatric cardiology, pediatric surgery) is an essential component of shock management and may influence outcome.

Critical Concepts

Expert Consultation

When treating a child in shock, providers must obtain consultation from appropriate experts as soon as possible.

Summary: Initial Management Principles

Table 70 summarizes initial shock management principles discussed in this section.

Table 70. Fundamentals of Initial Shock Management

Positioning the child

- Stable—Allow to remain with caregiver in a position of comfort
- Unstable—If hypotensive, place in supine position unless breathing is compromised

Optimizing arterial O_2 content

- Administer a high concentration of O_2 via a nonrebreathing mask
- Consider blood transfusion in cases of significant blood loss or other causes of severe anemia
- Consider use of continuous positive airway pressure, noninvasive positive airway pressure, or mechanical ventilation with positive end-expiratory pressure

Supporting ventilation as indicated (invasive or noninvasive)

Establishing vascular access

- Consider IO access early

Beginning fluid resuscitation

- Give an isotonic crystalloid bolus of 20 mL/kg over 5 to 20 minutes (5-10 minutes with severe, hypotensive, hypovolemic shock); repeat 20 mL/kg boluses as needed to restore blood pressure and tissue/organ perfusion. Reassess the child after each bolus
- For trauma and hemorrhage, administer PRBCs if the child does not respond to isotonic crystalloid
- Modify bolus fluid therapy to deliver 5 to 10 mL/kg over 10 to 20 minutes if you suspect cardiogenic shock or severe myocardial dysfunction

(continued)

(continued)

Monitoring

- SpO$_2$
- Heart rate
- Blood pressure
- Level of consciousness
- Temperature
- Urine output

Performing frequent reassessment

- Evaluate trends
- Determine response to therapy

Conducting laboratory studies

- To identify shock etiology and severity
- To evaluate organ dysfunction secondary to shock
- To identify metabolic derangements
- To evaluate the response to therapy

Administering pharmacologic support—see Table 69: Vasoactive Therapy Used in the Treatment of Shock

- To increase heart rate
- To improve myocardial function or redistribute cardiac output (increase contractility, reduce or increase SVR, improve organ perfusion)
- To correct metabolic derangements
- To manage pain and anxiety

Obtain subspecialty consultation

Fluid Therapy

The primary objective of fluid therapy in shock is to restore intravascular volume and tissue perfusion. Rapid fluid resuscitation is required for hypovolemic and distributive shock, including septic shock. Cardiogenic and obstructive shock, as well as special conditions such as severe poisonings or fluid loss with DKA, may dictate alternative approaches to fluid resuscitation.

In general, boluses of isotonic crystalloid will expand intravascular volume. Blood and blood products are generally not used for volume expansion in children with shock unless shock is due to hemorrhage. Blood products may also be indicated for correction of some coagulopathies.

Isotonic Crystalloid Solutions

Isotonic crystalloid solutions, such as normal saline or lactated Ringer's, are the preferred initial fluids for volume replacement in the management of shock. They are inexpensive, readily available, and do not cause sensitivity reactions.

Foundational Facts

Fluid Used for Initial Fluid Resuscitation

For most children with shock, isotonic crystalloids are recommended as the initial resuscitation fluid.

Critical Concepts

Quantity of Crystalloid Solution in Shock Resuscitation

Because isotonic crystalloids are distributed throughout the extracellular space, a large quantity of crystalloid solution may be needed to restore intravascular volume for children in shock. Rapid infusion of a large volume of fluid may be well tolerated by a healthy child, but may cause pulmonary and peripheral edema in a critically ill child. Reassessment after every fluid bolus is critical.

Colloid Solutions

Colloid solutions (eg, 5% albumin and fresh frozen plasma) may be alternatives to crystalloid solutions. However, they have disadvantages for the acute resuscitation of a child in shock. They are less widely available than crystalloid solutions and may take time to prepare. Blood-derived colloid solutions may cause sensitivity reactions. Synthetic colloids may cause coagulopathies; their use is usually limited to 20 to 40 mL/kg. As with crystalloids, excessive administration of colloids can lead to pulmonary edema, particularly in children with cardiac or renal disease. Despite these limitations, fresh frozen plasma may be used in specific circumstances, such as massive hemorrhage and blood administration (see "Indications for Blood Product Administration" later in this part).

Rate and Volume of Fluid Administration

Start fluid resuscitation for shock with 20 mL/kg of isotonic crystalloid administered as a bolus over 5 to 20 minutes. Repeat boluses of 20 mL/kg if needed to restore blood pressure and perfusion. The volume of fluid deficit is often difficult to predict from the child's history. Use clinical examination and supporting laboratory studies to identify the volume needed; it may be necessary to administer more than the estimated volume deficit. Reassess frequently and after administration of each bolus.

As noted above, *give fluid boluses rapidly* for hypotensive and septic shock. Children with septic shock may require 60 mL/kg or more of isotonic crystalloid solution during the first hour of therapy; as much as 200 mL/kg or more may be required in the first 8 hours of therapy.

If myocardial dysfunction or obstructive shock is present or suspected, *give smaller volumes of fluid more slowly*. Administer boluses of 5 to 10 mL/kg over 10 to 20 minutes and reassess after each bolus; stop bolus administration if the child develops signs of worsening respiratory status, rales, or other evidence of pulmonary edema or hepatomegaly. Obtain further diagnostic assessment and expert consultation (eg, echocardiogram) to confirm suspicions and guide the next interventions. Be prepared to provide support of airway, oxygenation, and ventilation with positive end-expiratory pressure as needed if pulmonary edema develops.

Modification of fluid resuscitation is appropriate for children in shock associated with DKA. Children with DKA may be significantly dehydrated, but often have high serum osmolality (caused by hyperglycemia). Rapid administration of crystalloid solution and reduction in serum osmolality may contribute to risk of cerebral edema. Therefore, fluid management in DKA is complex. Consider giving an initial bolus of isotonic crystalloid 10 to 20 mL/kg over 1 to 2 hours. This constitutes a fluid bolus, but it is atypical in that it is given over a longer period of time than the usual fluid bolus. However, if the patient with DKA is in hypotensive shock, the treatment approach should default to more aggressive bolus fluids for shock as per any other etiology of shock. Many institutions have local protocols about specific management of DKA and its associated metabolic, electrolyte, and fluid derangements. Expert consultation should be sought when possible. After giving a fluid bolus, reassess the patient.

Similarly, children who have ingested calcium channel blockers or β-adrenergic blockers may have myocardial dysfunction and are less tolerant of rapid volume expansion. When caring for children with severe febrile illness in settings with limited access to critical care resources (ie, mechanical ventilation and inotropic support), administration of bolus IV fluids should be undertaken with extreme caution because it may be harmful. Once again, providers should reassess the patient after every fluid bolus.

Table 71 gives a summary of fluid boluses and rates of delivery based on the underlying cause of shock.

Table 71. Guide to Fluid Boluses and Rates of Delivery Based on Underlying Cause of Shock

Type of Shock	Volume of Fluid	Approximate Rate of Delivery
Hypovolemic shock **Distributive shock**	20 mL/kg bolus (repeat as needed)	Over 5-10 minutes
Cardiogenic shock (nonpoisoning)	5-10 mL/kg bolus (repeat as needed)	Over 10-20 minutes
Poisonings (eg, calcium channel blocker or β-adrenergic blocker)	5-10 mL/kg (repeat as needed)	Over 10-20 minutes
Diabetic Ketoacidosis (DKA)		
DKA with compensated shock	10-20 mL/kg	Per local protocol; if used, give over at least 1-2 hours*

*See text above for details.

Rapid Fluid Delivery

IV fluid administration systems generally used for pediatric fluid therapy do not deliver fluid boluses as rapidly as required for management of some forms of shock. To facilitate rapid fluid delivery

- Place as large an IV catheter as possible, especially if blood or colloid administration is needed; ideally, insert 2 catheters
- Place an in-line 3-way stopcock in the IV tubing system
- Deliver fluid by using a 30- to 60-mL syringe to push fluids through the stopcock, or use a pressure bag (beware of risk of air embolism) or a rapid infusion device
- If IV access cannot be established, establish IO access

Standard Infusion Pumps Typically Cannot Deliver Bolus Fluids

Standard infusion pumps—even if set at the maximum infusion rate—do not provide a sufficiently rapid rate of fluid delivery, especially in larger children. For example, a 50-kg patient with septic shock should ideally receive 1 L of crystalloid in 5 to 10 minutes, but standard infusion pumps may have a maximum rate of 999 mL for the hourly rate.

Frequent Reassessment During Fluid Resuscitation

Frequent reassessment is essential during fluid resuscitation to manage shock effectively. Such reassessment should

- Assess the physiologic response to therapy after each fluid bolus
- Determine the need for further fluid boluses
- Assess for signs of detrimental effects (eg, pulmonary edema) during and after fluid resuscitation

Signs of physiologic improvement include improved perfusion, increase in blood pressure, slowing of heart rate (toward normal), decreased respiratory rate (toward normal), increased urine output, and improved mental status. If the child's condition does not improve or worsens after fluid boluses, try to identify the cause of the shock to help determine the next interventions. For example, persistently delayed capillary refill despite initial fluid administration may indicate ongoing hemorrhage or other fluid loss. Deterioration of the child's condition after fluid therapy may signal cardiogenic or obstructive shock. Increased work of breathing may indicate pulmonary edema.

Indications for Blood Product Administration

Administration of PRBCs is recommended for replacement of traumatic blood loss if the child's perfusion is inadequate despite administration of 2 to 3 boluses of 20 mL/kg of isotonic crystalloid. Under these circumstances, administer 10 mL/kg PRBCs as soon as available.

Fully crossmatched blood is generally not available in emergencies because most blood banks require about 1 hour for the crossmatching process. Crossmatched blood may become available for children who are stabilized with crystalloid but have ongoing blood losses. Priorities for the type of blood or blood products used in order of preference are

- Crossmatched
- Type specific
- Type O-negative (O[−] preferred for females and either O[+] or O[−] for males)

Unmatched, type-specific blood may be used if ongoing blood loss results in hypotension despite administration of crystalloid. Most blood banks can supply type-specific blood within 10 minutes. Type-specific blood is ABO and Rh compatible, but, unlike fully crossmatched blood, may have other antibodies that are incompatible with the patient's blood.

Use type O blood if there is an immediate need for blood administration to prevent circulatory collapse or cardiopulmonary arrest, because it can be administered to children of any blood type. O-negative blood is preferred for females of childbearing age to avoid Rh sensitization. Either O-negative or O-positive blood may be administered to males.

Complications of Rapid Administration of Blood Products

Rapid infusion of cold blood or blood products, particularly in large volume, may produce several complications, including

- Hypothermia
- Myocardial dysfunction
- Ionized hypocalcemia

Hypothermia may adversely affect cardiovascular function and coagulation and may compromise several metabolic functions, including metabolism of citrate, which is present in stored blood. Inadequate citrate clearance, in turn, causes ionized hypocalcemia. The combined effects of hypothermia and ionized hypocalcemia can result in significant myocardial dysfunction and hypotension.

To minimize these problems, warm blood and blood products, if possible, with an approved commercial blood-warming device before or during rapid IV administration. Prepare calcium for administration if the child becomes hypotensive during rapid transfusion; in some cases, it may be beneficial to administer calcium empirically to prevent hypocalcemia.

Glucose

Monitor blood glucose concentration as a component of shock management. Hypoglycemia is a common finding in critically ill children. It can result in brain injury if not rapidly identified and effectively treated. In one pediatric study, hypoglycemia was present in 18% of children who received resuscitative care in an emergency department for decreased level of consciousness, status epilepticus, respiratory failure, cardiopulmonary failure, or cardiac arrest. For more details, see Losek JD. *Ann Emerg Med*. 2000;35:43-46 in the Suggested Reading List on the Student Website.

Glucose Monitoring

Measure serum glucose concentration in all critically ill infants and children (eg, altered mental status, respiratory compromise, shock) as soon as possible. The serum glucose concentration can be measured from capillary, venous, or arterial blood samples with a point-of-care device or by laboratory analysis. Small infants and chronically ill children have higher glucose utilization rates and limited stores of glycogen. This limited supply may be rapidly depleted during episodes of physiologic stress, resulting in hypoglycemia. Infants receiving non–glucose-containing IV fluids are at increased risk for developing hypoglycemia.

Critical Concepts

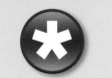

Identify Hypoglycemia

In all critically ill or injured children, perform a rapid glucose test to rule out hypoglycemia as a cause of or a contributing factor to shock or decreased level of consciousness.

Hyperglycemia, also frequently present in seriously ill or injured children, may result from a relative insulin-resistant state induced by high concentrations of endogenous catecholamines and cortisol. Although controlling serum glucose concentration within a narrow range through use of an insulin infusion improved survival in critically ill adult and pediatric patients, tight glucose control was also associated with more frequent episodes of hypoglycemia. See Van den Berghe et al. *Crit Care Med*. 2003;31:359-366 and Vlasselaers et al. *Lancet*. 2009;373:547-556 in the Suggested Reading List on the Student Website for details. There are insufficient data to support routine use of this tight control of glucose concentration in critically ill children. Consider treating hyperglycemia in high-risk groups, such as brain-injured children, while monitoring closely to prevent hypoglycemia.

Diagnosis of Hypoglycemia

Hypoglycemia may be difficult to recognize clinically because some children have no outward signs or symptoms (ie, asymptomatic hypoglycemia). Others may show nonspecific clinical signs (eg, poor perfusion, diaphoresis, tachycardia, hypothermia, irritability or lethargy, hypotension). These clinical signs are also common to many other conditions, including hypoxemia, ischemia, or shock.

Clinical Signs of Hypoglycemia
• Poor perfusion
• Diaphoresis
• Tachycardia
• Hypothermia
• Irritability or lethargy
• Hypotension

Although single threshold values are not applicable to every patient, the following lowest acceptable glucose concentrations can be used to define hypoglycemia:

Age	Consensus Definition of Hypoglycemia, mg/dL
Preterm neonates	<45
Term neonates	
Infants	<60
Children	
Adolescents	

The reported low range of normal glucose is typically related to sample measurements obtained in nonstressed, fasting infants and children. It is difficult to extrapolate these thresholds to the glucose concentration required by a stressed, critically ill, or injured child.

Management of Hypoglycemia

If the glucose concentration is low and the child has minimal symptoms and normal mental status, you may administer glucose orally (eg, with orange juice or other glucose-containing fluid). If the concentration is very low or the child is symptomatic, you should give IV glucose at a dose of 0.5 to 1 g/kg. IV dextrose is commonly administered as $D_{25}W$ (2-4 mL/kg) or $D_{10}W$ (5-10 mL/kg). Dextrose is the same substance as glucose. Reassess the serum glucose concentration after dextrose administration. Provide a continuous infusion of glucose-containing IV fluid to prevent recurrent hypoglycemia.

Do not routinely infuse dextrose-containing fluids for volume resuscitation of shock. This can cause hyperglycemia, increase the serum osmolality, and produce an osmotic diuresis that will further exacerbate hypovolemia and shock. Electrolyte imbalances (eg, hyponatremia) can also develop.

Management According to Type of Shock

Effective management of shock targets treatment to the etiology of the shock. For the purposes of the PALS Provider Course, shock is categorized into 4 types, based on the underlying cause. However, this classification method oversimplifies the physiologic state seen in individual patients. Some children with shock have elements of hypovolemic, distributive, and cardiogenic shock, with 1 type being dominant. Any child with severe shock may develop characteristics of myocardial dysfunction and maldistribution of blood flow. For a more comprehensive discussion of shock by etiology, see "Part 8: Recognition of Shock."

Management of the following types of shock is discussed in this section:

- Hypovolemic
- Distributive
- Cardiogenic
- Obstructive

Management of Hypovolemic Shock

Rapid administration of isotonic crystalloids is the primary therapy for hypovolemic shock. Children with hypovolemic shock who receive an appropriate volume of fluid within the first hour of resuscitation have the best chance for survival and recovery. Timely administration of fluid is key to preventing deterioration from compensated hypovolemic shock to hypotensive and refractory shock.

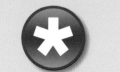

Critical Concepts

Timely Fluid Resuscitation in Hypovolemic Shock

It is important to provide rapid, adequate fluid resuscitation for hypovolemic shock. Avoid the common errors of inadequate or delayed administration of fluid resuscitation.

Other components in effective management of hypovolemic shock are

- Identifying the type of volume loss (nonhemorrhagic vs hemorrhagic)
- Replacing volume deficit
- Preventing and replacing ongoing losses (eg, bleeding, GI losses)
- Restoring acid-base balance
- Correcting metabolic derangements

Determining Adequate Fluid Resuscitation

Dehydration is defined as a loss of water with varying loss of electrolytes leading to a hypertonic (hypernatremic), isotonic, or hypotonic (hyponatremic) state. The losses can be from some combination of the interstitial, intracellular, and intravascular compartments; the relative loss from each component helps determine clinical symptoms. Severity of dehydration is generally related to the percentage of total body water loss (ie, percent dehydration), but the percentage is not consistent across all age groups because the relative proportion of fluid loss based on total body weight is size dependent.

Adequate fluid resuscitation in hypovolemic shock is determined by the

- Extent of volume depletion
- Type of volume loss (eg, blood, electrolyte-containing fluid, or electrolyte-and-protein–containing fluid)

The extent of volume depletion may be underestimated and undertreated. In many cases, volume loss is compounded by inadequate fluid intake. Use vital signs and physical examination to assess the child's response to each fluid bolus. The clinical parameters used to help determine the percentage of dehydration include

- General appearance
- Presence or absence of tears and appearance of eyes (normal vs sunken)
- Moisture of mucous membranes
- Skin elasticity
- Respiratory rate and depth
- Heart rate
- Blood pressure
- Capillary refill time
- Urine output
- Mental status

Clinically significant dehydration in children is generally associated with at least 5% volume depletion (ie, 5% or greater loss in body weight) corresponding to a fluid deficit of 50 mL/kg or greater. Therefore, treating a child with clinically evident dehydration with administration of a single 20 mL/kg bolus of isotonic crystalloid may be insufficient. Conversely, it is usually unnecessary to completely correct the estimated deficit within the first hour. After perfusion is restored and the child is no longer in shock, the total fluid deficit may be corrected over the next 24 to 48 hours.

Although all forms of hypovolemic shock are initially treated with rapid infusion of isotonic crystalloid, early identification of the type of volume loss can optimize further treatment. Fluid losses may be classified as nonhemorrhagic and hemorrhagic. Nonhemorrhagic losses include electrolyte-containing fluids (eg, diarrhea, vomiting, osmotic diuresis associated with DKA) and protein-and-electrolyte–containing fluids (eg, losses associated with burns and peritonitis).

Nonhemorrhagic Hypovolemic Shock

Common sources of nonhemorrhagic fluid loss are gastrointestinal (ie, vomiting and diarrhea), urinary (eg, diabetes insipidus [DI]), and capillary leak (eg, burns). Hypovolemia caused by nonhemorrhagic fluid loss is generally classified in terms of percent loss of body weight (Table 72). Correlation of blood pressure and fluid deficits is imprecise. As a general rule, however, shock may be observed in children with fluid deficits of 50 to 100 mL/kg (particularly in hyponatremic dehydration), but it is more consistently observed with deficits of 100 mL/kg or greater.

Table 72. Stages and Signs of Dehydration

Severity of Dehydration	Infant Estimated Weight Loss (mL/kg)*	Adolescent Estimated Weight Loss (mL/kg)*	Clinical Signs	Pitfalls in Assessment
Mild	5% (50)	3% (30)	• Dry mucous membranes • Oliguria	• Oral mucosa may be dry in chronic mouth breathers • Frequency and amount of urine are difficult to assess during diarrhea, especially with infants wearing diapers
Moderate	10% (100)	5% to 6% (50-60)	• Poor skin turgor • Sunken fontanel • Marked oliguria • Tachycardia • Quiet tachypnea	• Affected by sodium concentration; increased sodium concentration better maintains intravascular volume • Fontanel open only in infants • Oliguria is affected by fever, sodium concentration, and underlying disease
Severe	15% (150)	7% to 9% (70-90)	• Marked tachycardia • Weak to absent distal pulses • Narrow pulse pressure • Increased respiratory rate • Anuria • Hypotension and altered mental status (late findings)	• Clinical signs are affected by fever, sodium concentration, and underlying disease; increased sodium concentration better maintains intravascular volume

*mL/kg refers to the estimated corresponding fluid deficit normalized to body weight.
Modified with permission from Roberts KB. Fluid and electrolytes: parenteral fluid therapy. *Pediatr Rev.* 2001;22(11):380-387.

Rapidly infuse 20 mL/kg boluses of isotonic crystalloid to effectively treat children with hypovolemic shock secondary to dehydration. Failure to improve after at least 3 boluses (ie, 60 mL/kg) of isotonic crystalloid indicates that

- The extent of fluid losses may be underestimated
- The type of fluid replacement may need to be altered (eg, need for colloid or blood)
- There are ongoing fluid losses (eg, occult bleeding)
- Your initial assumption about the etiology of the shock may be incorrect (ie, consider alternative or combined types of shock)

Ongoing fluid losses (eg, diarrhea, burns) must be replaced in addition to correcting existing fluid deficits. Colloid is not routinely indicated as the initial treatment of hypovolemic shock. Albumin and other colloids, however, have been used successfully for volume replacement in children with large "third-space" losses or albumin deficits.

Hemorrhagic Hypovolemic Shock

Hemorrhagic hypovolemic shock is classified according to an estimated percent of total blood volume loss (Table 73).

In children, the dividing line between mild and compensated vs moderate or severe hypotensive hemorrhagic shock is thought to correlate with an acute loss of about 30% of blood volume. The estimated total blood volume of a child is 75 to 80 mL/kg; a 30% blood volume loss, therefore, represents a blood loss of about 25 mL/kg.

Table 73. Systemic Responses to Blood Loss in Pediatric Patients

System	Mild Blood Volume Loss (<30%)	Moderate Blood Volume Loss (30%-45%)	Severe Blood Volume Loss (>45%)
Cardiovascular	Increased heart rate; weak, thready peripheral pulses; normal systolic blood pressure (80-90 + 2 x age in years); normal pulse pressure	Markedly increased heart rate; weak, thready central pulses; low normal systolic blood pressure (70-80 + 2 x age in years); narrowed pulse pressure	Tachycardia followed by bradycardia; very weak or absent central pulses; absent peripheral pulses; hypotension (<70 + 2 x age in years); narrowed pulse pressure (or undetectable diastolic blood pressure)
Central nervous system	Anxious; irritable; confused	Lethargic; dulled response to pain*	Comatose
Skin	Cool, mottled; prolonged capillary refill	Cyanotic; markedly prolonged capillary refill	Pale and cold
Urine output†	Low to very low	Minimal	None

*The child's dulled response to pain with this degree of blood loss (30% to 45%) may be indicated by a decreased response to IV catheter insertion.
†After initial decompression by urinary catheter. Low normal is 2 mL/kg per hour (infant), 1.5 mL/kg per hour (younger child), 1 mL/kg per hour (older child), and 0.5 mL/kg per hour (adolescent). Intravenous contrast can falsely elevate urinary output.
Reproduced from American College of Surgeons Committee on Trauma. Pediatric trauma. In: *Advanced Trauma Life Support for Doctors: ATLS Student Course Manual.* 9th ed. Chicago, IL: American College of Surgeons; 2012:257.

Fluid resuscitation in hemorrhagic shock begins with rapid infusion of isotonic crystalloid in boluses of 20 mL/kg. Because isotonic crystalloids are distributed throughout the extracellular space, it may be necessary to give up to 3 boluses of 20 mL/kg (60 mL/kg) of fluid to replace a 25% loss of blood volume; approximately 3 mL of crystalloid is needed for every 1 mL of blood lost. If the child remains hemodynamically unstable despite 2 to 3 boluses of 20 mL/kg isotonic crystalloid, consider a transfusion of PRBCs.

Critical Concepts

3 mL to 1 mL Rule

For fluid resuscitation in hemorrhagic shock, give about 3 mL of isotonic crystalloid for every 1 mL of blood lost.

For blood replacement, use PRBCs in 10 mL/kg boluses. Whole blood (20 mL/kg) can be given in place of PRBCs, but it is harder and more time-consuming to obtain. Also, the risk of transfusion reaction is significantly increased if the blood is not crossmatched. To minimize adverse effects, warm the blood if a blood-warming device is available, especially when transfusing rapidly.

Indications for transfusion in hemorrhagic shock include

- Crystalloid-refractory hypotension or poor perfusion
- Known significant blood loss

Crystalloid-refractory hemorrhagic shock is defined as persistent hypotension despite administration of 40 to 60 mL/kg crystalloid. Children with rapid hemorrhage may demonstrate a normal or low initial hemoglobin concentration. Transfuse blood for a low hemoglobin concentration because anemia increases the risk of tissue hypoxia from inadequate arterial O_2 content and O_2 delivery.

Medication Therapy

Vasoactive agents are not routinely indicated for the management of hypovolemic shock. Moribund children with profound hypovolemic shock and hypotension may require short-term administration of vasoactive agents, such as epinephrine, to restore cardiac contractility and vascular tone once adequate fluid resuscitation is provided.

Acid-Base Balance

Early in the progression of hypovolemic shock, the child may develop tachypnea and respiratory alkalosis. However, the alkalosis does not completely correct the metabolic (lactic) acidosis produced by hypovolemic shock. A child with long-standing or severe shock may have severe acidosis because the child eventually develops fatigue or cardiorespiratory failure. Children with head or chest injuries may not demonstrate compensatory tachypnea.

Persistent acidosis and poor perfusion are indications of inadequate resuscitation or, in hemorrhagic shock, of ongoing blood loss. Sodium bicarbonate is not recommended for the treatment of metabolic acidosis secondary to hypovolemic shock. As long as fluid resuscitation improves perfusion and end-organ function, metabolic acidosis is well tolerated and will correct gradually. Sodium bicarbonate administration is indicated if the metabolic acidosis is caused by significant bicarbonate losses from renal or gastrointestinal losses (ie, a non–anion gap metabolic acidosis) because it is difficult to compensate for an ongoing bicarbonate loss.

Specific Treatment Considerations

Follow the initial management principles (Table 70) in addition to the considerations specific to hypovolemic shock shown in Table 74.

Table 74. Management of Hypovolemic Shock: Specific Treatment Considerations

Initiate fluid resuscitation as quickly as possible.

- *In all patients,* rapidly infuse isotonic crystalloid (normal saline or lactated Ringer's) in 20 mL/kg boluses; repeat as needed.
- In patients with crystalloid-refractory hemorrhagic shock, give a transfusion of PRBCs, 10 mL/kg.
- If loss of protein-containing fluids is documented or suspected (low albumin concentration), consider administration of colloid-containing fluids if the child fails to respond to crystalloid resuscitation.

Correct metabolic derangements.

Identify the type of volume loss (hemorrhagic or nonhemorrhagic) to determine best treatment.

Control any external hemorrhage with direct pressure; measure and replace ongoing losses (eg, continued nonhemorrhagic losses with diarrhea).

Consider other laboratory studies:

- Complete blood cell count
- Type and crossmatch
- Arterial blood gas with particular attention to the base deficit
- Electrolyte panel to calculate anion gap, glucose, and ionized calcium
- Serum or plasma lactate concentration
- Diagnostic imaging to identify the source of bleeding or volume loss

Management of Distributive Shock

Initial management of distributive shock focuses on expanding intravascular volume to correct hypovolemia and fill the expanded dilated vascular space. Use vasoactive agents if the child remains hypotensive or poorly perfused despite rapid bolus fluid administration or if the diastolic pressure remains low with a wide pulse pressure.

This section discusses management of the following types of distributive shock:

- Septic shock
- Anaphylactic shock
- Neurogenic shock

Management of Septic Shock

The clinical, hemodynamic, and metabolic changes observed in septic shock result from the host's response to an infection, including the release or activation of inflammatory mediators. The primary goals in the initial management of septic shock are

- Restoration of hemodynamic stability
- Support of organ function
- Identification and control of infection

Fundamental principles of management include increasing tissue O_2 delivery by optimizing cardiac output and arterial O_2 content and minimizing O_2 consumption.

Identify and Intervene

Septic Shock

Early identification of septic shock is key to initiating resuscitation and preventing development of multisystem organ failure and cardiac arrest. Hemodynamic support to maintain O_2 delivery can reduce pediatric morbidity and mortality from septic shock.

Overview of Pediatric Septic Shock Algorithm

The recommended treatment approach to restore hemodynamic stability for septic shock in children is presented in the Pediatric Septic Shock Algorithm (Figure 40). It outlines 3 phases requiring rapid recognition, stabilization/resuscitation, and critical care management, as follows:

- **Early detection of signs of septic shock,** which may include alteration in mental status, heart rate, temperature, and perfusion. Note that systolic or diastolic hypotension may or may not be present.
- **Initial Stabilization/Resuscitation**
  - **Within 10 to 15 minutes** of recognition of signs of shock, support airway, oxygenation, and ventilation, monitor heart rate and pulse oximetry, and establish vascular access.
  - **Within the first hour** of onset of shock, administer antibiotics, give fluid boluses (repeating, as needed, to correct shock), and initiate vasoactive drug therapy if shock persists despite administration of fluid boluses.
  - **Reassess child during and after each fluid bolus.** Stop rapid fluid bolus administration if rales, respiratory distress, or hepatomegaly develop. If additional boluses are needed to treat shock, it may be necessary to administer smaller boluses over longer intervals. See text below for additional details.
  - **Critical Care:** If signs of shock persist, critical care expertise is needed to establish hemodynamic monitoring, continue initial vasoactive drug therapy, and titrate additional drug therapy, as needed, to treat shock.

Once shock has been effectively treated, further management includes continued monitoring and support of organ function, treatment of the source of the infection, and evaluation of the child's clinical course and therapy.

Pediatric Septic Shock Algorithm

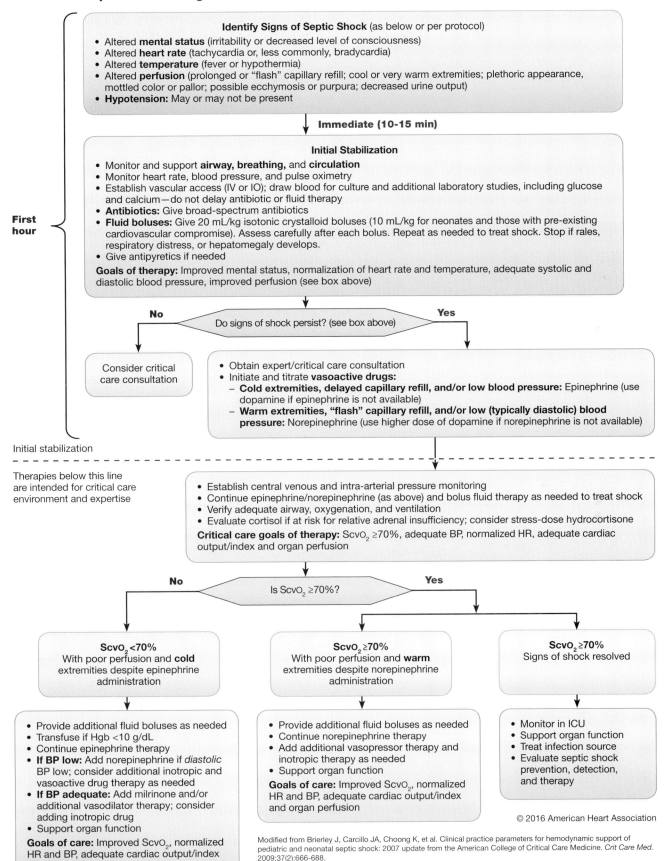

Figure 40. The Pediatric Septic Shock Algorithm.

Initial Stabilization/ Resuscitation for Septic Shock

Adequate treatment during the first hour after the onset of symptoms is critical to maximize survival for a child in septic shock. Support adequate airway, oxygenation, and ventilation. Initial components of management of septic shock are

- Administer antibiotics within 1 hour of first medical contact (if possible, draw blood sample for culture before antibiotic administration, but do not delay antibiotics)
- Initiate fluid resuscitation within 10 to 15 minutes of the recognition of shock; give boluses of 20 mL/kg (10 mL/kg for neonates and those with preexisting heart disease) of isotonic crystalloid; repeat as needed to treat shock
- Reassess frequently and after each fluid bolus; stop fluid boluses if rales, respiratory distress, or hepatomegaly develop
- Identify and correct metabolic derangements, including glucose, calcium, and possible absolute or relative adrenal insufficiencies
- Perform diagnostic assessments (eg, lactate concentration, base deficit, and central venous O_2 saturation [$ScvO_2$]) to identify the severity of shock and monitor response to fluid therapy
- Support organ system perfusion and function

The child with persistent shock despite fluid boluses has fluid-refractory shock and requires rapid initiation of vasopressors within the first hour of therapy. Rapid, appropriate fluid bolus administration is a priority. Inadequate intravascular volume rapidly leads to low stroke volume and hypotension. A child in septic shock often requires a large volume of fluid to restore perfusion. It may be necessary to rapidly infuse 3 or 4 boluses (20 mL/kg each) of isotonic crystalloid solution. Titrate the volume and rate of fluid administration during and after each bolus by assessing the child's mental status, heart rate, temperature, blood pressure, and organ perfusion (including presence and quality of peripheral pulses, capillary refill, skin temperature and color, and urine output).

The spirit of the recommendations about fluid therapy for treatment of septic shock is a continued emphasis on fluid resuscitation for both compensated (detected by physical examination) and decompensated (hypotensive) septic shock. Moreover, emphasis is also placed on the use of individualized patient evaluation before the administration of IV fluid boluses, including physical examination by a clinician and frequent reassessment to determine the appropriate volume of fluid resuscitation. The clinician should also integrate clinical signs with patient and locality-specific information about prevalent diseases, vulnerabilities (such as severe anemia and malnutrition), and available critical care resources.

When caring for children with severe febrile illness (such as those included in the FEAST trial) in settings with limited access to critical care resources (ie, mechanical ventilation and inotropic support), administration of bolus intravenous fluids should be undertaken with extreme caution because it may be harmful (see Maitland et al. *N Engl J Med.* 2011;364[26]:2483-2495 for details).

Monitor for signs of increased respiratory distress and pulmonary edema, such as rales/ crackles, which may result from increased vascular permeability. If such signs develop, stop rapid bolus fluid administration. The child requires supplementary O_2 and may require endotracheal intubation and mechanical ventilation with positive end-expiratory pressure. If additional fluid boluses are needed, smaller volumes should be given more slowly (eg, 5 to 10 mL/kg over 10 to 20 minutes).

Pulmonary edema may also develop with cardiogenic shock, which often is manifested by hepatomegaly, cardiomegaly, and poor myocardial contractility. In both instances, you may need to reduce the volume and rate of fluid administration.

Draw blood samples for blood culture. As noted, administer the first dose of broad-spectrum antibiotics within 1 hour after first medical contact. Do not delay antimicrobial therapy to wait for blood cultures or to perform other diagnostic assessments such as lumbar puncture.

Anticipate the possible need for vasopressors and stress-dose hydrocortisone. Order these drugs from the pharmacy early so that they will be at the bedside. They should be immediately available if the shock is fluid refractory or if adrenal insufficiency is suspected. Vasopressors can be administered via peripheral venous or IO access, so initiation of vasopressor therapy should not await transfer to a critical care unit. Because delay in initiation of vasoactive support has been associated with increased length of stay and mortality in pediatric septic shock, it is important to begin vasoactive drug therapy within the first hour if shock persists despite bolus fluid administration (see below).

Identify and correct metabolic derangements immediately. Hypoglycemia and ionized hypocalcemia are commonly seen in septic shock and may contribute to myocardial dysfunction.

Use diagnostic assessments (eg, lactate concentration, base deficit, and $ScvO_2$) to identify the severity of shock and monitor the response to fluid therapy.

Managing Fluid-Refractory Septic Shock

If severe shock persists despite rapid administration of isotonic crystalloid fluid boluses, start treatment for fluid-refractory septic shock with vasoactive drug therapy. Vasoactive drug therapy is recommended within the first hour of therapy as follows:

- Administer vasoactive therapy to improve tissue perfusion and blood pressure. Typically epinephrine is administered to the child with fluid-refractory septic shock and cold extremities, because a recent randomized study conducted among such children suggests improved outcomes when epinephrine is used as the initial vasopressor (see Ventura AM et al. *Crit Care Med.* 2015;43[11]:2292-2302)
- Administer additional fluid boluses of 20 mL/kg isotonic crystalloid as needed; consider giving a colloid-containing fluid
- Consider endotracheal intubation and early assisted ventilation with supplementary O_2 and PEEP as needed

After initial stabilization/resuscitation, including administration of antibiotics, fluid boluses, and vasoactive therapy within the first hour of care, evaluate heart rate, blood pressure, and peripheral perfusion to determine the next intervention. If heart rate, blood pressure, and perfusion are returning to normal, arrange admission or transfer to an appropriate pediatric facility. If the child remains hypotensive or poorly perfused, proceed to the next level in the algorithm. Initiate consultation with a pediatric critical care unit or transport team. Continue fluid and vasoactive therapy while preparing for admission or transfer.

Critical Care of Septic Shock

Once critical care expertise is available for the child with persistent shock despite initial fluid bolus and vasoactive drug therapy, additional hemodynamic monitoring can be established and additional vasoactive drugs and fluid boluses can be provided.

- Establish central venous and intra-arterial pressure monitoring
- Monitor central venous oxygen saturation ($ScvO_2$) and the difference between arterial and central venous oxygen saturation, and assess the child's heart rate, blood pressure, and perfusion
- Analyze laboratory data (eg, serum glucose, calcium, lactate)
- Continue epinephrine/norepinephrine and add additional vasoactive drugs as needed
- Provide fluid boluses as needed to treat shock; assess the child frequently and after each fluid bolus
- Evaluate cortisol if the child is at risk for relative adrenal insufficiency; consider stress-dose hydrocortisone administration

Vasoactive and inotropic drug therapy is initially guided by assessment of $ScvO_2$, if available, and evaluation of the child's blood pressure, perfusion of extremities (including the quality of peripheral pulses and color and temperature of extremities), and organ perfusion, including level of consciousness and urine output. The goal of critical care therapy is to establish an $ScvO_2$ of 70% or greater with no signs of shock.

It is not always clear from the physical examination whether a child has vasodilation or vasoconstriction. For example, some children with cool extremities may have vasodilation but be poorly perfused because of low stroke volume and poor cardiac function. The reasons for specific drug selection according to type of shock are described below.

Throughout the management of septic shock, it is important to support organ function, serum electrolytes, acid-base balance, and lactate, glucose, and calcium concentrations. In titrating drug and fluid therapy, goals of care are to improve the child's $ScvO_2$, cardiac output/index, blood pressure, and organ perfusion.

Shock With Cold Extremities and ScvO₂ of 70% or Less

Because these children often have sluggish capillary refill and evidence of vasoconstriction, extremities are typically cool with pallor or mottling and delayed capillary refill. Urine output is typically decreased. Additional fluid boluses are often needed. If the child has a hemoglobin level lower than 10 mg/dL, transfusion will increase oxygen-carrying capacity, oxygen content, and oxygen delivery.

Epinephrine is the preferred vasoactive agent to treat shock with cold extremities. It has potent inotropic effects that can improve stroke volume. The epinephrine dose is titrated to support blood pressure and systemic perfusion. At low infusion doses, epinephrine can lower SVR (from its β-adrenergic effects). At higher infusion rates, epinephrine can increase SVR (from its α-adrenergic action). An infusion dose of epinephrine of 0.3 mcg/kg per minute or higher usually produces a predominant α-adrenergic effect. Epinephrine may increase lactate concentration by stimulating lactate production in skeletal muscle. Additional vasoactive drugs (including milrinone and even vasodilators) may be needed.

If the child has a low blood pressure, the α-adrenergic vasoconstrictive effects of norepinephrine may be effective in increasing the blood pressure, particularly if diastolic hypotension is present. Additional vasoactive or inotropic drugs may be added and titrated to improve cardiac output/index and blood pressure.

If the child has an adequate blood pressure and persistent signs of shock, milrinone may improve cardiac output and produce some vasodilation. Milrinone has inotropic effects because it inhibits phosphodiesterase, the enzyme that inactivates cyclic adenosine monophosphate (cyclic AMP), the intracellular messenger responsible for many of the sympathomimetic effects produced by catecholamines. It also has vasodilatory effects. If poor perfusion persists, other inotropes and vasodilators (eg, sodium nitroprusside) may be useful for improving tissue perfusion.

Shock With Warm Extremities and ScvO₂ of 70% or Greater

Norepinephrine is the vasoactive agent of choice for the child with fluid-refractory septic shock who presents in shock with warm extremities and an $ScvO_2$ 70% or greater but with poor perfusion or hypotension. Norepinephrine is chosen for its potent α-adrenergic vasoconstricting effects, which can raise diastolic blood pressure by increasing SVR. It is also chosen for its ability to increase cardiac contractility with little change in heart rate. This can restore blood pressure by increasing SVR, venous tone, and stroke volume.

A vasopressin infusion may be useful in the setting of norepinephrine-refractory shock. Vasopressin antagonizes the mechanisms of sepsis-mediated vasodilation. It acts synergistically with endogenous and exogenous catecholamines in stabilizing blood pressure, but it has no effect on cardiac contractility.

Correction of Adrenal Insufficiency

A child in septic shock with fluid-refractory and epinephrine- or norepinephrine-resistant shock may have adrenal insufficiency. If you suspect adrenal insufficiency, or a patient is at known risk for adrenal insufficiency (ie, history of steroid use), give hydrocortisone 1 to 2 mg/kg IV bolus early. If possible, obtain a baseline cortisol concentration before administration, and obtain expert consultation for any additional evaluation and management.

Therapeutic End Points

Titrate vasoactive agents in septic shock to therapeutic end points, including

- $ScvO_2$ 70% or greater and cardiac index 3.3 to 6.0 L/min/m² (see Brierley et al. *Crit Care Med.* 2009;37[2]:666-688 in the Suggested Reading List on the Student Website for details)
- Normalized heart rate (declining from very rapid rate toward normal)
- Adequate blood pressure
- Good distal pulses and perfusion with capillary refill 2 seconds or less
- Improved level of consciousness/responsiveness
- Appropriate urine output
- Improving metabolic acidosis and lactate concentration

Strict adherence to end points is recommended to avoid excessive vasoconstriction in key organs.

Poststabilization Care

Once signs of shock are resolved, the child requires continued monitoring and support of organ function. The source infection must be eliminated. In addition, the healthcare team should evaluate the cause of the infection to determine if it could have been prevented (and how) and the speed of the recognition of the septic shock (could it have been improved), and identify any potential improvements that could be made to increase the efficiency and effectiveness of shock resuscitation for future patients with septic shock.

Management of Anaphylactic Shock

Management of anaphylactic shock focuses on treatment of life-threatening cardiopulmonary problems and reversal or blockade of the mediators released as part of the uncontrolled allergic response. Primary therapy is administration of epinephrine to reverse the effects of histamine and other allergic mediators. The epinephrine dose may be repeated if needed. Angioedema (tissue swelling resulting from a marked increase in capillary permeability) may result in complete upper airway obstruction, so providers should anticipate the need for very early airway intervention with assisted ventilation. The epinephrine may prevent or reverse hypotension, and fluid resuscitation may also be effective in restoring blood pressure and supporting effective perfusion. For details, see recommendations for treatment of anaphylaxis in the emergency department published in Campbell RL et al. *Ann Allergy Asthma Immunol*. 2014;113:599-608, included in the Suggested Reading List on the Student Website.

Specific Treatment Considerations

Consider the initial general management of shock outlined in Table 70 in addition to the following specific treatments for anaphylactic shock as indicated (Table 75).

Table 75. Management of Anaphylactic Shock: Specific Treatment Considerations

- Place the patient supine, administer oxygen, and maintain airway.
- Epinephrine: First-line treatment
  - IM epinephrine or epinephrine by autoinjector (pediatric or adult, depending on the child's size) is the most important agent for the treatment of anaphylaxis.
  - A second dose or an epinephrine infusion may be needed after 10-15 minutes in severe anaphylaxis, frequently a low-dose infusion (<0.05 mcg/kg per minute) is effective.
- Administer isotonic crystalloid fluid boluses as needed to support circulation.
- Albuterol
  - Administer albuterol as needed for bronchospasm by metered dose inhaler, intermittent nebulizer, or continuous nebulizer.
- Antihistamines
  - H_1 blocker (ie, diphenhydramine)
  - Consider an H_2 blocker (ie, ranitidine or famotidine).
  - *Note:* The combination of both an H_1 and H_2 blocker may be more effective than either given alone.
- Corticosteroids
  - Methylprednisolone or equivalent corticosteroid

For hypotension refractory to intramuscular epinephrine and fluid, use vasopressors as indicated.

- Epinephrine infusion; titrate as needed

Observation is indicated for identification and treatment of late-phase symptoms. Late-phase symptoms may occur in 25% to 30% of children several hours after acute-phase symptoms. The likelihood of late-phase symptoms increases in proportion to the severity of acute-phase symptoms.

Management of Neurogenic Shock

Children with neurogenic shock typically present with hypotension, bradycardia, and sometimes hypothermia. Minimal response to fluid resuscitation is commonly observed. Blood pressure is characterized by a low diastolic blood pressure with a wide pulse pressure because of loss of vascular tone. Children with spinal shock may be more sensitive to variations in ambient temperature and may require supplementary warming or cooling.

Specific Treatment Considerations

The initial management principles for shock outlined in Table 70 may be considered in addition to the following specific treatments for neurogenic shock as indicated (Table 76).

Table 76. Management of Neurogenic Shock: Specific Treatment Considerations

Position the child flat or head down to improve venous return.

Administer a trial of fluid therapy (isotonic crystalloid) and assess response.

For fluid-refractory hypotension, use vasopressors (eg, norepinephrine, epinephrine) as indicated.

Provide supplementary warming or cooling as needed.

Management of Cardiogenic Shock

Cardiogenic shock is a condition of inadequate tissue perfusion that results from myocardial dysfunction. Initially, cardiogenic shock may resemble hypovolemic shock, so identifying a cardiogenic etiology may be difficult. If you suspect cardiogenic shock, consider a slow administration (10 to 20 minutes) of a relatively small fluid bolus (ie, 5 to 10 mL/kg) while carefully monitoring the child for response. Cardiogenic shock is probably present if the child does not improve, the child's respiratory function deteriorates, or the child develops signs of pulmonary edema. Evidence of venous congestion (eg, elevated central venous pressure, distended jugular veins, or hepatomegaly) and cardiomegaly (on chest x-ray) are also suggestive of a cardiac etiology of shock.

Main Objectives

A main objective in the management of cardiogenic shock is to improve the effectiveness of cardiac function and cardiac output by increasing the efficiency of ventricular ejection. Another main objective is to minimize metabolic demand.

Many children with cardiogenic shock have high preload and do not require additional fluid therapy. Others may require a cautious fluid bolus to increase preload. The most effective way to increase stroke volume in these patients is to reduce afterload (SVR) rather than give an inotropic agent. Inotropes may increase cardiac contractility but will also increase myocardial O_2 demand. However, children who are already hypotensive may require fluid therapy and inotropic support before they will tolerate afterload reduction. Specific management includes

- Cautious fluid administration and monitoring
- Laboratory and other diagnostic studies
- Medications
- Mechanical circulatory support

Consult a pediatric critical care or pediatric cardiology specialist at the earliest opportunity. This will help to establish a diagnosis (eg, echocardiogram), guide ongoing therapy, and facilitate direct transfer to definitive care.

Cautious Fluid Administration and Monitoring

Large heart size on the chest x-ray in a child with evidence of shock and poor cardiac output is the hallmark of cardiogenic shock with adequate intravascular volume. Obtain an echocardiogram for more objective and accurate data about preload and cardiac function.

You should not give large or rapid fluid boluses to a child with cardiogenic shock. The boluses can worsen heart function and increase fluid in the lungs. If objective data or the child's history (eg, vomiting and poor intake) are consistent with inadequate preload, you may give a small fluid bolus *cautiously*. Remember the following:

- Give small isotonic fluid boluses (5-10 mL/kg)
- Give fluid boluses over relatively longer periods of time (eg, 10 to 20 minutes instead of 5 to 10 minutes)
- Monitor the child closely during fluid infusion
  - Assess for respiratory function frequently
  - Watch for development of pulmonary edema and deterioration in pulmonary function

Give supplementary O_2. Be prepared to provide assisted ventilation. Noninvasive positive pressure support may reduce the need for mechanical ventilation by decreasing the work of breathing and improving oxygenation.

Consider establishing central venous access to facilitate measurement of central venous pressure as an index of preload status and to assess right ventricular end-diastolic pressure and to provide access for multiple infusions. Central venous access also allows monitoring of $ScvO_2$ as an objective measurement of the adequacy of O_2 delivery relative to metabolic demand. Invasive monitoring with a pulmonary artery catheter, an option in the pediatric intensive care unit, is not critical to the diagnosis of cardiogenic shock.

Laboratory and Other Diagnostic Studies

Obtain laboratory studies to assess the impact of shock on end-organ function. No single laboratory study is completely sensitive or specific for cardiogenic shock. Appropriate studies often include

- An arterial blood gas to determine the magnitude of metabolic acidosis and adequacy of oxygenation and ventilation
- Hemoglobin concentration to ensure that O_2-carrying capacity is adequate
- Lactate concentration and $ScvO_2$ as indicators of the adequacy of O_2 delivery relative to metabolic demand
- Cardiac enzymes and thyroid function tests

Other useful studies include the following:

Study	Use
Chest x-ray	Provides information about cardiac size, pulmonary vascular markings, pulmonary edema, and coexistent pulmonary pathology
Electrocardiogram	May detect arrhythmia, myocardial injury, ischemic heart disease, or evidence of drug toxicity
Echocardiogram	May be diagnostic, revealing congenital heart disease, akinetic or dyskinetic ventricular wall motion or valvular dysfunction; also provides objective measurement of ventricular chamber volume (ie, preload) and function

Medications

If the child is normotensive, medication therapy consists of diuretics and vasodilators or inodilators. Diuretics are indicated when the child has evidence of pulmonary edema or systemic venous congestion. Vasodilators and inodilators are typically given by continuous infusion.

Children with cardiogenic shock may require medications to increase cardiac output by improving contractility. Most also require agents to reduce peripheral vascular resistance. This includes vasodilators, inotropes, and phosphodiesterase enzyme inhibitors (ie, inodilators). Milrinone is the preferred drug in many centers. For a detailed discussion of these agents, see "Medication Therapy" in in this Part.

Increased metabolic demand, particularly increased myocardial O_2 demand, plays a role in the vicious cycle of cardiogenic shock. Reducing metabolic demand is a critical component in the management of cardiogenic shock. Use ventilatory support and antipyretics to reduce metabolic demand. Analgesics and sedatives reduce O_2 consumption but also reduce the endogenous stress response that is helping redistribute blood flow to compensate for low cardiac output. Give these agents in small doses. Monitor the child carefully for evidence of potential respiratory depression or hypotension.

Mechanical Circulatory Support

Children with cardiogenic shock who do not respond to medical management may benefit from mechanical circulatory support if the cause of shock is potentially reversible. Extracorporeal life support can provide temporary maintenance of cardiac output, oxygenation, and ventilation while the underlying cause of cardiopulmonary failure is treated. Forms of extracorporeal life support include extracorporeal membrane oxygenation and ventricular assist devices. One specific etiology of cardiogenic shock for which extracorporeal membrane oxygenation may be considered is acute fulminant myocarditis with high risk of imminent cardiac arrest. Extracorporeal life support is usually available only in tertiary pediatric centers that have the resources and expertise to manage children with acute cardiopulmonary failure.

Specific Treatment Considerations

Follow the initial management principles for shock outlined in Table 70 in addition to the following considerations specific to cardiogenic shock (Table 77).

Table 77. Management of Cardiogenic Shock: Specific Treatment Considerations

- Administer supplementary O_2 and consider need for noninvasive positive pressure or mechanical ventilation.
- Give 5-10 mL/kg isotonic crystalloid infusion slowly (over 10-20 minutes); repeat PRN.
- Assess frequently for pulmonary edema.
- Be prepared to assist ventilation.
- Obtain expert consultation early.

Order laboratory and other studies to determine underlying cause and degree of cardiac and end-organ dysfunction.

Administer pharmacologic support (eg, vasodilators, phosphodiesterase enzyme inhibitors, inotropes, analgesics, antipyretics).

Consider mechanical circulatory support.

Management of Obstructive Shock

Management of obstructive shock is specific to the type of obstruction. This section discusses management of

- Cardiac tamponade
- Tension pneumothorax
- Ductal-dependent congenital heart lesions
- Massive pulmonary embolism

Main Objectives

The early clinical presentation of obstructive shock may resemble hypovolemic shock. A reasonable initial approach may include administering a fluid challenge (10-20 mL/kg isotonic crystalloid). Rapid identification of obstructive shock by using the secondary assessment and diagnostic assessments is critical to effective treatment. The main objectives in the management of obstructive shock are to

- Correct the cause of obstruction of cardiac output
- Restore tissue perfusion

Identify and Intervene

Obstructive Shock

Because children with obstructive shock can rapidly progress to cardiopulmonary failure and then cardiac arrest, immediate identification and correction of the underlying cause of the obstruction may be lifesaving.

General Management Principles

In addition to considerations specific to the etiology of the obstruction, follow the initial management principles outlined in the section Fundamentals of Shock Management.

Specific Management of Cardiac Tamponade

Cardiac tamponade is caused by accumulation of fluid, blood, or air in the pericardial space. This accumulation limits systemic venous return, impairs ventricular filling, and reduces cardiac output. Favorable outcome requires rapid identification and immediate treatment of tamponade. Children with cardiac tamponade may improve temporarily with fluid administration to augment cardiac output and tissue perfusion until pericardial drainage can be performed.

Consult appropriate specialists (eg, pediatric critical care, pediatric cardiology, pediatric surgery) early. Elective pericardial drainage (pericardiocentesis), often guided by echocardiography or fluoroscopy, should be performed by specialists who are trained and skilled in the procedure. Emergency pericardiocentesis may be performed in the setting of impending or actual pulseless arrest when there is a strong suspicion of pericardial tamponade.

Specific Management of Tension Pneumothorax

Tension pneumothorax is characterized by the accumulation of air under pressure in the pleural space with compression of the lung on the involved side and mediastinal shift to the other side of the chest. This prevents the lungs from expanding properly and applies pressure on the heart and great veins, compromising venous return and cardiac output. Favorable outcome depends on immediate diagnosis and urgent treatment. A tension pneumothorax should be identified through clinical examination, and treatment should not await confirmation with a chest radiograph.

Treatment of a tension pneumothorax is immediate needle decompression followed by thoracostomy for chest tube placement as soon as possible. A trained provider can quickly perform an emergency needle decompression by inserting an 18- to 20-gauge over-the-needle catheter over the top of the child's third rib (second intercostal space) in the midclavicular line. A gush of air is a sign that needle decompression has been successful. This indicates relief of pressure buildup in the pleural space.

Specific Management of Ductal-Dependent Lesions

Ductal-dependent lesions are a group of congenital cardiac abnormalities. These abnormalities result in pulmonary or systemic blood flow that must pass through an open/patent ductus arteriosus. The infant can deteriorate rapidly once the ductus begins to close during the first days or weeks of life.

Congenital heart defects with ductal-dependent pulmonary blood flow usually include a severe obstruction to pulmonary blood flow from the right ventricle, so all pulmonary blood flow then must pass from the aorta through the ductus arteriosus and into the lungs. When the ductus begins to close, the infant becomes profoundly cyanotic and hypoxemic.

Congenital heart defects with ductal-dependent systemic blood flow usually consist of an obstruction to outflow through or from the left side of the heart into the aorta. In such patients, systemic blood flow must pass from the right ventricle and pulmonary artery through the ductus into the aorta. In these patients, when the ductus starts to close, signs of shock develop with severe deterioration in systemic perfusion.

For any infant with ductal-dependent pulmonary or systemic blood flow, immediate treatment with continuous infusion of prostaglandin E_1 (PGE_1) can restore ductal openness/patency and may be lifesaving.

Other management actions for ductal-dependent obstructive lesions are

- Ventilatory support with O_2 administration
- Expert consultation to direct therapy
- Echocardiography to establish diagnosis and guide therapy
- Administration of inotropic agents to improve myocardial contractility
- Judicious administration of fluids to improve cardiac output
- Correction of metabolic derangements, including metabolic acidosis

Specific Management of Massive Pulmonary Embolism

Massive pulmonary embolism is a sudden block in the main or large-branch pulmonary artery. This block is usually caused by a blood clot that has traveled to the lungs from another part of the body. The block also can result from other substances, including fat, air, amniotic fluid, catheter fragment, or injected matter. Blood flow through the pulmonary circulation to the left side of the heart is obstructed, resulting in decreased left ventricular filling and inadequate cardiac output.

Initial treatment is supportive, including administration of O_2, ventilatory assistance, and fluid therapy if the child is poorly perfused. Consult a specialist who can perform echocardiography, a computed tomography scan with IV contrast, or angiography to confirm the diagnosis. Anticoagulants (eg, heparin, enoxaparin) are the definitive treatment for most children with pulmonary embolism who are not in shock. Because anticoagulants do not act immediately to relieve obstruction, consider fibrinolytic agents (eg, recombinant tissue plasminogen activator) in children with severe cardiovascular compromise.

Computed tomography angiography is the diagnostic assessment of choice because it can be rapidly obtained and does not require an invasive angiogram. Additional diagnostic studies that might be useful are an arterial blood gas, CBC, D-dimer, electrocardiography, chest x-ray, ventilation-perfusion scan, and echocardiography.

Management of Shock Flowchart

Management of Shock Flowchart	
• Oxygen	• IV/IO access
• Pulse oximetry	• BLS as indicated
• ECG monitor	• Point-of-care glucose testing

Hypovolemic Shock Specific Management for Selected Conditions	
Nonhemorrhagic	**Hemorrhagic**
• 20 mL/kg NS/LR bolus, repeat as needed • Consider colloid	• Control external bleeding • 20 mL/kg NS/LR bolus, repeat 2 or 3x as needed • Transfuse PRBCs as indicated

Distributive Shock Specific Management for Selected Conditions		
Septic	**Anaphylactic**	**Neurogenic**
Management Algorithm: • Septic Shock	• IM epinephrine (or autoinjector) • Fluid boluses (20 mL/kg NS/LR) • Albuterol • Antihistamines, corticosteroids • Epinephrine infusion	• 20 mL/kg NS/LR bolus, repeat PRN • Vasopressor

Cardiogenic Shock Specific Management for Selected Conditions	
Bradyarrhythmia/Tachyarrhythmia	**Other (eg, CHD, Myocarditis, Cardiomyopathy, Poisoning)**
Management Algorithms: • Bradycardia • Tachycardia With Poor Perfusion	• 5 to 10 mL/kg NS/LR bolus, repeat PRN • Vasoactive infusion • Consider expert consultation

Obstructive Shock Specific Management for Selected Conditions			
Ductal-Dependent (LV Outflow Obstruction)	**Tension Pneumothorax**	**Cardiac Tamponade**	**Pulmonary Embolism**
• Prostaglandin E$_1$ • Expert consultation	• Needle decompression • Tube thoracostomy	• Pericardiocentesis • 20 mL/kg NS/LR bolus	• 20 mL/kg NS/LR bolus, repeat PRN • Consider thrombolytics, anticoagulants • Expert consultation

Figure 41. Management of Shock Flowchart.

Resources

Resources for Management of Circulatory Emergencies

Intraosseous Access

Intraosseous (IO) cannulation is a relatively simple and effective method of rapidly establishing vascular access for emergency fluids or medications. It provides access to a noncollapsible marrow venous plexus, which serves as a rapid, safe, and reliable route for administration of drugs, crystalloids, colloids, and blood during resuscitation. IO access can be achieved in children of all ages, often in about 30 to 60 seconds. In certain circumstances (eg, cardiac arrest or severe shock with severe vasoconstriction), it may be the *initial* vascular access attempted. Any medication that can be administered IV can be given by the IO route. Fluids and medications delivered via an IO catheter can reach the central circulation within seconds. If peripheral vascular access cannot be readily obtained in a child with compensated or hypotensive shock, be prepared to establish IO access as soon as it is needed.

Sites for IO Access

Many sites are appropriate for IO infusion. The proximal tibia, just below the growth plate, is often used. Other sites are the distal tibia just above the medial malleolus, the distal femur, and the anterior-superior iliac spine. Newer devices, such as the IO drill, are approved for use in the humerus in older children, adolescents, and adults.

Contraindications

Contraindications to IO access include

- Fractures and crush injuries near the access site
- Conditions with fragile bones (eg, osteogenesis imperfecta)
- Previous attempts to establish IO access in the same bone

Avoid IO cannulation if infection is present in the overlying tissues.

Procedure (Proximal Tibia)

Use the following procedure to establish IO access (Table 78).

Table 78. Procedure to Establish IO Access

Step	Action
1	• To establish access in the proximal tibia, position the leg with slight external rotation. • Identify the tibial tuberosity just below the knee joint; the insertion site is the flat part of the tibia, about 1 to 3 cm (about 1 finger's width) below and medial to this bony prominence (Figure 42). Always use universal precautions when attempting vascular access. Disinfect the overlying skin and surrounding area.
2	• Leave the stylet in the needle during insertion to prevent the needle from becoming clogged with bone or tissue. • Stabilize the leg on a firm surface; do not place your hand behind the leg. *Note:* If a standard IO needle or bone marrow needle is not available, a large-bore (at least 18-gauge) standard hypodermic needle can be substituted, but the lumen may become clogged with bone or bone marrow during insertion. Short, wide-gauge spinal needles with internal stylets can be used in an emergency, but they tend to bend easily. A hemostat can be used to help stabilize the needle during insertion.
3	• Insert the needle through the skin over the anteromedial surface of the tibia perpendicular to the tibia; this avoids injury to the growth plate. • Use a twisting motion with gentle but firm pressure. • Continue inserting the needle through the cortical bone until there is a sudden decrease in resistance as the needle enters the marrow space. If the needle is placed correctly, it should stand easily without support.

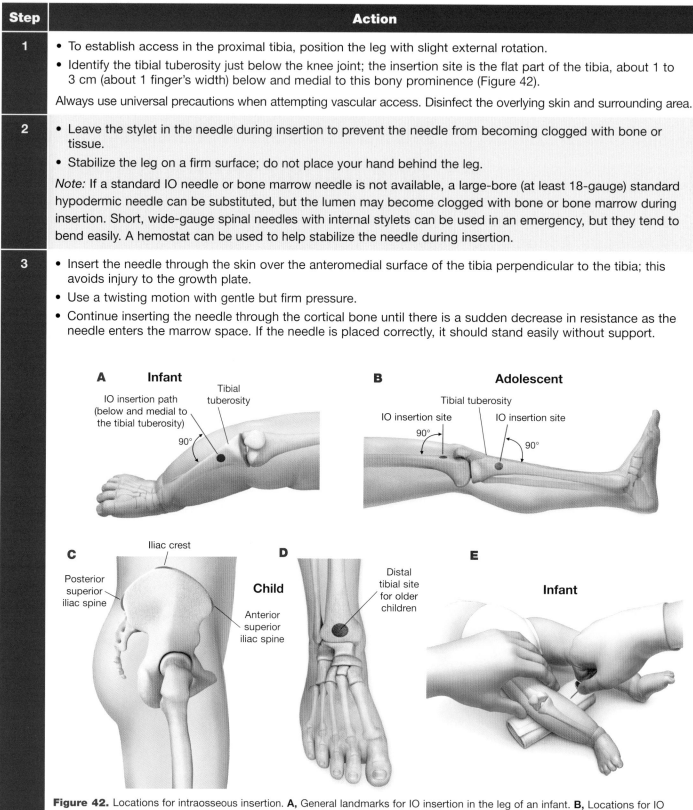

Figure 42. Locations for intraosseous insertion. **A,** General landmarks for IO insertion in the leg of an infant. **B,** Locations for IO insertion in the proximal tibia and distal femur in older children. **C,** Location for IO insertion in the iliac crest. **D,** Location for IO insertion in the distal tibia. **E,** Technique for immobilizing the leg while twisting the IO needle into the leg of an infant.

(continued)

(continued)

Step	Action
4	• Remove the stylet and attach a syringe. • Aspiration of bone marrow and blood into the hub of the needle confirms correct placement; blood may be sent to the lab for analysis (Note: Blood or bone marrow may not always be aspirated despite correct needle placement). • Infuse a small volume of saline. It should infuse easily. Check for swelling at the insertion site or posteriorly, behind the insertion site. (Swelling occurs if the needle was inserted too deeply and penetrated through the posterior cortical bone).
5	To stabilize the needle, place tape over the flange; you also may place gauze padding on both sides of the needle for support.
6	Tape IV tubing to the skin to avoid tension on the tubing that might displace the needle.
7	Fluid can be infused by a syringe attached to a 3-way stopcock or by pressure infusion. When using a pressurized fluid bag, make sure no air gets into the system.
8	Any medication that can be administered IV can be given by the IO route, including vasoactive drug infusions such as epinephrine. Follow all bolus medications with a saline flush.

After IO Insertion

After IO needle/catheter insertion, do the following:

Check the site and the underside of the leg for signs of swelling and IO needle displacement; fluids or drugs delivered via a displaced needle can cause severe complications (eg, tissue necrosis, compartment syndrome).

IO needles are intended for short-term use, generally less than 24 hours. Replacement with long-term vascular access is usually accomplished in an intensive care setting.

Color-Coded Length-Based Resuscitation Tape

Use a color-coded length-based tape (Table 79) to select the correct size of resuscitation supplies and to determine the child's weight (if not known) for calculating drug doses.

Table 79. Color-Coded Length-Based Resuscitation Tape

Equipment	GRAY* 3-5 kg	PINK Small Infant 6-7 kg	RED Infant 8-9 kg	PURPLE Toddler 10-11 kg	YELLOW Small Child 12-14 kg	WHITE Child 15-18 kg	BLUE Child 19-23 kg	ORANGE Large Child 24-29 kg	GREEN Adult 30-36 kg
Resuscitation bag		Infant/child	Infant/child	Child	Child	Child	Child	Child	Adult
Oxygen mask (NRB)		Pediatric	Pediatric	Pediatric	Pediatric	Pediatric	Pediatric	Pediatric	Pediatric/adult
Oral airway (mm)		50	50	60	60	60	70	80	80
Laryngoscope blade (size)		1 Straight	1 Straight	1 Straight	2 Straight	2 Straight	2 Straight or curved	2 Straight or curved	3 Straight or curved
ET tube (mm)†		3.5 Uncuffed 3.0 Cuffed	3.5 Uncuffed 3.0 Cuffed	4.0 Uncuffed 3.5 Cuffed	4.5 Uncuffed 4.0 Cuffed	5.0 Uncuffed 4.5 Cuffed	5.5 Uncuffed 5.0 Cuffed	6.0 Cuffed	6.5 Cuffed
ET tube insertion length (cm)	3 kg 9-9.5 4 kg 9.5-10 5 kg 10-10.5	10.5-11	10.5-11	11-12	13.5	14-15	16.5	17-18	18.5-19.5
Suction catheter (F)		8	8	10	10	10	10	10	10-12
BP cuff	Neonatal #5/infant	Infant/child	Infant/child	Child	Child	Child	Child	Child	Small adult
IV catheter (ga)		22-24	22-24	20-24	18-22	18-22	18-20	18-20	16-20
IO (ga)		18/15	18/15	15	15	15	15	15	15
NG tube (F)		5-8	5-8	8-10	10	10	12-14	14-18	16-18
Urinary catheter (F)	5	8	8	8-10	10	10-12	10-12	12	12
Chest tube (F)		10-12	10-12	16-20	20-24	20-24	24-32	28-32	32-38

Abbreviations: BP, blood pressure; ET, endotracheal; F, French; IO, intraosseous; IV, intravenous; NG, nasogastric; NRB, nonrebreathing.

*For Gray column, use Pink or Red equipment sizes if no size is listed.

†Per *2010 AHA Guidelines*, in the hospital cuffed or uncuffed tubes may be used.

Adapted from *Broselow™ Pediatric Emergency Tape*. Distributed by Armstrong Medical Industries Inc., Lincolnshire, IL. Copyright 2007 Vital Signs Inc. Courtesy and © Becton, Dickinson and Company. Reprinted with permission.

Part 10

Recognition of Arrhythmias

Overview

This Part discusses the recognition of arrhythmias, such as bradycardia (slow heart rate) and tachycardia (fast heart rate) with a palpable pulse and adequate or inadequate perfusion in infants and children.

Learning Objective

After studying this Part, you should be able to

- Differentiate between unstable and stable patients with arrhythmias

Preparation for the Course

You will be expected to identify bradycardic and tachycardic rhythms in an infant or child with a pulse and poor or adequate perfusion.

Bradycardia Definitions

Bradycardia is a heart rate that is slow in comparison with a normal heart rate range for the child's age, level of activity, and clinical condition. See Table 8: Normal Heart Rates in Part 3.

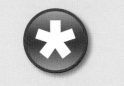

Critical Concepts

Symptomatic Bradycardia and Cardiopulmonary Compromise

Symptomatic bradycardia is a heart rate slower than normal for the child's age (usually less than 60/min) associated with cardiopulmonary compromise.

Cardiopulmonary compromise is defined as hypotension, acutely altered mental status [ie, decreased level of consciousness]), and signs of shock.

Bradycardia is an ominous sign of impending cardiac arrest in infants and children, especially if it is associated with hypotension or evidence of poor tissue perfusion. If, despite adequate oxygenation and ventilation, the heart rate is less than 60/min in an infant or child with signs of poor tissue perfusion, begin CPR.

Evaluating Heart Rate and Rhythm

Consider the following when evaluating the heart rate and rhythm in any seriously ill or injured child:

- The child's typical heart rate and baseline rhythm
- The child's level of activity and clinical condition (including baseline cardiac function)

Children with congenital heart disease may have underlying conduction abnormalities. Interpret the child's heart rate and rhythm by comparing them to the child's baseline heart rate and rhythm. Children with poor baseline cardiac function are more likely to become symptomatic from arrhythmias than children with normal cardiac function.

Tissue hypoxia is the leading cause of symptomatic bradycardia in children. Therefore, symptomatic bradycardia in children is usually the result of (rather than the reason for) progressive hypoxemia and respiratory failure or shock. Priorities in initial assessment and management should be to support the airway and provide adequate oxygenation and ventilation.

Bradycardia may be classified as

- Primary bradycardia
- Secondary bradycardia

Primary bradycardia is the result of congenital or acquired heart conditions that slow the spontaneous depolarization rate of the heart's normal pacemaker cells or slow conduction through the heart's conduction system. Causes of primary bradycardia include

- Congenital abnormality of the heart pacemaker or conduction system
- Surgical injury to the pacemaker or conduction system
- Cardiomyopathy
- Myocarditis

Secondary bradycardia is the result of noncardiac conditions that alter the normal function of the heart (ie, slow the sinus node pacemaker or slow conduction through the atrioventricular [AV] junction). Causes of secondary bradycardia include

- Hypoxia
- Acidosis
- Hypotension
- Hypothermia
- Drug effects

Recognition of Bradycardia

Signs and Symptoms of Bradycardia

Cardiac output (the volume of blood pumped by the heart per minute) is the product of stroke volume (the volume of blood pumped with each ventricular contraction) and heart rate (number of times the ventricles contract per minute):

Cardiac Output = Stroke Volume × Heart Rate

When heart rate decreases, cardiac output can only be maintained by an increase in stroke volume. Because the heart's ability to increase stroke volume is limited during infancy and early childhood, cardiac output typically declines with bradycardia. An extremely slow heart rate results in critically low cardiac output that can be life threatening and lead to cardiopulmonary compromise. The signs of cardiopulmonary compromise associated with bradycardia are

- Hypotension
- Altered mental status: decreased level of consciousness or irritability
- Shock: poor end-organ perfusion with or without hypotension

Additional signs can include

- Respiratory distress or failure
- Chest pain or vague feeling of discomfort in older children
- Sudden collapse

ECG Characteristics of Bradycardia

The electrocardiographic (ECG) characteristics of bradycardia include

Heart rate	Slow compared with normal heart rate for age
P waves	May or may not be visible
QRS complex	Narrow or wide (depending on the origin of the rhythm and/or location of injury to the conduction system)
P wave and QRS complex	May be unrelated (ie, AV dissociation)

See "Rhythm Recognition Review" in the Appendix for examples.

Types of Bradyarrhythmias

Bradycardia that is associated with a rhythm disturbance is called a *bradyarrhythmia*. Two common types of bradycardia in children are sinus bradycardia and AV block. These are discussed in detail in the next section. Other types of bradyarrhythmias are sinus node arrest with atrial, junctional, or ventricular escape rhythms. These are more complex rhythms and are not discussed in the PALS Provider Course.

Sinus Bradycardia

Sinus bradycardia is a sinus node depolarization rate that is slower than normal for the child's age (see Table 8: Normal Heart Rates in Part 3). Sinus bradycardia is not necessarily problematic. It is often present in healthy children at rest when metabolic demands of the body are relatively low (eg, during sleep). Well-conditioned athletes often have sinus bradycardia because they have high stroke volume and increased vagal tone. However, sinus bradycardia can also develop in response to hypoxia, hypotension, and acidosis. As discussed above, it is often the result of progressive respiratory failure or shock and indicates impending cardiac arrest. Sinus bradycardia also may result from drug effects. Therefore, evaluation of sinus bradycardia always must involve assessment of the clinical status of the child.

Rarely, children have a primary bradycardia with an intrinsic disorder of the sinus node that impairs the ability of the sinus node to depolarize at an adequate rate. These children usually have a history of surgery for complex congenital heart disease. Additional causes of sinus node disorders include congenital abnormalities of the conduction system, cardiomyopathy, and myocarditis.

AV Block

AV block is a disturbance of electrical conduction through the AV node. AV block is classified as follows and in Table 80:

- *First degree:* A prolonged PR interval representing slowed conduction through the AV node (Figure 43A)
- *Second degree:* Block of some, but not all, atrial impulses before they reach the ventricles. This block can be further classified as Mobitz type I or Mobitz type II second-degree AV block.
  - Mobitz type I AV block (also known as *Wenckebach phenomenon*) typically occurs at the AV node. It is characterized by progressive prolongation of the PR interval until an atrial impulse is not conducted to the ventricles (Figure 43B). The P wave corresponding to that atrial impulse is not followed by a QRS complex. The cycle of progressive lengthening of the PR interval until failure of conduction of the atrial impulse to the ventricles often repeats.
  - Mobitz type II second-degree AV block (Figure 43C) occurs below the level of the AV node. It is characterized by nonconduction of some atrial impulses to the ventricle without any change in the PR interval of the conducted impulses. Often there is a consistent ratio of atrial to ventricular depolarizations, typically 2 P waves to 1 QRS complex.
- *Third degree:* None of the atrial impulses conduct to the ventricles. This block may also be referred to as *complete heart block* or *complete AV block* (Figure 43D).

Table 80. AV Block Classification

Type	Causes	Characteristics	Symptoms
First degree	• *Note:* May be present in healthy children • Enhanced vagal tone • Myocarditis • Electrolyte disturbances (eg, hyperkalemia) • Hypoxemia • Myocardial infarction • Cardiac surgery • Drugs (eg, calcium channel blockers, β-adrenergic blockers, digoxin) • Acute rheumatic fever • Intrinsic AV nodal disease	Prolonged PR interval	Asymptomatic

(continued)

(continued)

Type	Causes	Characteristics	Symptoms
Second-degree Mobitz type I (Wenckebach phenomenon)	• *Note:* May be present in healthy children • Drugs (eg, calcium channel and β-adrenergic blockers, digoxin) • Any condition that stimulates vagal (parasympathetic) tone • Myocardial infarction	Progressive prolongation of the PR interval until a P wave is not followed by a QRS complex; the cycle often repeats.	Occasionally, may cause presyncope (light-headedness)
Second-degree Mobitz type II	• Typically results from intrinsic conduction system abnormalities • Rarely caused by increased parasympathetic tone or drugs • Cardiac surgery • Myocardial infarction	Some, but not all, P waves are blocked before they reach the ventricle. The PR interval is constant. Often, every other P wave is conducted (2:1 block).	May cause • Sensed irregularities of heartbeat (palpitations) • Presyncope (light-headedness) • Syncope
Third degree	• Extensive conduction system disease or injury, including myocarditis • Cardiac surgery • Congenital complete heart block • Myocardial infarction • Can also result from increased parasympathetic tone, toxic drug effects, or severe hypoxia/acidosis	• No relationship between P waves and QRS complexes • No atrial impulses reach ventricles • Ventricular rhythm maintained by a slower pacemaker	Most frequent symptoms are • Fatigue • Light-headedness • Syncope

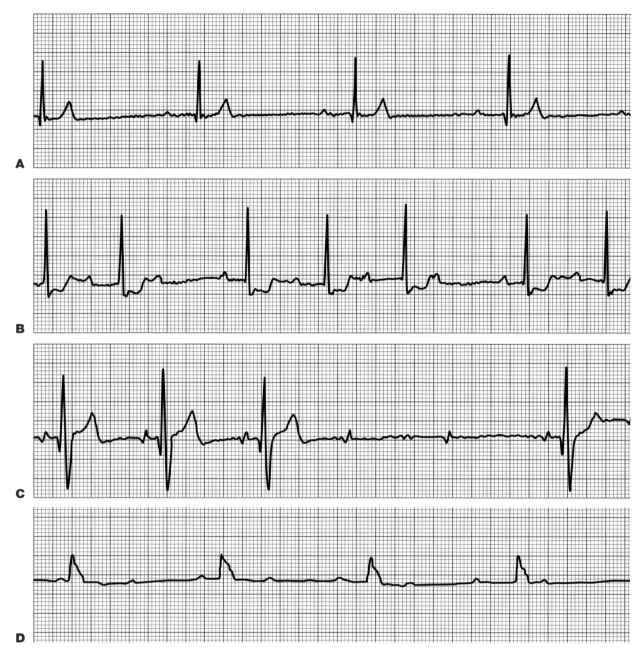

Figure 43. Examples of AV block. **A,** Sinus bradycardia with first-degree AV block. **B,** Second-degree AV block Mobitz type I (Wenckebach phenomenon). **C,** Second-degree AV block Mobitz type II. **D,** Third-degree AV block.

Tachyarrhythmias

Tachycardia is a heart rate that is fast compared with the normal heart rate for the child's age. See Table 8: Normal Heart Rates in Part 3. Sinus tachycardia is a normal response to stress or fever.

Tachyarrhythmias are rapid abnormal rhythms originating either in the atria or the ventricles of the heart. Tachyarrhythmias can be tolerated without symptoms for a variable period of time, especially if cardiac function is good. However, tachyarrhythmias can also cause acute hemodynamic compromise such as shock or deterioration to cardiac arrest. Rapid deterioration is more likely to occur if cardiac function is poor when the arrhythmia develops.

Recognition of Tachyarrhythmias

Signs and Symptoms

Tachyarrhythmias may cause nonspecific signs and symptoms that differ according to the age of the child. Clinical findings may include palpitations, light-headedness, and syncope. In infants who are at home, the tachyarrhythmia may be undetected for long periods (eg, for hours or days) until cardiac output is significantly compromised and the infant develops signs of congestive heart failure such as irritability, poor feeding, and rapid breathing. Episodes of extremely rapid heart rate may be life threatening if cardiac output is compromised. When a tachyarrhythmia develops in a child with poor baseline cardiovascular function, clinical signs can develop quickly and deterioration can be rapid.

Signs of hemodynamic instability associated with tachyarrhythmias are

- Hypotension
- Altered mental status (ie, decreased level of consciousness)
- Signs of shock (poor end-organ perfusion) with or without hypotension

Additional signs may include

- Sudden collapse with rapid, weak pulses
- Respiratory distress/failure

Effect on Cardiac Output

An increased heart rate can produce increased cardiac output, up to a point. If that point is exceeded (ie, the heart rate is extremely rapid), stroke volume decreases because diastole is shortened and there is insufficient time for filling of the ventricles during diastole. Cardiac output then decreases substantially. In addition, coronary perfusion (blood flow to the heart muscle) occurs chiefly during diastole; the decrease in duration of diastole that occurs with a very rapid heart rate reduces coronary perfusion. Finally, a fast heart rate increases myocardial O_2 demand. In infants, prolonged episodes of rapid heart rate (supraventricular tachycardia [SVT]) can cause myocardial dysfunction, leading to congestive heart failure (CHF). In any child, an extremely rapid heart rate can result in inadequate cardiac output and, ultimately, cardiogenic shock.

Classification of Tachycardia and Tachyarrhythmias

Tachycardia and tachyarrhythmias are classified according to the width of the QRS complex; the arrhythmias are divided into those with narrow (0.09 second or less) vs wide (greater than 0.09 second) QRS complexes (Table 81).

Table 81. Classification of Tachycardia and Tachyarrhythmias

Narrow Complex (≤0.09 second)	Wide Complex (>0.09 second)
• Sinus tachycardia • Supraventricular tachycardia • Atrial flutter	• Ventricular tachycardia • Supraventricular tachycardia with aberrant intraventricular conduction

Sinus Tachycardia

Sinus tachycardia (ST) is a sinus node depolarization rate faster than normal for the child's age. It typically develops in response to the body's need for increased cardiac output or O₂ delivery. ST is a normal physiologic response and is not considered an arrhythmia (Figure 44). In ST, the heart rate is not fixed but varies with activity and other factors (eg, the child's sleep/awake state, temperature) that influence O₂ demand.

Common causes of ST include exercise, pain, anxiety, tissue hypoxia, hypovolemia (hemorrhagic and nonhemorrhagic fluid loss), shock, fever, metabolic stress, injury, toxins/poisons/drugs, and anemia. Cardiac tamponade, tension pneumothorax, and thromboembolism are less common causes of ST.

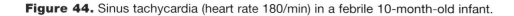

Figure 44. Sinus tachycardia (heart rate 180/min) in a febrile 10-month-old infant.

ECG Characteristics of ST

ECG characteristics of ST include the following:

Heart rate	Beat-to-beat variability with changes in activity or stress level • Usually <220/min in infants • Usually <180/min in children
P waves	Present/normal
PR interval	Constant, normal duration
R-R interval	Variable
QRS complex	Narrow (≤0.09 second)

Supraventricular Tachycardia

SVT is an abnormally fast rhythm originating above the ventricles. In infants and children, the most common cause is a reentry mechanism that occurs through an accessory pathway or within the AV node. SVT is the most common tachyarrhythmia that causes cardiovascular compromise during infancy. In addition to an accessory pathway reentry or AV nodal reentry, other mechanisms that can cause SVT are atrial flutter and ectopic atrial focus.

Two outdated terms for SVT are *paroxysmal atrial tachycardia* and *paroxysmal supraventricular tachycardia*. SVT was labeled "paroxysmal" because it occurs episodically (in paroxysms). The rapid rhythm starts and stops suddenly, often without warning.

Clinical Presentation of SVT

SVT (Figure 45) is a rapid, regular rhythm that often appears abruptly and may be episodic. During episodes of SVT, cardiopulmonary function is influenced by the child's age, duration of the tachycardia, baseline ventricular function, and ventricular rate. In infants with normal ventricular function, SVT may be present but undetected for long periods (hours or days) until cardiac output is significantly impaired. However, if baseline myocardial function is impaired (eg, in a child with congenital heart disease or cardiomyopathy), SVT can produce signs of shock in a short time.

In infants, SVT is often diagnosed when symptoms of CHF develop. *Common signs and symptoms of SVT in infants* include irritability; poor feeding; rapid breathing; unusual sleepiness; vomiting; and pale, mottled, gray, or cyanotic skin. *Common signs and symptoms of SVT in older children* include palpitations, shortness of breath, chest pain or discomfort, light-headedness, and fainting.

SVT is initially well tolerated in most infants and older children. However, it can lead to CHF and clinical evidence of shock when baseline myocardial function is impaired (eg, in a child with congenital heart disease or cardiomyopathy) or in an infant having prolonged episodes over hours to days. Ultimately, SVT can cause cardiovascular collapse.

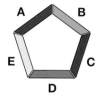

Signs

SVT may be identified as the result of its effect on systemic perfusion. SVT with cardiopulmonary compromise can produce the signs and symptoms listed in Table 82.

Table 82. Signs and Symptoms of SVT With Cardiopulmonary Compromise

Airway	Usually open/patent unless level of consciousness is significantly impaired
Breathing	• Tachypnea • Increased work of breathing • Crackles (or "wheezing" in infants) if CHF develops • Grunting if CHF develops
Circulation	• Tachycardia beyond the typical range for ST and characterized by fixed rate and/or abrupt onset • Delayed capillary refill time • Weak peripheral pulses • Cool extremities • Diaphoretic, pale, mottled, gray, or cyanotic skin • Hypotension • Jugular venous distension (difficult to observe in young children) or hepatomegaly if CHF develops
Disability	• Altered mental status • Sleepiness or lethargy • Irritability
Exposure	Defer evaluation of temperature until ABCs are supported

ECG Characteristics of SVT

ECG characteristics of SVT include the following:

Heart rate	No beat-to-beat variability with activity • Usually ≥220/min in infants • Usually ≥180/min in children
P waves	Absent or abnormal (may appear after the QRS complex)
PR interval	Because P waves are usually absent, PR interval cannot be determined; in ectopic atrial tachycardia, a short PR interval may be seen
R-R interval	Often constant
QRS complex	Usually narrow; wide complex uncommon

Narrow-QRS-complex SVT: In greater than 90% of children with SVT, the QRS complex is narrow (Figure 45), ie, 0.09 second or less.

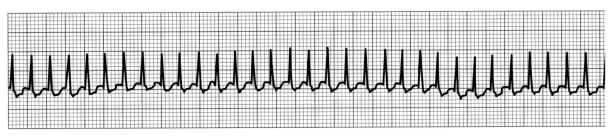

Figure 45. SVT in a 10-month-old infant.

Wide-QRS-complex SVT: SVT with aberrant intraventricular conduction (uncommon in the pediatric age group) produces a wide QRS complex (ie, greater than 0.09 second). This form of SVT most often occurs as a result of rate-related bundle branch block (within the ventricles) or preexisting bundle branch block. It also may be caused by an accessory pathway in which electrical impulses are conducted from the atria to the ventricles through the accessory pathway rather than through the AV node. The impulse then returns to the atria through the AV node (or through a different accessory pathway).

It can be difficult to differentiate SVT with aberrant conduction from ventricular tachycardia (VT). This usually requires careful analysis of at least one 12-lead ECG. Both SVT with aberrant conduction and VT can cause similar hemodynamic instability, have similar rates, and have wide QRS complexes (greater than 0.09 second). In the pediatric age group, unless patient history or previous ECGs suggest the likelihood of SVT with aberrant conduction (eg, preexisting bundle branch block), assume that a tachycardia with a wide QRS complex is due to VT.

Comparison of ST and SVT

It may be difficult to differentiate SVT with shock from shock resulting from another etiology with compensatory ST. The characteristics in Table 83 may aid in differentiating ST from SVT. Note that signs of heart failure and other signs and symptoms of poor perfusion may be absent early after the onset of SVT.

Table 83. Characteristics of ST and SVT

Characteristic	ST	SVT
History	Gradual onset Compatible with ST (eg, history of fever, pain, dehydration, hemorrhage)	Abrupt onset or termination or both Infant: Symptoms of CHF Child: Sudden onset of palpitations
Physical examination	Signs of underlying cause of ST (eg, crackles, fever, hypovolemia, anemia)	Infant: Signs of CHF (eg, rales, hepatomegaly, edema)
Heart rate	Infant: Usually <220/min Child: Usually <180/min	Infant: Usually ≥220/min Child: Usually ≥180/min

(continued)

(continued)

Characteristic	ST	SVT
Monitor	Variability in heart rate with changes in level of activity or stimulation; slowing of heart rate with rest or treatment of underlying cause (eg, administration of IV fluids for hypovolemia)	Minimal or no variability in heart rate with changes in level of activity or stimulation
ECG	P waves present/normal/upright in leads I/aVF	P waves absent/abnormal/inverted (negative) in leads II/III/aVF; if present, they usually follow the QRS complex
Chest x-ray	Usually small heart and clear lungs unless ST is caused by pneumonia, pericarditis, or underlying heart disease	Signs of CHF (eg, enlarged heart, pulmonary edema) may be present

P waves may be difficult to identify in both ST and SVT once the ventricular rate exceeds 200/min.

Atrial Flutter

Atrial flutter is a narrow-complex tachyarrhythmia that can develop in newborn infants with normal hearts (Figure 46). It also can develop in children with congenital heart disease, especially after cardiac surgery. A reentrant mechanism typically is present in children with enlarged atria or with anatomic barriers resulting from cardiac surgery (eg, atriotomy scars or surgical anastomoses). A reentry circuit within the atria allows a wave of depolarization to travel in a circle within the atria. Because the AV node is not part of the circuit, AV conduction may be variable. The atrial rate can exceed 300/min, whereas the ventricular rate is slower and may be irregular. Classically, a "sawtooth" pattern of the P waves is present on the ECG.

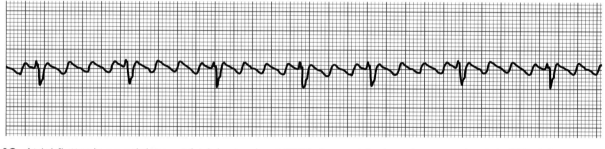

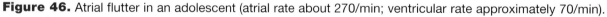

Figure 46. Atrial flutter in an adolescent (atrial rate about 270/min; ventricular rate approximately 70/min).

Ventricular Tachycardia

VT is a wide-QRS-complex tachyarrhythmia generated within the ventricles (Figure 47.) VT is uncommon in children. When VT with pulses is present, the ventricular rate may vary from near normal to greater than 200/min. Rapid ventricular rates compromise ventricular filling, stroke volume, and cardiac output and may deteriorate into pVT or ventricular fibrillation (VF).

Most children who develop VT have underlying heart disease (or have had surgery for heart disease), long QT syndrome, or myocarditis/cardiomyopathy. They may have a family history of a sudden, unexplained death in a child or young adult, suggesting cardiomyopathy or an inherited cardiac ion "channelopathy." Other causes of VT in children include electrolyte disturbances (eg, hyperkalemia, hypocalcemia, hypomagnesemia) and drug toxicity (eg, tricyclic antidepressants, cocaine, methamphetamines).

ECG Characteristics of VT

ECG characteristics of VT include the following:

Ventricular rate	At least 120/min and regular
QRS complex	Wide (>0.09 second)
P waves	Often not identifiable; when present, may not be related to QRS (AV dissociation); at slower rates, atria may be depolarized in a retrograde manner, resulting in a 1:1 ventricular-to-atrial association
T waves	Typically opposite in polarity from QRS

It may be difficult to differentiate SVT with aberrant conduction from VT. Fortunately, aberrant conduction is present in less than 10% of children with SVT. In general, the healthcare provider should initially assume that a wide-complex rhythm is VT unless the child is known to have aberrant conduction or previous episodes of wide-QRS-complex SVT.

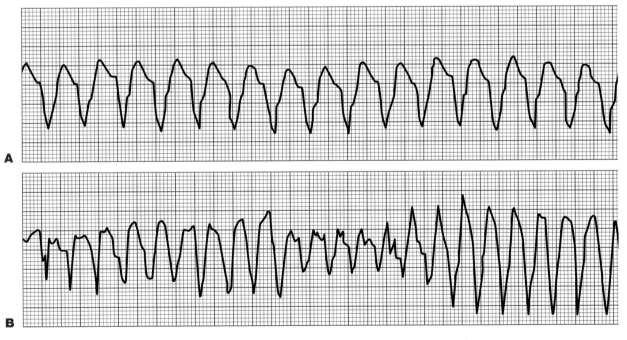

A

B

Figure 47. Ventricular tachycardia; **A,** Monomorphic. **B,** Polymorphic (torsades de pointes).

Polymorphic VT, Including Torsades de Pointes

VT may be monomorphic (QRS complexes are uniform in appearance) or polymorphic (QRS complexes vary in appearance). If the ventricular rate is slow enough, the patient with monomorphic VT can maintain pulses. In contrast, polymorphic VT is typically associated with loss of pulses at onset or within a very short time after onset. Torsades de pointes is a distinctive form of polymorphic VT. The term *torsades de pointes* is French and means "turning on a point." In torsades de pointes, the QRS complexes change in polarity and amplitude, appearing to rotate around the ECG isoelectric line (Figure 47B). The ventricular rate can range from 150 to 250/min. Torsades de pointes can be seen in conditions associated with a prolonged QT interval, including congenital long QT syndrome and drug toxicity. The prolonged QT interval is identified during sinus rhythm; it cannot be evaluated during the tachycardia. A rhythm strip may show the child's baseline QT prolongation because torsades de pointes sometimes occurs in bursts that convert spontaneously to sinus rhythm.

Conditions and agents that predispose to torsades de pointes include

- Long QT syndromes (often congenital and inherited)
- Hypomagnesemia
- Hypokalemia
- Antiarrhythmic drug toxicity (ie, Class IA, quinidine, procainamide, disopyramide; Class IC, encainide, flecainide; Class III, sotalol, amiodarone)
- Other drug toxicities (eg, tricyclic antidepressants, calcium channel blockers, phenothiazines)

It is important to recognize that VT, especially polymorphic VT (including torsades de pointes), can rapidly deteriorate to VF. The long QT syndromes and other inherited arrhythmia syndromes (ie, channelopathies) are associated with sudden death from either primary VF or torsades de pointes. Polymorphic VT not associated with a prolonged QT interval during sinus rhythm is treated as generic VT.

Management of Arrhythmias

Overview

This Part discusses the management of bradycardia (slow heart rate) with a pulse and poor perfusion and tachycardia (fast heart rate) with a palpable pulse and adequate or inadequate perfusion. Providers should quickly treat symptomatic tachyarrhythmias before they result in shock or cardiac arrest.

Learning Objective

After studying this Part, you should be able to

- Describe clinical characteristics of instability in patients with arrhythmias

Preparation for the Course

You will be expected to manage a child as outlined in the algorithms for bradycardia with a pulse and poor perfusion, tachycardia with a pulse and poor perfusion, and tachycardia With a Pulse and Poor Perfusion.

Principles of Management of Pediatric Arrhythmias

Whenever the child has an abnormal heart rate or rhythm, you must quickly determine if the arrhythmia is causing hemodynamic instability or other signs of deterioration. The signs of instability in a patient with arrhythmia include the following:

- Respiratory distress or failure
- Shock with poor end-organ perfusion, which may occur with or without hypotension
- Irritability or a decreased level of consciousness
- Chest pain or a vague feeling of discomfort in older children
- Sudden collapse

Priorities in the initial management of arrhythmias are the same as they are for all critically ill children: support the ABCs—airway, breathing, and circulation—and treat the underlying cause.

Management: Pediatric Bradycardia With a Pulse and Poor Perfusion

The Pediatric Bradycardia With a Pulse and Poor Perfusion Algorithm (Figure 48) outlines the steps for evaluation and management of the child presenting with symptomatic bradycardia (bradycardia with a pulse and poor perfusion). See the Critical Concepts box "Symptomatic Bradycardia and Cardiopulmonary Compromise" in Part 10 for more information about symptomatic bradycardia and cardiopulmonary compromise. In the text that follows, box numbers refer to the corresponding boxes in this algorithm.

Pediatric Bradycardia With a Pulse and Poor Perfusion Algorithm

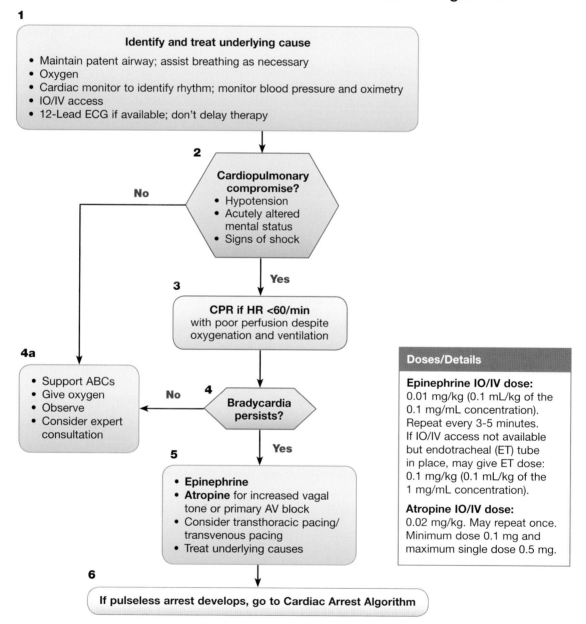

1

Identify and treat underlying cause

- Maintain patent airway; assist breathing as necessary
- Oxygen
- Cardiac monitor to identify rhythm; monitor blood pressure and oximetry
- IO/IV access
- 12-Lead ECG if available; don't delay therapy

2

Cardiopulmonary compromise?
- Hypotension
- Acutely altered mental status
- Signs of shock

No →

Yes ↓

3

CPR if HR <60/min
with poor perfusion despite oxygenation and ventilation

4a
- Support ABCs
- Give oxygen
- Observe
- Consider expert consultation

No ←

4

Bradycardia persists?

Yes ↓

5
- **Epinephrine**
- **Atropine** for increased vagal tone or primary AV block
- Consider transthoracic pacing/ transvenous pacing
- Treat underlying causes

6

If pulseless arrest develops, go to Cardiac Arrest Algorithm

Doses/Details

Epinephrine IO/IV dose:
0.01 mg/kg (0.1 mL/kg of the 0.1 mg/mL concentration). Repeat every 3-5 minutes. If IO/IV access not available but endotracheal (ET) tube in place, may give ET dose: 0.1 mg/kg (0.1 mL/kg of the 1 mg/mL concentration).

Atropine IO/IV dose:
0.02 mg/kg. May repeat once. Minimum dose 0.1 mg and maximum single dose 0.5 mg.

© 2016 American Heart Association

Figure 48. The Pediatric Bradycardia With a Pulse and Poor Perfusion Algorithm.

Identify and Treat Underlying Causes (Box 1)

Once you identify symptomatic bradycardia with cardiopulmonary compromise, initial management may include the following, but priorities are immediate oxygenation and ventilation (Table 84).

Table 84. Management of Symptomatic Bradycardia With Cardiopulmonary Compromise

Airway	Support the airway (position the child or allow the child to assume a position of comfort) or open the airway (perform manual airway maneuver) if needed.
Breathing	• Give O_2 in high concentration—use a nonrebreathing mask if available. • Assist ventilation as indicated (eg, bag-mask ventilation). • Attach a pulse oximeter to assess oxygenation.
Circulation	• Monitor blood pressure and assess perfusion. • Attach a monitor/defibrillator (with transcutaneous pacing capability if available). • Establish vascular access (IV or IO). • Check electrode pad position and skin contact to ensure that there are no artifacts and that the ECG tracing is accurate. • Record a 12-lead ECG if available (do not delay therapy). • Obtain appropriate laboratory studies (eg, potassium, glucose, ionized calcium, magnesium, blood gas for pH, toxicology screen).

A child with primary bradycardia may benefit from evaluation by a pediatric cardiologist. However, do not delay initiation of emergency treatment, including high-quality CPR, if symptoms are present.

Reassess (Box 2)

Reassess to determine if bradycardia and cardiopulmonary compromise continue despite adequate oxygenation and ventilation.

Critical Concepts

Reassess for Cardiopulmonary Compromise

Reassess the child for signs of cardiopulmonary compromise, including

• Hypotension
• Altered mental status: acutely decreased level of consciousness
• Shock: signs of poor perfusion with or without hypotension

Bradycardia and Cardiopulmonary Compromise?	Management
No	Go to Box 4a. Support ABCs as needed, administer supplementary O_2, and perform frequent reassessments. Consider expert consultation.
Yes	Go to Box 3. Perform CPR if heart rate is <60/min with continued signs of poor perfusion, despite adequate oxygenation and ventilation.

If Adequate Respiration and Perfusion (Box 4a)

If pulses, perfusion, and respirations are adequate, no emergency treatment is needed. Monitor and continue evaluation.

If Bradycardia and Cardiopulmonary Compromise Persist, Perform CPR (Box 3)

If bradycardia is associated with cardiopulmonary compromise (Critical Concepts box "Reassess for Cardiopulmonary Compromise") and if heart rate is less than 60/min despite effective oxygenation and ventilation, perform chest compressions and ventilation (CPR). If the bradycardia persists, proceed with medication therapy and possible pacing (Box 5). Reassess the child frequently in response to each therapy provided.

Foundational Facts

Perform High-Quality CPR

During CPR, push fast (100-120 compressions/min), push hard (at least one third the depth of the anteroposterior diameter of the chest or about 2 inches in the child or about 1½ inches in an infant), allow complete chest recoil after each compression, minimize interruptions in chest compressions, and avoid excessive ventilation.

Reassess Rhythm (Box 4)

Reassess to determine if bradycardia and cardiopulmonary compromise continue despite provision of oxygenation, ventilation, and CPR.

Bradycardia and Cardiopulmonary Compromise?	Management
No	Go to Box 4a. Support ABCs as needed, administer supplementary O_2, and perform frequent reassessment. Consider expert consultation.
Yes	Go to Box 5. Administer medications and consider cardiac pacing.

Administer Medications (Box 5)

If bradycardia and cardiopulmonary compromise continue despite oxygenation, ventilation, and CPR, administer epinephrine. Consider atropine.

Epinephrine

Epinephrine is indicated for symptomatic bradycardia that persists despite effective oxygenation and ventilation. Epinephrine has both α- and β-adrenergic activity. β-adrenergic activity increases heart rate and cardiac contractility, and α-adrenergic activity causes vasoconstriction. The effects of epinephrine and other catecholamines may be reduced by acidosis and hypoxia. This makes support of the airway, ventilation, oxygenation, and perfusion (with chest compressions) essential.

Epinephrine	
Route	**Dose**
IV/IO	0.01 mg/kg (0.1 mL/kg)
Endotracheal	0.1 mg/kg (0.1 mL/kg)
Repeat every 3 to 5 minutes as needed	

For persistent bradycardia, consider a continuous infusion of epinephrine (0.1 to 0.3 mcg/kg per minute). A continuous epinephrine infusion may be useful, particularly if the child has responded to a bolus of epinephrine. Titrate the infusion dose to clinical response.

Atropine

Atropine sulfate is a parasympatholytic (or anticholinergic) drug that accelerates sinus or atrial pacemakers and enhances atrioventricular (AV) conduction. Administer atropine instead of epinephrine for bradycardia caused by increased vagal tone, cholinergic drug toxicity (eg, organophosphates), or complete AV block. Atropine (and pacing) are preferred over epinephrine as the first-choice treatment of symptomatic AV block due to primary bradycardia. Atropine is not indicated for AV block from secondary bradycardia (ie, treatable causes such as hypoxia or acidosis). The rationale for using atropine rather than epinephrine in these situations is that epinephrine can cause ventricular arrhythmias if the myocardium is chronically abnormal or hypoxic/ischemic. If the child does not respond to atropine, use epinephrine.

Atropine may be used for the treatment of second-degree AV block (Mobitz types I and II) and third-degree AV block. The healthcare provider should recognize, however, that symptomatic AV block may not respond to atropine and the child may require pacing.

| **Atropine** ||
Route	**Dose**
IV/IO	0.02 mg/kg; minimum 0.1 mg, maximum 0.5 mg
	May repeat dose once, in 5 minutes
	Note: Larger doses may be required for organophosphate poisoning.
ET *Note:* IV/IO administration is preferred, but if it is not available, atropine can be administered by ET tube. Because absorption of atropine given by the endotracheal route is unreliable, a larger dose (2-3 times the IV dose) may be required.	0.04 to 0.06 mg/kg

Tachycardia may follow administration of atropine, but atropine-induced tachycardia is generally well tolerated in the pediatric patient.

Consider Cardiac Pacing (Box 5)

Temporary cardiac pacing may be lifesaving in selected cases of bradycardia caused by complete heart block or abnormal sinus node function. For example, pacing is indicated for AV block after surgical correction of congenital heart disease.

Treat Underlying Causes (Box 5)

Identify and treat potentially reversible causes and special circumstances that can cause bradycardia. The 2 most common potentially reversible causes of bradycardia are hypoxia and increased vagal tone. Be aware that after heart transplantation, sympathetic nerve fibers are no longer attached to the heart, so the response to sympathomimetic drugs may be unpredictable. For the same reason, anticholinergic drugs such as atropine may be ineffective. Early cardiac pacing may be indicated in such patients.

Treat potentially reversible causes of bradycardia as shown in Table 85.

Table 85. Treatment of Causes of Bradycardia

Reversible Cause	**Treatment**
Hypoxia	Give high-concentration supplementary O_2 with assisted ventilation as necessary.
Hydrogen ion (acidosis)	Provide ventilation to treat respiratory acidosis secondary to hypercarbia; consider sodium bicarbonate in severe metabolic acidosis.

(continued)

(continued)

Reversible Cause	Treatment
Hyperkalemia	Restore normal potassium concentration.
Hypothermia	Warm the child as needed, but avoid hyperthermia if the patient has experienced a cardiac arrest.
Heart block	For AV block, consider atropine, chronotropic drugs, and electrical pacing; obtain expert consultation.
Toxins/poisons/drugs	Treat with a specific antidote and provide supportive care. Some toxicologic causes of bradyarrhythmias are • Cholinesterase inhibitors (organophosphates, carbamates, and nerve agents) • Calcium channel blockers • β-adrenergic blockers • Digoxin and other cardiac glycosides • Clonidine and other centrally acting α_2-adrenergic agonists • Opioids • Succinylcholine
Trauma	Head trauma: Bradycardia in a child with head trauma is an ominous sign of high intracranial pressure. Provide oxygenation and ventilation. A brief period of mild hyperventilation may occasionally be used as temporizing rescue therapy in response to signs of impending herniation (eg, irregular respirations or apnea, bradycardia, hypertension, unequal or dilated pupil[s] not responsive to light, decerebrate or decorticate posturing). Obtain immediate expert assistance for relief of increased intracranial pressure.

Pulseless Arrest (Box 6)

If pulseless cardiac arrest develops, start CPR. Proceed according to the Pediatric Cardiac Arrest Algorithm (see "Part 4: Recognition and Management of Cardiac Arrest").

Management of Tachyarrhythmias

Pulseless Arrest (Box 6) Initial Management Questions

Answer the following questions to direct your initial management of a critically ill or injured child with a rapid heart rate:

Does the child have a pulse (or signs of circulation)?

Pulse or Signs of Circulation	Management
Absent	Initiate the Pediatric Cardiac Arrest Algorithm (see "Part 4: Recognition and Management of Cardiac Arrest"). *Note:* Because the accuracy of a pulse check is poor, recognition of cardiac arrest may require that you identify the *absence of signs of circulation* (ie, the child is unresponsive, is not breathing or only gasping). With invasive monitoring of arterial pressure, absence of arterial waveform is observed.
Present	Proceed with one of the tachycardia algorithms.

Is perfusion adequate or poor?

Perfusion	Management
Poor	Follow the Pediatric Tachycardia With a Pulse and Poor Perfusion Algorithm for emergency treatment.
Adequate	Follow the Pediatric Tachycardia With a Pulse and Adequate Perfusion Algorithm. Consider consulting a pediatric cardiologist.

Is the QRS complex narrow or wide?

Rhythm	Management
Narrow complex (≤0.09 second)	Consider the differential of sinus tachycardia vs supraventricular tachycardia.
Wide complex (>0.09 second)	Consider the differential of supraventricular tachycardia vs VT, but treat as presumed VT unless the child has known aberrant conduction.

Initial Management Priorities

As soon as you recognize a tachyarrhythmia in an infant or child, assess for signs of hypotension, altered mental status, shock (ie, poor perfusion), or life-threatening hemodynamic instability. Initial management priorities include the following:

- Support the ABCs and oxygenation as needed.
- Establish monitoring: attach monitor/defibrillator and pulse oximeter.
- Establish vascular access.
- Obtain a 12-lead ECG (but do not delay urgent intervention).
- Obtain laboratory studies (eg, potassium, glucose, ionized calcium, magnesium, blood gas to assess pH and cause of pH changes) as appropriate. *Note:* Do not delay urgent intervention for these studies.
- Assess neurologic status.
- Anticipate the need for medications depending on the type of rhythm disturbance (ie, supraventricular vs ventricular).
- Simultaneously try to identify and treat reversible causes.

Do Not Delay Emergency Treatment for Tachycardia

Seek expert consultation from a pediatric cardiologist for evaluation of children with tachyarrhythmias. However, do not delay emergency treatment.

Emergency Interventions

Specific emergency interventions used to treat tachyarrhythmias with pulses are dictated by the severity of the child's condition. Treatments also vary based on the width of the observed QRS complex (narrow vs wide). Interventions may include the following:

- Vagal maneuvers (if the child with a narrow-complex tachycardia is stable or while preparations are made for synchronized cardioversion)
- Cardioversion
- Medication therapy
- Other interventions

Vagal Maneuvers

In normal infants and children, the heart rate decreases when the vagus nerve is stimulated. In patients with supraventricular tachycardia (SVT), vagal stimulation may terminate the tachycardia by slowing conduction through the AV node. Several maneuvers can stimulate vagal activity. The success rates of these maneuvers in terminating tachyarrhythmias vary, depending on the child's age, level of cooperation, and underlying condition.

Critical Concepts

Vagal Maneuvers

Ice to the face is a vagal maneuver that can be performed in infants and children of all ages (Figure 49). Fill a small plastic bag with a mixture of ice and water. Apply it to the upper half of the child's face for 15 to 20 seconds. Do not occlude the nose or mouth.

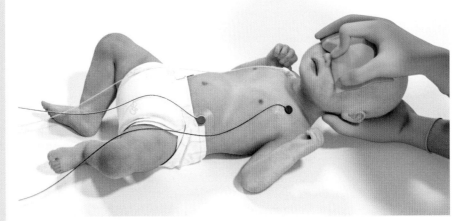

Figure 49. Vagal maneuvers. Ice water is applied to the upper half of the infant's face for vagal stimulation in an attempt to terminate SVT. Note that the bag of ice water does not cover the nose or mouth and does not obstruct ventilation.

- Children old enough to cooperate can perform a Valsalva maneuver by blowing through a narrow straw
- Carotid sinus massage may also be performed safely and easily in older children
- Do not use ocular pressure because it may produce retinal injury

Be sure to support the child's airway, breathing, and circulation. If possible, obtain a 12-lead ECG before and after the maneuver; record and monitor the ECG continuously during the maneuver. *If the child is stable* and the rhythm does not convert, you may repeat the attempt. If the second attempt fails, select another method or provide medication therapy. *If the child is unstable,* attempt vagal maneuvers only while making preparations for pharmacologic or electrical cardioversion. Do not delay definitive treatment to perform vagal maneuvers.

Cardioversion

Electrical cardioversion is painful. Whenever possible, establish vascular access and provide procedural sedation and analgesia before cardioversion, especially in a hemodynamically stable infant or child. If the child's condition is unstable, do not delay synchronized cardioversion to achieve vascular access. Sedation in the setting of an arrhythmia carries increased risk. When procedural sedation is given in this setting, providers must carefully select medications to minimize hemodynamic effects.

The next section discusses the following important concepts about cardioversion:

- Definition of synchronized cardioversion
- Potential problems with synchronized shocks
- Indications for the use of synchronized cardioversion
- Energy doses

Synchronized Cardioversion

Manual defibrillators are capable of delivering both unsynchronized and synchronized shocks. If the shock is unsynchronized, it is delivered at any time in the cardiac cycle. Unsynchronized shocks are used for defibrillation because the cardiac arrest rhythms have no QRS. Synchronized shocks are used for cardioversion from SVT and VT with a pulse. If the shock is synchronized, shock delivery is timed to coincide with the R wave of the patient's QRS complex. The goal is to prevent VF that could result from delivery of the shock during the vulnerable period of the T wave. When you press the shock button to deliver a synchronized shock, the defibrillator/cardioverter may seem to pause before it delivers a shock because it is waiting to synchronize shock delivery with the next QRS complex. See the Critical Concepts box "Cardioversion (for Unstable SVT or VT With a Pulse)" later in this Part for a description of the procedure.

Potential problems: In theory, synchronization is simple. The operator pushes the sync button on the defibrillator, charges the device, and delivers the shock. However, in practice there can be potential problems, such as

- In most units, the sync button must be activated each time synchronized cardioversion is attempted. Most devices will default to an unsynchronized shock immediately after delivery of a synchronized shock.
- If the R waves of a tachycardia are undifferentiated or of low amplitude, the monitor sensors may be unable to identify them and therefore will not deliver the shock. If this occurs, increase the gain of the ECG lead being monitored or select a different ECG lead.
- Synchronization may take extra time (eg, if it is necessary to attach separate ECG electrodes or if the operator is unfamiliar with the equipment).

Indications: Synchronized cardioversion is used for

- Hemodynamically unstable patients (poor perfusion, hypotension, or heart failure) with tachyarrhythmias (SVT, atrial flutter, VT), but with palpable pulses
- Elective cardioversion, under the direction of a pediatric cardiologist, for children with hemodynamically stable SVT, atrial flutter, or VT with a pulse

Energy dose: In general, cardioversion requires less energy than defibrillation does. Start with an energy dose of 0.5 to 1 J/kg for cardioversion of SVT or VT with a pulse. If the initial dose is ineffective, increase the dose to 2 J/kg. The experienced provider may increase the shock dose more gradually (eg, 0.5 J/kg, and then 1 J/kg, followed by 2 J/kg for subsequent doses). If the rhythm does not convert to sinus rhythm, reevaluate the diagnosis of SVT vs sinus tachycardia (ST).

Critical Concepts

Cardioversion (for Unstable SVT or VT With a Pulse)

Consider expert consultation for suspected VT.

1. Turn on defibrillator.

2. Set *lead switch* to *paddles* (or *lead I, II,* or *III* if monitor leads are used).

3. Select adhesive pads or paddles. Use the largest pads or paddles that can fit on the patient's chest without touching each other.

4. If using paddles, apply conductive gel or paste. Be sure cables are attached to defibrillator.

5. Consider sedation.

6. Select *synchronized* mode.

7. Look for markers on R waves indicating that *sync* mode is operative. If necessary, adjust monitor gain until sync markers occur with each R wave.

8. Select energy dose:
   Initial dose: 0.5 to 1 J/kg
   Subsequent doses: 2 J/kg

9. Announce "Charging defibrillator," and press *charge* on defibrillator controls or apex paddle.

10. When defibrillator is fully charged, state firm chant, such as "I am going to shock on three." Then count. "All clear!"

11. After confirming all personnel are clear of the patient, press the *shock* button on the defibrillator or press both paddle *discharge* buttons simultaneously. Hold paddles in place until shock is delivered.

12. Check the monitor. If tachycardia persists, prepare to attempt cardioversion again.

13. Reset the *sync* mode and increase the energy dose. You must reset the *sync* mode after each synchronized cardioversion, because most defibrillators default back to unsynchronized mode after delivery of a synchronized shock. This default allows an immediate defibrillation (nonsynchronized) shock if the cardioversion produces VF.

Note: If VF develops, immediately begin CPR and prepare to deliver an unsynchronized shock as soon as possible. See the Critical Concepts box "Manual Defibrillation (for VF or pVT)" in Part 4.

Medication Therapy

Table 86 reviews common agents used in the management of tachyarrhythmias.

Table 86. Medication Therapy Used in the Pediatric Tachycardia With a Pulse and Adequate Perfusion and Pediatric Tachycardia With a Pulse and Poor Perfusion Algorithms

Drug	Indications/Precautions	Dosage/Administration
Adenosine	**Indications** • Drug of choice for the treatment of SVT • Effective for SVT caused by reentry at the AV node (both accessory pathway and AV nodal reentry mechanisms) • May be helpful in distinguishing atrial flutter from SVT • Not effective for treatment of atrial flutter, atrial fibrillation, or tachycardias caused by mechanisms other than reentry through the AV node **Mechanism of Action** • Blocks conduction through the AV node temporarily (for about 10 seconds) **Precautions** • A common cause of adenosine cardioversion "failure" is that the drug is administered too slowly or with inadequate IV flush. • A brief period (10-15 seconds) of bradycardia (asystole or third-degree heart block) may ensue after administration of adenosine (Figure 50); consider warning caregiver and patient, if age appropriate, that bradycardia can be very uncomfortable.	**Dose** • With continuous ECG monitoring, administer 0.1 mg/kg (maximum initial dose 6 mg) as a rapid IV bolus. • If the drug is effective, the rhythm will convert to sinus rhythm within 15 to 30 seconds of administration (Figure 50). • If there is no effect, give 1 dose of 0.2 mg/kg (maximum second dose 12 mg); this dose is more likely to be needed when the drug is administered into a peripheral (rather than central) vein. • Decrease the initial dose by approximately 75% for patients receiving carbamazepine or dipyridamole or those with transplanted hearts (see Thajudeen et al. *J Am Heart Assoc.* 2012;1:e001461 in the Suggested Reading List on the Student Website for details). **Administration** • Because adenosine has a short half-life (<10 seconds), administer as rapidly as possible. • The drug is rapidly taken up by vascular endothelial cells and red blood cells and metabolized by an enzyme on the surface of red blood cells (adenosine deaminase). • To enhance delivery to the site of action in the heart, use a rapid flush technique (5-10 mL normal saline). • Adenosine may be given by the IO route.

(continued)

(continued)

Drug	Indications/Precautions	Dosage/Administration
Amiodarone	**Indications** • Effective for the treatment of a wide variety of atrial and ventricular tachyarrhythmias in children • May be considered in the treatment of hemodynamically stable SVT refractory to vagal maneuvers and adenosine • Safe and effective for hemodynamically unstable VT in children **Mechanism of Action** • Inhibits α-and β-adrenergic receptors, producing vasodilation and AV nodal suppression (this slows conduction through the AV node) • Inhibits the outward potassium current so it prolongs the QT duration • Inhibits sodium channels, which slows conduction in the ventricles and prolongs QRS duration **Precautions** • Drug effects may be beneficial in some patients but may also increase the risk for polymorphic VT (torsades de pointes) by prolonging the QT interval. • Rare but significant acute side effects of amiodarone include bradycardia, hypotension, and polymorphic VT. • Use with caution if hepatic failure is present. • Because the pharmacology of amiodarone is complex, and it has slow and incomplete oral absorption, long half-life, and potential for long-term adverse effects, a pediatric cardiologist or similarly experienced provider should direct long-term amiodarone therapy.	**Dose** • For supraventricular and ventricular arrhythmias with poor perfusion, a loading dose of 5 mg/kg infused over 20 to 60 minutes is recommended (maximum single dose: 300 mg). Because this drug can cause hypotension and decrease cardiac contractility, a slower rate of delivery is recommended for treatment of a perfusing rhythm than for cardiac arrest. Providers must weigh the potential for causing hypotension against the need to achieve a rapid drug effect. • Repeat doses of 5 mg/kg may be given up to a maximum of 15 mg/kg per day as needed (should not exceed the maximum recommended adult cumulative daily dose of 2.2 g over 24 hours). **Administration** • Rapid administration of amiodarone may cause vasodilation and hypotension; it may also cause heart block or polymorphic VT. • Monitor blood pressure frequently during administration. • Seek expert consultation when using amiodarone. • Routine use of amiodarone in combination with another agent that prolongs the QT interval (eg, procainamide) is not recommended.

(continued)

(continued)

Drug	Indications/Precautions	Dosage/Administration
Procainamide	**Indications** • Can be used to treat a wide range of atrial and ventricular arrhythmias in children, including SVT and VT • Can terminate SVT that is resistant to other drugs • May be considered for treatment of hemodynamically stable SVT refractory to vagal maneuvers and adenosine • Effective in the treatment of atrial flutter and atrial fibrillation • May be used to treat or suppress VT **Mechanism of Action** • Blocks sodium channels so it prolongs the effective refractory period of both the atria and ventricles and depresses conduction velocity within the conduction system • By slowing intraventricular conduction, prolongs QT, QRS, and PR intervals **Precautions** • Paradoxically shortens the effective refractory period of the AV node and increases AV nodal conduction; may cause increased heart rate when used to treat ectopic atrial tachycardia and atrial fibrillation • Can cause hypotension in children through its potent vasodilator effect • Reduce dose for patients with poor renal or cardiac function	**Dose** • Infuse a loading dose of 15 mg/kg over 30 to 60 minutes with continuous ECG monitoring and frequent blood pressure monitoring. **Administration** • Procainamide must be given by slow infusion to avoid toxicity from heart block, hypotension, and prolongation of the QT interval (which predisposes to VT or torsades de pointes). • Monitor blood pressure frequently during administration. • Procainamide, like amiodarone, may increase the risk of polymorphic VT (torsades de pointes). • Routine use of procainamide in combination with another agent (eg, amiodarone) that prolongs the QT interval is not recommended without expert consultation. **Other** • Seek expert consultation when using procainamide. • Despite a long history of use, there are limited data in children comparing the effectiveness of procainamide with other antiarrhythmic agents.

Other Interventions

Many other interventions (eg, digoxin, short-acting β-blockers, overdrive pacing) have been used for treatment of SVT in children but should be reserved for expert consultation.

Verapamil, a calcium channel blocking agent, *should not be used routinely* to treat SVT in infants because refractory hypotension and cardiac arrest have been reported after administration. Use verapamil with caution in children because it may cause hypotension and myocardial depression. If using verapamil in children 1 year or older, infuse the drug in a dose of 0.1 mg/kg (up to 5 mg) over at least 2 minutes with continuous ECG monitoring.

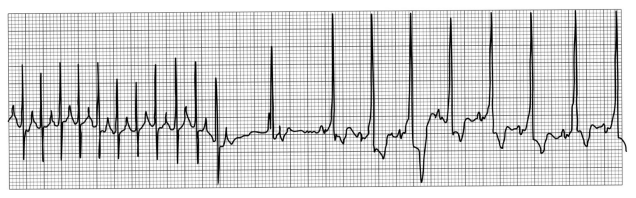

Figure 50. SVT converting to sinus rhythm with administration of adenosine.

Summary of Emergency Interventions

The specific emergency interventions listed in Table 87 are used to treat tachyarrhythmias with pulses, based on the width of the observed QRS complex (narrow vs wide).

Table 87. Emergency Interventions for Tachyarrhythmias With Pulses

Intervention	Narrow-Complex Tachyarrhythmia	Wide-Complex Tachyarrhythmia
Vagal maneuvers	Used for SVT	Used for SVT
Synchronized cardioversion	Used for • SVT • Atrial flutter (seek expert consultation)	Used for VT with palpable pulses
Medication therapy	Used for SVT: • Adenosine • Amiodarone (seek expert consultation) • Procainamide (seek expert consultation) • Verapamil for children ≥1 year of age (seek expert consultation) Drugs used for other SVT with a pulse (eg, atrial flutter): Seek expert consultation	Used for VT with palpable pulses: • Amiodarone (seek expert consultation) • Procainamide (seek expert consultation) • Lidocaine Drug used for torsades de pointes: • Magnesium Drugs used for SVT with abnormal/aberrant intraventricular conduction: • Adenosine • Amiodarone (seek expert consultation) • Procainamide (seek expert consultation)

Pediatric Tachycardia With a Pulse and Adequate Perfusion Algorithm

The Pediatric Tachycardia With a Pulse and Adequate Perfusion Algorithm (Figure 51) outlines the steps for assessment and management of a child presenting with symptomatic tachycardia and adequate perfusion. Box numbers in the text refer to the corresponding boxes in the algorithm.

Pediatric Tachycardia With a Pulse and Adequate Perfusion Algorithm

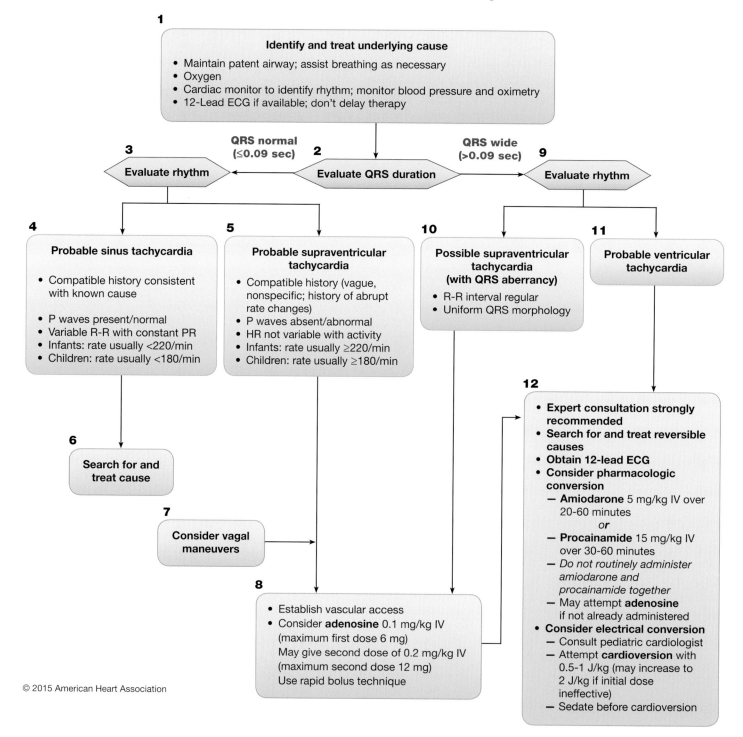

© 2015 American Heart Association

Figure 51. The Pediatric Tachycardia With a Pulse and Adequate Perfusion Algorithm.

Initial Management (Box 1)

When systemic perfusion is adequate, you have more time to evaluate the rhythm and the child. Begin the initial management steps, which may include the following:

- Assess and support the airway, oxygenation, and ventilation as needed
- If O_2 is needed, provide it with a nonrebreathing mask
- Evaluate the presence and strength of peripheral pulses
- Attach a continuous ECG monitor/defibrillator and a pulse oximeter
- Obtain a 12-lead ECG if practical

Evaluate QRS Duration (Box 2)

Evaluate QRS duration to determine the type of arrhythmia.

QRS Duration	Probable Arrhythmia	Proceed in Algorithm
Normal/narrow (≤0.09 second)	ST or SVT	Boxes 3, 4, 5, 6, 7, 8
Wide (>0.09 second)	Probable VT vs SVT with aberrant conduction	Boxes 9, 10, 11, 12

Normal QRS: ST or SVT? (Boxes 3-5)

If QRS duration is normal (0.09 second or less) (Box 3), evaluate the rhythm and try *to determine if the rhythm represents ST or SVT.*

Signs and symptoms consistent with ST (Box 4) include the following:

- History is compatible with ST, consistent with a known cause (eg, the child has fever, dehydration, pain).
- P waves are present and normal.
- Heart rate varies with activity or stimulation.
- R-R is variable, but PR is constant.
- Heart rate is less than 220/min in an infant or less than 180/min in a child.

Signs and symptoms consistent with SVT (Box 5) include the following:

- There is a history of vague or nonspecific symptoms or palpitations, sudden onset, no history compatible with ST (eg, no fever, dehydration, or other identifiable cause of ST).
- P waves are absent or abnormal.
- Heart rate does not vary with activity or stimulation.
- Heart rate is 220/min or greater in an infant or 180/min or greater in a child.

Treatment of ST (Box 6)

Treatment of ST is directed at the cause of ST. Because ST is a clinical sign of a problem, don't attempt to decrease the heart rate by pharmacologic or electrical interventions. Instead, search for and treat the cause. Continuous ECG monitoring will confirm a decrease in heart rate to more normal levels if treatment of the underlying cause is effective.

Treat Cause of SVT (Boxes 7 and 8)

Vagal Maneuvers

Consider vagal maneuvers (Box 7). In the stable patient with SVT, try the following:

- Place a bag with ice water over the upper half of the infant's face (without obstructing the airway)
- Ask an older child to try to blow through an obstructed straw
- Perform carotid sinus massage in older children

Monitor and record the ECG continuously before, during, and after attempted vagal maneuvers. If the maneuvers fail, they can be attempted a second time. Do not apply ocular pressure. For more information, see the Critical Concepts box "Vagal Maneuvers" in this Part.

Adenosine

For SVT resistant to vagal maneuvers, establish vascular access and administer adenosine (Box 8). Adenosine is the drug of choice for most common forms of SVT caused by a reentrant pathway involving the AV node.

Adenosine	
Route	**Dose**
IV/IO	0.1 mg/kg (maximum first dose 6 mg)
	If the first dose is ineffective, you may give 1 dose of 0.2 mg/kg (maximum second dose 12 mg).

Use a rapid bolus with a *rapid flush* 2-syringe technique (5-10 mL normal saline).

Wide QRS, Possible VT vs SVT (Boxes 9, 10, and 11)

If QRS duration is wide (greater than 0.09 second), the rhythm is either VT or, less likely, SVT with aberrant intraventricular conduction. In infants and children, treat wide-complex tachycardia as presumed VT unless the child is known to have aberrant conduction.

If the wide QRS-complex tachyarrhythmia has a uniform QRS morphology and regular R-R interval and the child remains hemodynamically stable, consider giving a dose of adenosine (Box 9). If the arrhythmia is VT, adenosine will not be effective but will do no harm. Adenosine is effective in the unusual situation of SVT with aberrancy.

Pharmacologic Conversion vs Electrical Conversion (Box 12)

If a child with a wide-complex tachycardia is hemodynamically stable, early consultation with a pediatric cardiologist or other provider with appropriate expertise is strongly recommended.

Pharmacologic Conversion

Establish vascular access and consider administering *one* of the following medications:

Medication	Route	Dosage and Administration
Amiodarone	IV/IO	5 mg/kg over 20 to 60 minutes
Procainamide	IV/IO	15 mg/kg over 30 to 60 minutes

Seek expert consultation when giving amiodarone or procainamide. Do not routinely administer amiodarone and procainamide together or with other medications that prolong the QT interval. If these initial efforts do not terminate the rapid rhythm, reevaluate the rhythm.

If not already administered, consider adenosine, because a wide-complex tachycardia could be SVT with aberrant ventricular conduction (Box 12).

Electrical Cardioversion

If SVT or a wide-complex tachycardia does not respond to medication therapy and the child remains hemodynamically stable, it is best to consult a pediatric cardiologist before proceeding with synchronized cardioversion. Base the decision of whether to proceed on the provider's experience. If you proceed with synchronized cardioversion, administer a sedative and analgesic. After the child is sedated, start with an energy dose of 0.5 to 1 J/kg. If the initial dose is ineffective, increase the dose to 2 J/kg. An experienced provider may increase the shock dose more gradually (eg, 0.5 J/kg, and then 1 J/kg, and then all remaining shocks at 2 J/kg). *Record and monitor the ECG before, during, and after each cardioversion attempt.* Obtain a 12-lead ECG after cardioversion.

Pediatric Tachycardia With a Pulse and Poor Perfusion Algorithm

The Pediatric Tachycardia With a Pulse and Poor Perfusion Algorithm (Figure 52) outlines the steps for assessment and management of the child presenting with symptomatic tachycardia and poor perfusion. Box numbers in the text refer to the corresponding boxes in the algorithm.

Pediatric Tachycardia With a Pulse and Poor Perfusion Algorithm

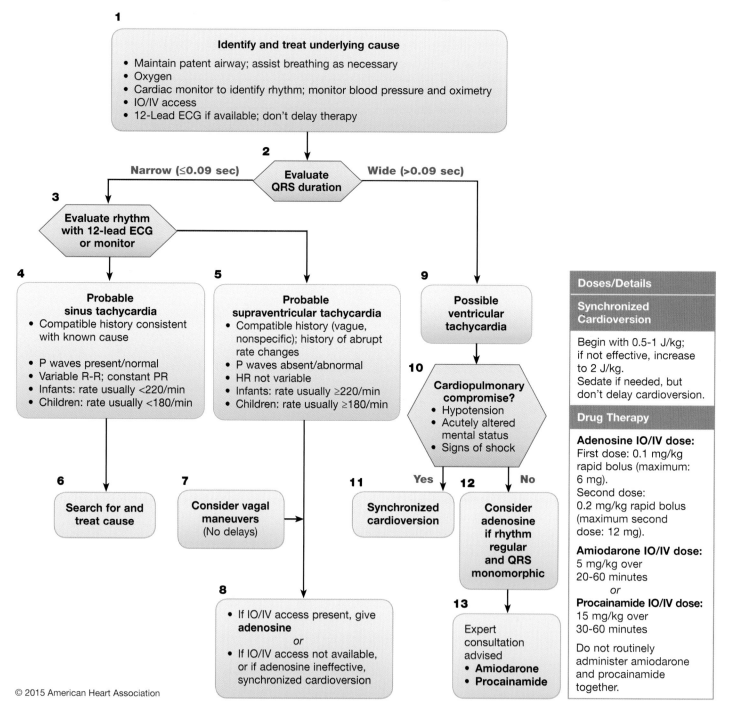

© 2015 American Heart Association

Figure 52. The Pediatric Tachycardia With a Pulse and Poor Perfusion Algorithm.

Initial Management (Box 1)

In a child with tachycardia and palpable pulses but signs of hemodynamic compromise (ie, poor perfusion, weak pulses), begin initial management steps (Box 1) while attempting to identify and correct the underlying cause. Initial management interventions may include the following:

- Maintain open/patent airway, assist breathing, and provide O_2 as needed
- Attach monitors for cardiac rhythm, O_2 saturation, and blood pressure
- Establish IV/IO access
- Obtain a 12-lead ECG if available and if it does not delay other care

Evaluate QRS Duration (Box 2)

Quickly evaluate QRS duration to determine the type of arrhythmia. Although a 12-lead ECG may be useful, initial therapy does not require precise ECG diagnosis of the tachyarrhythmia causing poor perfusion. You can measure QRS width from a rhythm strip.

QRS Duration	Probable Arrhythmia	Proceed in Algorithm
Normal (≤**0.09 second**)	ST or SVT	Boxes 3, 4, 5, 6, 7, 8
Wide (>**0.09 second**)	VT	Boxes 9, 10, 11, 12, 13

Normal QRS: ST or SVT? (Boxes 3-5)

If QRS duration is normal, evaluate the rhythm and try to *determine if the rhythm represents ST or SVT* (Box 3).

- Signs and symptoms consistent with ST (Box 4) include the following:
- History is compatible with ST or consistent with a known cause (eg, the child has fever, dehydration, pain)
- P waves are present and normal
- Heart rate varies with activity or stimulation
- R-R is variable, but PR is constant
- Heart rate is less than 220/min in an infant or less than 180/min in a child

Signs and symptoms consistent with SVT (Box 5) include the following:

- History of vague or nonspecific symptoms or palpitations, sudden onset, no history compatible with ST (eg, no fever, dehydration, or other identifiable cause of ST)
- P waves are absent or abnormal
- Heart rate does not vary with activity or stimulation
- Heart rate is 220/min or greater in an infant or 180/min or greater in a child

Treat Cause of ST (Box 6)

Treatment of ST is directed at the cause of ST. Because ST is a clinical sign of a problem, do not attempt to decrease the heart rate by pharmacologic or electrical interventions. Instead, search for and treat the cause. Continuous ECG monitoring will confirm a decrease in heart rate to more normal levels if treatment of the underlying cause is effective.

Treatment of SVT (Boxes 7 and 8)

Vagal Maneuvers

Consider vagal maneuvers (Box 7) only while making preparations for pharmacologic or electrical cardioversion. Do not delay definitive treatment to perform vagal maneuvers.

- Place a bag of ice water over the upper half of the infant's face (without obstructing the nose or mouth)
- Have a child try to blow through an obstructed straw
- Perform carotid sinus massage in older children

Monitor and record the ECG continuously before, during, and after these attempted vagal maneuvers. Do not apply ocular pressure. For more information, see the Critical Concepts box "Vagal Maneuvers" earlier in this Part.

Adenosine

If vascular access (IV/IO) and medications are readily available, administer adenosine (Box 8).

Adenosine	
Route	**Dose**
IV/IO	0.1 mg/kg (maximum first dose 6 mg)
	If the first dose is ineffective, you may give 1 dose of 0.2 mg/kg (maximum second dose 12 mg).

Use a rapid bolus with a *rapid flush* 2-syringe technique (5-10 mL normal saline).

Synchronized Cardioversion (Box 8)

If IV/IO access is not readily available or if adenosine is ineffective, attempt synchronized cardioversion. Provide procedural sedation if it will not delay cardioversion. Start with an energy dose of 0.5 to 1 J/kg. If the initial dose is ineffective, increase the dose to 2 J/kg. An experienced provider may increase the shock dose more gradually (eg, 0.5 J/kg, and then 1 J/kg, then followed by 2 J/kg). *Record and monitor the ECG continuously before, during, and immediately after each cardioversion attempt.*

If neither intervention is effective, proceed to Box 13. It is advisable to obtain expert consultation before using amiodarone or procainamide.

Wide QRS, Possible VT (Box 9)

If QRS duration is wide (greater than 0.09 second), treat the rhythm as presumed VT unless the child is known to have aberrant conduction (Box 9).

Treatment of Wide-Complex Tachycardia With Poor Perfusion (Box 13)

Treat a wide-complex tachycardia with pulses but poor perfusion urgently with synchronized cardioversion, using a starting energy dose of 0.5 to 1 J/kg. Increase the dose to 2 J/kg if the initial dose is ineffective. An experienced provider may increase the shock dose more gradually (eg, 0.5 J/kg, and then 1 J/kg, followed by 2 J/kg). If possible, provide sedation and analgesia before cardioversion, but do not delay cardioversion if the child is hemodynamically unstable. Selection and administration of sedatives require expertise to avoid creating or worsening hemodynamic instability.

Because a wide-complex tachycardia could also represent SVT with aberrant intraventricular conduction, consider giving a dose of adenosine first *if it does not delay cardioversion*. Adenosine is not effective but will do no harm if the tachyarrhythmia is VT; adenosine is effective in the unusual situation of SVT with aberrancy.

Refractory Wide-Complex Tachycardia (Box 13)

If a wide-complex tachycardia is refractory to cardioversion, consultation with a pediatric cardiologist is strongly recommended before using amiodarone or procainamide.

Consider administration of *one* of the following medications:

Medication	Route	Dosage and Administration
Amiodarone	IV/IO	5 mg/kg over 20 to 60 minutes
Procainamide	IV/IO	15 mg/kg over 30 to 60 minutes

Amiodarone or procainamide can be used for the treatment of wide-complex SVT (unresponsive to adenosine) and VT in children. Both medications must be given by a slow (amiodarone over 20 to 60 minutes, procainamide over 30 to 60 minutes) IV infusion with careful monitoring of blood pressure. Do not routinely administer amiodarone and procainamide together or with other medications that prolong the QT interval.

Part 12

Post–Cardiac Arrest Care

Overview

As soon as return of spontaneous circulation (ROSC) develops after cardiac arrest or resuscitation from severe shock or respiratory failure, a systematic approach to assessment and support of the respiratory, cardiovascular, and neurologic systems and targeted temperature management is critical. Although effective resuscitation is a major focus of the PALS Provider Course, ultimate outcome is often determined by the subsequent care the child receives. This includes safe transport to a center with expertise in caring for seriously ill or injured children.

One objective of optimal post–cardiac arrest care is to avoid common causes of both early and late morbidity and mortality. Early mortality can be caused by hemodynamic instability and respiratory complications. Late morbidity and mortality can result from multiorgan failure or brain injury or both.

The extent of post–cardiac arrest evaluation and management is influenced by the PALS provider's scope of practice and available resources.

Learning Objective

After completing this Part, you should be able to

- Implement post–cardiac arrest care

Preparation for the Course

During the course you will learn about the phases of post–cardiac arrest care. This will include optimizing oxygenation, ventilation, and perfusion, stabilizing cardiopulmonary function, and providing neurologic care, including targeted temperature management.

Goals of Therapy

For optimal post–cardiac arrest care, identify and treat organ system dysfunction. This includes

- Providing adequate oxygenation and ventilation
- Supporting tissue perfusion and cardiovascular function
- Avoiding hypotension
- Correcting acid-base and electrolyte imbalances
- Maintaining adequate glucose concentration
- Providing targeted temperature management: avoiding hyperthermia and considering need for therapeutic hypothermia
- Ensuring adequate analgesia and sedation

Post–cardiac arrest management consists of 2 general phases to stabilize the child.

The first phase is immediate post–cardiac arrest management. During this phase you will continue to provide advanced life support for immediate life-threatening conditions and focus on the ABCs:

- **A**irway and **B**reathing: Assess and support airway, oxygenation, and ventilation. At this time, you will typically use diagnostic equipment and assessments—such as monitoring end-tidal CO_2 by capnography, arterial blood gas analysis, and chest x-ray—to further establish the adequacy of oxygenation and ventilation and to confirm endotracheal (ET) tube position in the mid-trachea.
- **C**irculation: Assess and maintain adequate blood pressure and perfusion. Treat arrhythmias. Diagnostic assessments—such as lactate concentration, venous O_2 saturation, and base deficit—provide information on adequacy of tissue perfusion. As you proceed with evaluation, identify and treat any reversible or contributing causes of the arrest or critical illness.

In the second phase of post–cardiac arrest management, provide broader multiorgan supportive care, including targeted temperature management. After the child is stabilized, coordinate transfer or transport to a tertiary care setting as appropriate.

Primary Goals

The primary goals of post–cardiac arrest management are to

- Optimize and stabilize airway, oxygenation, ventilation, and cardiopulmonary function with emphasis on restoring and maintaining vital organ perfusion and function (especially of the brain)
- Prevent secondary organ injury
- Identify and treat the cause of acute illness
- Institute measures that may improve long-term, neurologically intact survival
- Minimize the risk of deterioration of the child during transport to the next level of care

Systemic Approach

Assess the child by using the Systematic Approach (see "Part 3: Systematic Approach to the Seriously Ill or Injured Child"). In addition to repeated *primary assessments,* your evaluation will often include the secondary assessment as well as diagnostic assessments. The *secondary assessment* is a review of patient history and a focused physical examination. *Diagnostic assessments* include invasive and noninvasive monitoring and appropriate laboratory and nonlaboratory tests.

This Part discusses evaluation and management of the following systems during the post–cardiac arrest period:

- Respiratory system
- Cardiovascular system
- Neurologic system

Respiratory System

Management Priorities

Continue to monitor and support the child's airway, oxygenation, and ventilation. Look for clinical signs and objective measurements of adequate oxygenation and ventilation. (See "Part 6: Recognition of Respiratory Distress and Failure" for more information on assessment of the respiratory system.) During resuscitation, high-flow O_2, inhaled medications, and ET intubation may be required. In the post–cardiac arrest phase, elective intubation may be appropriate to achieve airway control and support the child during diagnostic studies, such as a computed tomography scan. If the child is being manually ventilated, transition to mechanical ventilation.

The goals of respiratory management in the immediate post–cardiac arrest period are listed in Table 88.

Table 88. Goals of Respiratory Management in Immediate Post–Cardiac Arrest Period

Goal	Considerations
Maintain adequate oxygenation (generally an O_2 saturation ≥94% but <100%) to reduce the risk of reperfusion injury	Once ROSC is achieved, titrate O_2 administration to target normoxemia while ensuring that hypoxemia is strictly avoided. Maintain an O_2 saturation ≥94%, avoiding hypoxemia, but <100%, to avoid hyperoxia (an O_2 saturation of 100% can correspond to a Po_2 of anywhere between 80 and approximately 500 mm Hg). Determining optimal Pao_2 and O_2 saturation requires evaluation of the child's arterial O_2 content, as it is an important determinant of tissue O_2 delivery. If the child is anemic, tissue O_2 delivery may be better maintained by achieving a high Pao_2 and O_2 saturation. In comparison, an O_2 saturation ≥94% but <100% is typically adequate in a child with a normal hemoglobin concentration and normal O_2 consumption and no cyanotic heart disease. Thus, oxygen is titrated to a value appropriate to the specific patient condition.
Maintain adequate ventilation and $Paco_2$ appropriate to the patient	It is reasonable to target a $Paco_2$ that is appropriate to each child's clinical condition and to limit exposure to severe hyper- or hypocapnia. For example, for most patients with neurologic injury, a normal $Paco_2$ is desirable to avoid hypocapnia (hypocarbia) or hypercapnia (hypercarbia). However, in children with asthma and respiratory failure, rapid correction of hypercarbia is unnecessary. Conversely, in children with congenital heart disease and pulmonary hypertension, hypercarbia must be avoided. Efforts to achieve normocarbia with mechanical ventilation in a child with asthma could result in complications such as pneumothorax.

General Recommendations

General recommendations for assessment and management of the respiratory system may include those listed in Table 89.

Table 89. General Recommendations for Assessment and the Management of the Respiratory System

Assessment and Management of the Respiratory System	
Assessment	

Monitoring	• Continuously monitor the following parameters (at a minimum):
	  – SpO_2 and heart rate by pulse oximetry (compare pulse oximetry heart rate with ECG and pulse rate to ensure that pulse oximeter values are accurate)
	  – Heart rate and rhythm
	  – If the patient is intubated, monitor end-tidal CO_2 by capnography if equipment and expertise are available, or intermittently confirm exhaled CO_2 by colorimetric device. Always monitor exhaled CO_2 by either capnography or colorimetric device during intrahospital and interhospital transport to aid in immediate detection of inadvertent extubation.
	• If the child is already intubated, verify tube position, openness/patency, and security.
	• After proper tube position is confirmed, ensure that the tube is well taped and that tube position at the lip or gum is documented.
	Providers must use both clinical assessment and confirmatory devices (such as monitoring of exhaled CO_2) to verify proper tube placement immediately after intubation, during transport, and when the child is moved (eg, from gurney to bed).

Physical examination	• Observe for adequate and equal chest rise bilaterally and auscultate for abnormal or asymmetric breath sounds. • Monitor for evidence of respiratory compromise (eg, tachypnea, increased work of breathing, agitation, decreased responsiveness, poor air exchange, cyanosis) or inadequate respiratory effort.
Laboratory tests	• Obtain an arterial sample for arterial blood gas analysis if possible. If the child is mechanically ventilated, obtain the arterial blood gas 10 to 15 minutes after establishing initial ventilator settings; ideally, correlate blood gases with capnographic end-tidal CO_2 to enable noninvasive monitoring of ventilation.
Other tests	• Obtain a chest x-ray to verify correct depth of the ET tube insertion and position in the mid-trachea, and to identify pulmonary conditions that may require specific treatment (eg, pneumothorax, aspiration).

(continued)

(continued)

Assessment and Management of the Respiratory System
Management

Oxygenation	• If the child is not intubated, provide supplementary O_2 with a partial or a nonrebreathing mask until you confirm adequate SpO_2. • After ROSC, adjust inspired O_2 concentration to achieve an SpO_2 ≥94% but <100%, (ie, 94% to 99%). • If the child has an SpO_2 of <90% while receiving 100% inspired O_2, consider noninvasive ventilatory support or ET intubation with mechanical ventilation and positive end-expiratory pressure. • If the child has a cyanotic cardiac lesion, adjust the O_2 saturation goal to the child's baseline SpO_2 and clinical status.
Ventilation	• Assist ventilation as needed, targeting a normal $PaCO_2$ (ie, 35 to 45 mm Hg) if the child's lung function was previously normal. Remember that normalization of $PaCO_2$ may not be appropriate in all situations. Avoid routine hyperventilation in children with neurologic problems unless there are signs of impending cerebral herniation. Limit exposure to severe hypercapnia or hypocapnia.
Respiratory failure	• Intubate the trachea if O_2 administration and other interventions do not achieve adequate oxygenation and ventilation. Intubate if needed to maintain an open/patent airway and adequate oxygenation and ventilation in the child with decreased level of consciousness. In some patients, CPAP or noninvasive ventilation may be adequate. • Use appropriate ventilator settings. • Verify ET tube position, openness/patency, and security; retape if needed before transport. • Assess for a large glottic air leak. Consider reintubation with a cuffed tube or a larger uncuffed tube if the glottic air leak prevents adequate chest rise, oxygenation, or ventilation. Weigh the risk of removing the advanced airway against the benefit of improving tidal volume, oxygenation, and ventilation. • If a cuffed ET tube is in place and is inflated, check the cuff pressure (goal for most tubes is <20 to 25 cm H_2O; follow the manufacturer's recommendations) or assess for the presence of a minimal glottic air leak at an inspiratory pressure of <20 to 25 cm H_2O. • Insert a gastric tube to relieve and help prevent gastric inflation. *Use the "DOPE" mnemonic to troubleshoot acute deterioration in a mechanically ventilated patient. (See the Critical Concepts box "Sudden Deterioration in an Intubated Patient" in the "Resources for Management of Respiratory Emergencies" at the end of Part 7.)*

(continued)

(continued)

Assessment and Management of the Respiratory System

Analgesia and sedation	• Control pain with analgesics (eg, fentanyl or morphine) and anxiety with sedatives (eg, lorazepam or midazolam) when needed. • Administer sedation and analgesia to all responsive intubated patients. *Use lower doses of sedatives or analgesics if the child is hemodynamically unstable; titrate the dose while stabilizing hemodynamic function. When used in equipotent doses, morphine is more likely than fentanyl to cause hypotension because morphine causes histamine release.*

Neuromuscular blockade	• For the intubated patient with poor oxygenation and ventilation despite adequate sedation and analgesia, assess for acute causes of deterioration by using the DOPE mnemonic. Then consider neuromuscular blocking agents (eg, vecuronium, pancuronium) with sedation. Indications for use of neuromuscular blocking agents include
	
	  – High peak or mean airway pressure caused by high airway resistance or reduced lung compliance
	
	  – Patient ventilator asynchrony
	
	  – Difficult airway
	
	Neuromuscular blockade may reduce the risk of ET tube displacement. Be aware that neuromuscular blockers do not provide sedation or analgesia and will mask seizures. Neuromuscular blockers will also eliminate many signs of agitation that may signal inadequate oxygenation and ventilation. When using neuromuscular blockers, always ensure that the child is adequately sedated by evaluating for signs of stress, such as tachycardia, hypertension, pupil dilation, or tearing.

Cardiovascular System

Management Priorities

Ischemia resulting from cardiac arrest and subsequent reperfusion can cause circulatory dysfunction that can last for hours after ROSC. Compromised tissue perfusion and oxygenation from shock and respiratory failure can have secondary adverse effects on cardiovascular function. The goals of circulatory management are to maintain adequate blood pressure, cardiac output, and distribution of blood flow to restore or maintain tissue oxygenation and delivery of metabolic substrates. Management priorities are to

- Restore and maintain intravascular volume (preload)
- Treat myocardial dysfunction
- Control arrhythmias
- Maintain normal blood pressure and adequate systemic perfusion
- Maintain adequate SpO_2 and PaO_2
- Maintain adequate hemoglobin concentration
- Consider therapies to reduce metabolic demand (eg, support ventilation and reduce temperature)

This section includes

- General recommendations for advanced evaluation and management of the cardiovascular system
- The PALS Management of Shock After ROSC Algorithm
- Information about administration of maintenance fluids

Review "Part 8: Recognition of Shock" and "Part 9: Management of Shock" for more information about the pathophysiology of shock and the use of fluid therapy and medications to maintain cardiac output and tissue perfusion.

General Recommendations

General recommendations for assessment and management of the cardiovascular system may include those listed in Table 90.

Table 90. General Recommendations for Assessment and Management of the Cardiovascular System

Assessment and Management of the Cardiovascular System	
Assessment	

Monitoring	• Monitor the following frequently or continuously:
	  – Heart rate and rhythm by cardiac monitor
	  – Blood pressure and pulse pressure (noninvasively or invasively)
	  – SpO_2 by pulse oximetry
	  – Urine output by urinary catheter
	  – Temperature
	• In the critical care setting, also consider monitoring
	  – Central venous pressure by central venous catheter
	  – O_2 saturation by central venous catheter $ScvO_2$
	  – Trends in venous oxygenation by near infrared spectroscopy
	  – Cardiac function (eg, echocardiogram) or cardiac output by noninvasive monitoring
	
	Noninvasive blood pressure monitoring (ie, by automated blood pressure devices) is often unreliable in children with poor perfusion or frequent arrhythmias. Blood pressure monitoring with an indwelling arterial catheter and monitoring system is more reliable in these children, provided the catheter is open/patent and the transducer is appropriately zeroed and leveled.

Physical examination	• Repeat the physical examination (eg, evaluate quality of central and peripheral pulses, heart rate, capillary refill, blood pressure, extremity temperature and color) frequently until the child is stable. • Monitor end-organ function (eg, neurologic function, renal function, skin perfusion) to detect evidence of worsening circulatory function.

(continued)

(continued)

Assessment and Management of the Cardiovascular System

Laboratory tests	• Arterial or venous blood gas
	• Hemoglobin and hematocrit
	• Serum glucose, electrolytes, blood urea nitrogen (BUN), creatinine, calcium
	• Consider monitoring lactate and central venous O_2 saturation

In addition to pH, note the magnitude of any metabolic acidosis (base deficit). A persistent metabolic (lactic) acidosis suggests inadequate cardiac output and O_2 delivery. Serum electrolytes can help identify an anion gap acidosis. If the child has an elevated anion gap but normal lactate, consider other causes of acidosis, such as toxins or uremia.

The difference in O_2 saturation between an arterial and superior vena caval blood sample [$S(a-v)O_2$] provides information about the balance of oxygen supply vs demand. Assuming that O_2 consumption remains constant, a high $S(a-v)O_2$ difference (>35-40) suggests low oxygen delivery. This may be caused by a fall in cardiac output, or an atrial oxygen content. When oxygen delivery falls, there will be increased O_2 extraction in the tissues (ie, blood flow and O_2 delivery are decreased, so O_2 extraction must increase), producing a fall in the superior vena caval oxygen saturation.

Troponin concentrations are frequently elevated after cardiac arrest, especially if defibrillation was performed.

Nonlaboratory tests	• Perform a chest x-ray to evaluate ET tube insertion depth and position in the mid-trachea, assess heart size, and identify pulmonary edema or other pathology.
	• Evaluate a 12-lead ECG for arrhythmias or evidence of myocardial ischemia.
	• Consider echocardiography if there is concern about pericardial tamponade or myocardial dysfunction.

A small heart is often present with reduced cardiac preload or severe lung hyperinflation. A large heart may be associated with normal or increased cardiac preload, pericardial effusion, congestive heart failure, or when the patient is unable to take a deep breath (eg, with severe abdominal distension).

(continued)

(continued)

Assessment and Management of the Cardiovascular System	
Management	
Intravascular volume	• Establish secure vascular access (if possible, 2 catheters, either IV or IO). • Administer fluid boluses (10-20 mL/kg of isotonic crystalloid over 5-20 minutes) as needed to establish adequate intravascular volume. Smaller boluses of fluid (5-10 mL/kg) administered over 10 to 20 minutes may be appropriate in the setting of heart failure. Adjust the fluid administration rate to replace fluid deficits and meet ongoing requirements. Avoid excessive fluid administration in the presence of myocardial dysfunction or respiratory failure. • Consider the need for colloid or blood administration. • Calculate maintenance fluid requirements and administer as appropriate. **Do not use boluses of hypotonic or dextrose-containing fluids for volume resuscitation.** *See "Administration of Maintenance Fluids" later in this Part.*
Blood Pressure	• **Treat hypotension aggressively**, titrating volume and vasoactive medications as appropriate. • Post–cardiac arrest systolic blood pressure must be maintained above the fifth percentile for age (for children 1-10 years of age, estimated with the following formula: 70 mm Hg + (age in years × 2). • If hypotension is due to excessive vasodilation (eg, sepsis), early use of a vasopressor may be indicated. • The use of adrenergic agents during resuscitation may produce elevation in systemic vascular resistance and cause hypertension. Because the half-life of these agents is relatively short, assess for other causes of hypertension in the post–cardiac arrest phase (eg, pain, anxiety, seizures). *Treatment of hypotension is crucial to avoid secondary multisystem injury. See the PALS Management of Shock After ROSC Algorithm for more information about management of hypotensive and normotensive shock.*
Tissue oxygenation	• Provide supplementary O_2 in a sufficient concentration to ensure adequate oxygenation. • After ROSC following cardiac arrest, titrate O_2 to maintain adequate SpO_2 (94%-99%). • Support adequate perfusion. • Consider transfusion with packed red blood cells for patients with low hematocrit and signs of inadequate O_2 delivery.

(continued)

(continued)

Assessment and Management of the Cardiovascular System	
Metabolic demand	• Consider ET intubation and assisted ventilation to reduce the work of breathing. • Control pain with analgesia (eg, morphine, fentanyl). • Control agitation as needed with sedation (eg, lorazepam, midazolam); rule out hypoxemia, hypercarbia, or poor perfusion as potential causes of agitation. • Control fever with antipyretics. *Caution: Sedatives or analgesics may cause hypotension. Consider expert consultation before elective ET intubation. The use of sedatives or analgesics, ET intubation, and initiation of positive-pressure ventilation can all precipitate cardiovascular collapse in a child with poor myocardial function.*
Arrhythmias	• Monitor for tachyarrhythmias and bradyarrhythmias and treat aggressively. • If bradycardia develops, first ensure adequate oxygenation and ventilation; if the heart rate remains <60/min with signs of poor perfusion despite adequate oxygenation and ventilation, initiate CPR. • If arrhythmia persists, control with drugs or electrical therapy per algorithms. • Seek expert consultation for arrhythmia management. *See "Part 10: Recognition of Arrhythmias" and "Part 11: Management of Arrhythmias" for more information.*
Postarrest myocardial dysfunction	• Anticipate postarrest myocardial dysfunction in the first 24 hours after ROSC. • Consider vasoactive agents to improve contractility and/or decrease afterload if blood pressure is adequate. • Correct metabolic abnormalities that can contribute to poor myocardial function (eg, acidosis, hypocalcemia, hypoglycemia). • Consider positive-pressure ventilation (noninvasive ventilation or via ET tube) to improve left ventricular function. *Myocardial dysfunction is common in children after resuscitation from cardiac arrest. Postarrest myocardial dysfunction can produce hemodynamic instability and secondary organ injury and may precipitate another cardiac arrest.*

Treatment of Shock

After resuscitation from cardiac arrest or shock, hemodynamic compromise may result from a combination of

- Inadequate intravascular volume
- Decreased cardiac contractility
- Either increased or decreased systemic vascular resistance (SVR) or pulmonary vascular resistance

Children with cardiogenic shock typically have poor myocardial function and a compensatory increase in systemic and pulmonary vascular resistances in an attempt to maintain an adequate blood pressure. The increased SVR may become detrimental because it increases left ventricular afterload. Very low SVR most commonly occurs in children with early septic shock. When children with septic shock do not respond to bolus fluid administration (ie, the shock is fluid refractory), they may have high rather than low SVR and poor myocardial function, similar to cardiogenic shock.

Support of Systemic Perfusion

The parameters listed in Table 91 can be manipulated to optimize systemic perfusion.

Table 91. Parameters to Optimize Systemic Perfusion

Parameters to Optimize	Action (When Needed)
Preload	• Administer fluid bolus.
Contractility	• Administer inotropes or inodilators. • Correct hypoxia, electrolyte and acid-base imbalances, and hypoglycemia/hypocalcemia. • Treat poisonings (eg, administer antidotes if available).
Afterload (SVR)	• Administer vasopressors or vasodilators as appropriate.
Heart rate	• Administer chronotropes for bradycardia (eg, epinephrine). • Administer antiarrhythmics. • Correct hypoxia. • Consider pacing.

See the section "Pathophysiology of Shock" in Part 8 for a discussion of preload, afterload, and contractility.

Management of Shock After ROSC

The PALS Management of Shock After ROSC Algorithm (Figure 53) outlines evaluation and management steps after cardiac arrest. Box numbers in the text refer to the corresponding boxes in the algorithm.

Management of Shock After ROSC

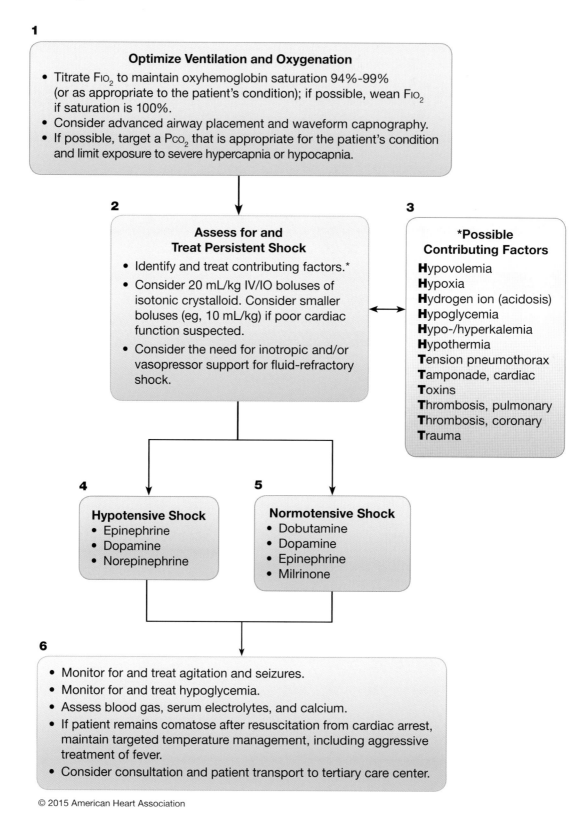

1

Optimize Ventilation and Oxygenation

- Titrate F_{IO_2} to maintain oxyhemoglobin saturation 94%-99% (or as appropriate to the patient's condition); if possible, wean F_{IO_2} if saturation is 100%.
- Consider advanced airway placement and waveform capnography.
- If possible, target a P_{CO_2} that is appropriate for the patient's condition and limit exposure to severe hypercapnia or hypocapnia.

2

Assess for and Treat Persistent Shock

- Identify and treat contributing factors.*
- Consider 20 mL/kg IV/IO boluses of isotonic crystalloid. Consider smaller boluses (eg, 10 mL/kg) if poor cardiac function suspected.
- Consider the need for inotropic and/or vasopressor support for fluid-refractory shock.

3

***Possible Contributing Factors**

Hypovolemia
Hypoxia
Hydrogen ion (acidosis)
Hypoglycemia
Hypo-/hyperkalemia
Hypothermia
Tension pneumothorax
Tamponade, cardiac
Toxins
Thrombosis, pulmonary
Thrombosis, coronary
Trauma

4

Hypotensive Shock
- Epinephrine
- Dopamine
- Norepinephrine

5

Normotensive Shock
- Dobutamine
- Dopamine
- Epinephrine
- Milrinone

6

- Monitor for and treat agitation and seizures.
- Monitor for and treat hypoglycemia.
- Assess blood gas, serum electrolytes, and calcium.
- If patient remains comatose after resuscitation from cardiac arrest, maintain targeted temperature management, including aggressive treatment of fever.
- Consider consultation and patient transport to tertiary care center.

© 2015 American Heart Association

Figure 53. The PALS Management of Shock After ROSC Algorithm.

Optimize Oxygenation and Ventilation (Box 1)

An important component of supporting cardiovascular function is achieving adequate oxygenation and ventilation. Titrate FiO_2 to maintain an O_2 saturation of 94% to 99%; wean O_2 concentration if saturation is 100%. Consider placement of an advanced airway and use of waveform capnography if not yet established.

Fluid Therapy (Box 2)

The first intervention to consider for treatment of shock is administration of a bolus of 10 to 20 mL/kg of isotonic crystalloid. If you suspect postarrest myocardial dysfunction, which occurs commonly, consider administering a smaller fluid bolus (5-10 mL/kg) over 10 to 20 minutes, and then reassess. *If the child demonstrates signs of poor cardiac function (eg, large liver, pulmonary edema, jugular venous distention, large heart on chest x-ray), carefully evaluate the need for fluid administration. Excessive fluid administration can worsen cardiopulmonary function.*

Reassess the child frequently and after each fluid bolus to determine response to therapy.

Possible Contributing Factors (Box 3)

Consider factors that may contribute to postarrest shock, including metabolic derangements and conditions such as hypovolemia and cardiac tamponade (H's and T's).

Hypotensive Shock (Box 4)

If the child remains hypotensive after bolus fluid administration, consider infusion of one or a combination of the following drugs:

Medication	Route	Dosage and Administration
Epinephrine	IV/IO	0.1-1 mcg/kg per minute
and/or		
Dopamine	IV/IO	10-20 mcg/kg per minute
and/or		
Norepinephrine	IV/IO	0.1-2 mcg/kg per minute

Ensure that cardiac preload is adequate; base your choice of drug on the most likely cause of hypotension (inadequate heart rate, poor contractility, excessive vasodilation, or a combination of factors). If the heart rate is abnormally low, catecholamine administration may increase the heart rate and cardiac output. However, when catecholamines cause extreme tachycardia, they increase myocardial O_2 demand.

Epinephrine

Epinephrine is a potent vasoactive agent that can either lower or increase SVR depending on the infusion dose. Low-dose infusions generally produce β-adrenergic effects (increased heart rate and contractility and vasodilation); higher doses generally produce α-adrenergic effects (vasoconstriction). Because there is great interpatient variability, titrate the drug to the desired clinical effect. Epinephrine may be preferable to dopamine in children (especially infants) with marked circulatory instability and hypotensive shock.

Dopamine

Titrate the dopamine infusion to treat shock associated with poor contractility and/or low SVR that is unresponsive to fluid administration. At doses greater than 5 mcg/kg per minute, dopamine typically stimulates cardiac β-adrenergic receptors, but this effect may not be as significant in infants and in patients with chronic congestive heart failure. Doses of 10 to 20 mcg/kg per minute typically increase SVR due to the α-adrenergic effect. Infusion rates greater than 20 mcg/kg per minute may result in excessive vasoconstriction.

Norepinephrine

Norepinephrine is a potent inotropic and peripheral vasoconstricting agent. Titrate the infusion to treat shock with low SVR (septic, anaphylactic, spinal) that is unresponsive to bolus fluid administration.

Normotensive Shock (Box 5)

If the child is normotensive but remains poorly perfused after bolus fluid administration, consider administration of one or a combination of the following drugs:

Medication	Route	Dosage and Administration
Dobutamine	IV/IO	2-20 mcg/kg per minute
and/or		
Dopamine	IV/IO	2-20 mcg/kg per minute
and/or		
Low-dose epinephrine	IV/IO	0.1-0.3 mcg/kg per minute
and/or		
Milrinone	IV/IO	Load with 50 mcg/kg over 10-60 minutes. Loading doses may cause hypotension Infusion: 0.25-0.75 mcg/kg per minute
and/or		
Inamrinone	IV/IO	Load with 0.75-1 mg/kg over 5 minutes; may repeat twice (maximum: 3 mg/kg total) Infusion: 5-10 mcg/kg per minute

Dobutamine

Dobutamine has a selective effect on $β_1$-adrenergic and $β_2$-adrenergic receptors and has intrinsic α-adrenergic blocking activity. It increases myocardial contractility and usually decreases SVR. Titrate an infusion to improve cardiac output. Monitor for extreme tachycardia.

Dopamine

See "Dopamine" in "Hypotensive Shock (Box 4)" earlier in this Part.

Low-Dose Epinephrine

See "Epinephrine" in "Hypotensive Shock (Box 4)" earlier in this Part.

Milrinone

Milrinone is an inodilator that augments cardiac output with little effect on heart rate and myocardial O_2 demand. Use an inodilator for treatment of myocardial dysfunction with increased systemic or pulmonary vascular resistance. You may need to administer additional fluids because the vasodilatory effects will expand the vascular space.

Compared with drugs like dopamine and norepinephrine, inodilators have a long half-life. In addition, whenever the infusion rate is changed, there will be a long delay in reaching a new steady-state hemodynamic effect (4.5 hours with milrinone). The adverse effects may persist for several hours after you stop the infusion.

Other Post–Cardiac Arrest Considerations (Box 6)

Multiple organ systems are affected after ROSC. Treat agitation and seizures with appropriate medications. Correct metabolic derangements, noting that treatment of metabolic acidosis is best accomplished by treating the underlying cause of the acidosis (ie, restore perfusion in shock). Provide targeted temperature management: consider therapeutic hypothermia for children who remain comatose and prevent or aggressively treat fever. Arrange for transfer to an appropriate pediatric critical care unit.

Administration of Maintenance Fluids

Maintenance Fluid Composition

After initial stabilization, adjust the rate and composition of IV fluids based on the patient's condition. If cardiovascular function is adequate, consider administration of maintenance fluids once intravascular volume has been restored and fluid deficits have been replaced. When you calculate the maintenance fluid requirements and plan for fluid administration, be sure to include the fluid administered with vasoactive drug infusions.

In the first hours after resuscitation, the appropriate composition of IV fluids is an isotonic crystalloid (0.9% NaCl or lactated Ringer's), with or without dextrose, based on the child's condition and age. Avoid hypotonic fluids in critically ill children in the post–cardiac arrest phase.

Specific components may be added to maintenance fluids based on the clinical condition:

- Dextrose should generally be included in IV fluids for infants and for children who are hypoglycemic or at risk for hypoglycemia.
- Potassium chloride (KCl) 10 to 20 mEq/L is typically added for children with adequate renal function and documented urine output once periodic monitoring of potassium is available. Do not add KCl to maintenance fluid in children with hyperkalemia, renal failure, muscle injury, or severe acidosis.

Maintenance Fluid Calculation by 4-2-1 Method

The 4-2-1 method is a practical approach to estimating hourly maintenance fluid requirements in children (Table 92).

Table 92. Estimation of Maintenance Fluid Requirements

Weight (kg)	Estimated Hourly Fluid Requirements	Sample Collection
<10	4 mL/kg per hour	8-kg infant: 4 mL/kg per hour × 8 kg = 32 mL/h
10-20	40 mL/h + **2** mL/kg per hour for each kilogram between 10 and 20 kg	15-kg child: 40 mL/h + 2 mL/kg per hour × 5 kg = 50 mL/h
>20	60 mL/h + **1** mL/kg per hour for each kilogram above 20 kg	30-kg child: 60 mL/h + 1 mL/kg per hour × 10 kg = 70 mL/h

An alternate calculation of maintenance hourly fluid rate for patients weighing greater than 20 kg is weight in kilograms + 40 mL/h.

Once you have calculated the estimated maintenance fluid requirements, adjust the actual rate of fluid administration to the child's clinical condition (eg, pulse, blood pressure, systemic perfusion, urine output) and level of hydration.

Neurologic System

Management Priorities

The goals of neurologic management during the post–cardiac arrest period are to preserve brain function and prevent secondary neuronal injury. Management priorities are to

- Maintain adequate brain perfusion
- Maintain normoglycemia
- Provide targeted temperature management: prevent or aggressively treat fever and consider therapeutic hypothermia if indicated
- Treat increased intracranial pressure
- Treat seizures; search for and treat cause

General Recommendations

General recommendations for assessment and management of the neurologic system are listed in Table 93.

Table 93. General Recommendations for Assessment and Management of the Neurologic System

Assessment and Management of the Neurologic System
Assessment

Monitoring	• Monitor temperature. • Monitor heart rate and systemic blood pressure. *In children with poor peripheral perfusion, reliable monitoring of core temperature requires invasive devices (rectal, bladder, esophageal thermometer).*
Physical examination	• Perform frequent, brief neurologic assessments (eg, Glasgow Coma Scale, pupil responses, gag reflex, corneal reflexes, oculocephalic reflexes). • Identify signs of impending cerebral herniation. • Identify seizure activity. • Identify abnormal neurologic findings, including abnormal movements (posturing/myoclonus/hyperreflexia). *Signs of impending cerebral herniation include unequal or dilated unresponsive pupils, posturing, hypertension, bradycardia, respiratory irregularities or apnea, and reduced response to stimulation. A sudden increase in intracranial pressure (ICP) (if monitoring is in place) is often observed. Other causes of central nervous system dysfunction are hypoxic-ischemic brain injury, hypoglycemia, convulsive or nonconvulsive seizures, toxins/drugs, electrolyte abnormalities, hypothermia, traumatic brain injury, stroke or intracranial hemorrhage, and central nervous system infection.* *See the section "Disability" in Part 3 for more information on neurologic assessment.*
Laboratory tests	• Perform point-of-care glucose testing; repeat measurement after treatment of hyperglycemia or hypoglycemia. • Obtain serum electrolytes, point-of-care glucose, and serum ionized calcium concentration if seizure activity is present; measure concentrations of anticonvulsant medications if the child was receiving these agents. • Consider toxicologic studies if poisoning or overdose is suspected. • Consider cerebral spinal fluid studies if central nervous system infection is suspected, but defer a lumbar puncture if the patient's cardiopulmonary status is not stable.

(continued)

(continued)

Assessment and Management of the Neurologic System	
Nonlaboratory tests	• Consider a computed tomography scan if central nervous system dysfunction or neurologic deterioration is present. • Consider an electroencephalogram (EEG) if nonconvulsive status epilepticus is suspected or seizures are a concern during administration or duration of effect of neuromuscular blockers. EEGs performed within the first 7 days after pediatric cardiac arrest may be considered in prognosticating neurologic outcome at the time of hospital discharge, but should not be used as the sole criterion.
Management	
Brain perfusion	• Optimize brain perfusion by supporting cardiac output and arterial O_2 content. • Avoid hyperventilation unless there are signs of impending cerebral herniation. *Support cardiac output by optimizing heart rate, preload, afterload, and contractility. See the section "Support of Systemic Perfusion" earlier in this Part for more information.*
Blood glucose	• Treat hypoglycemia. • Monitor glucose concentration. In general, try to avoid causing or worsening hyperglycemia. • In the critical care setting, consider treating persistent hyperglycemia; careful monitoring is needed to prevent hypoglycemia. *Although hyperglycemia is associated with poor outcome in critically ill children, the relative benefits of active treatment of hyperglycemia vs risks of hypoglycemia in critically ill children remains uncertain. In most animal studies, hyperglycemia at the time of cerebral ischemia produces a worse outcome, but the effect of hyperglycemia occurring after ROSC is less clear.*

(continued)

(continued)

Assessment and Management of the Neurologic System

Targeted Temperature Management	Provide targeted temperature management. This includes preventing or aggressively treating fever and considering therapeutic hypothermia.

Prevent/Treat Fever

- Prevent fever; adjust environmental temperature as needed (cooling devices may be used to maintain a target temperature and prevent fever).
- Aggressively treat fever (temperature 38°C or higher) with antipyretics and cooling devices or procedures.
- Do not actively rewarm a post–cardiac arrest patient who has a temperature between 32°C and 37°C after ROSC unless hypothermia is contributing to hemodynamic instability.

Fever adversely influences recovery from ischemic brain injury and is associated with poor outcome after resuscitation from cardiac arrest. Metabolic O_2 demand increases by 10% to 13% for each degree Celsius elevation of temperature above normal. Increased metabolic demand may worsen neurologic injury. Furthermore, fever increases the release of inflammatory mediators, cytotoxic enzymes, and neurotransmitters, which increase brain injury.

Therapeutic Hypothermia

- For infants and children remaining comatose after out-of-hospital cardiac arrest, it is reasonable either to maintain 5 days of continuous normothermia (36° to 37.5°C) or to maintain 2 days of initial continuous hypothermia (32° to 34°C), followed by 3 days of continuous normothermia.
- For infants and children remaining comatose after in-hospital cardiac arrest, there is insufficient evidence to recommend cooling over normothermia, but all patients should receive targeted temperature management that prevents or aggressively treats fever. During cooling, treatment or prevention of shivering is often required.
- Monitor for and treat complications of hypothermia, including diminished cardiac output, arrhythmia, infection, pancreatitis, coagulopathy, thrombocytopenia, hypophosphatemia, and hypomagnesemia.

Complications of therapeutic hypothermia include diminished cardiac output, arrhythmia, infection, pancreatitis, coagulopathy, thrombocytopenia, hypophosphatemia, and hypomagnesemia.

(continued)

(continued)

Assessment and Management of the Neurologic System

Increased ICP	• Elevate the head of bed to 30° if blood pressure is adequate and no spinal precautions are in place. • Keep head in midline. • Support adequate ventilation to maintain normocapnia. • If signs of impending cerebral herniation develop (eg, irregular respirations or apnea, bradycardia, hypertension, unequal or dilated pupil[s] not responsive to light, decerebrate or decorticate posturing), a brief period of mild hyperventilation may occasionally be used as temporizing rescue therapy. • Consider mannitol or hypertonic saline for acute herniation syndrome. • For children with neurosurgical conditions (eg, traumatic brain injury, intracranial hemorrhage), obtain expert consultation about indications for monitoring of ICP and/or neurosurgical intervention. *Prolonged hyperventilation is not effective to treat increased ICP, and excessive hyperventilation may worsen neurologic outcome. Hypocarbia results in cerebral vasoconstriction, reducing cerebral blood flow. Hyperventilation also reduces venous return and cardiac output, contributing to cerebral ischemia.*
Seizures	• Treat seizures aggressively. Therapeutic options include a benzodiazepine (eg, lorazepam, midazolam), fosphenytoin/phenytoin, levetiracetam or a barbiturate (eg, phenobarbital). Monitor blood pressure carefully if phenytoin or phenobarbital is used, because these drugs may cause hypotension. • Search for a correctable metabolic cause, such as hypoglycemia, hyponatremia, or hypocalcemia. • Consider toxins or metabolic disease as the etiology. • Consult a neurologist if available.

Life Is Why

Education Is Why

Heart disease is the No. 1 cause of death in the world—with more than 17 million deaths per year. That's why the AHA is continuously transforming our training solutions as science evolves, and driving awareness of how everyone can help save a life.

Appendix

BLS Competency Testing

BLS Skills Testing Checklists

The Child CPR and AED Skills Testing Checklist and the Infant CPR Skills Testing Checklist provide detailed descriptions of the CPR skills that you will be expected to perform. Your instructor will evaluate your CPR skills during the skills test on the basis of these descriptions.

If you perform a specific skill exactly as described in the critical performance criteria details, the instructor will check that specific skill as "passing." If you do not perform a specific skill exactly as it is described, the skill will not be checked off and you will require remediation in that skill.

Study the BLS skills testing checklists so that you will be able to perform each skill correctly.

Pediatric Advanced Life Support
Child CPR and AED
Skills Testing Checklist

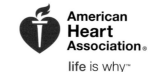

American Heart Association®

life is why™

American Academy of Pediatrics

DEDICATED TO THE HEALTH OF ALL CHILDREN™

Student Name _____ Date of Test _____

Hospital Scenario: "You are working in a hospital or clinic, and you see a child who has suddenly collapsed in the hallway. You check that the scene is safe and then approach the patient. Demonstrate what you would do next."

Prehospital Scenario: "You arrive on the scene for a child who is not breathing. No bystander CPR has been provided. You approach the scene and ensure that it is safe. Demonstrate what you would do next."

Assessment and Activation
- ☐ Checks responsiveness
- ☐ Checks breathing
- ☐ Shouts for help/Activates emergency response system/Sends for AED
- ☐ Checks pulse

Once student shouts for help, instructor says, "Here's the barrier device. I am going to get the AED."

Cycle 1 of CPR (30:2) *CPR feedback devices preferred for accuracy*

Child Compressions
- ☐ Performs high-quality compressions*:
  - Hand placement on lower half of sternum
  - 30 compressions in no less than 15 and no more than 18 seconds
  - Compresses at least one third the depth of the chest, about 2 inches (5 cm)
  - Complete recoil after each compression

Child Breaths
- ☐ Gives 2 breaths with a barrier device:
  - Each breath given over 1 second
  - Visible chest rise with each breath
  - Resumes compressions in less than 10 seconds

Cycle 2 of CPR (repeats steps in Cycle 1) *Only check box if step is successfully performed*
- ☐ Compressions
- ☐ Breaths
- ☐ Resumes compressions in less than 10 seconds

Rescuer 2 says, "Here is the AED. I'll take over compressions, and you use the AED."

AED (follows prompts of AED)
- ☐ Powers on AED
- ☐ Correctly attaches pads
- ☐ Clears for analysis
- ☐ Clears to safely deliver a shock
- ☐ Safely delivers a shock

Resumes Compressions
- ☐ Ensures compressions are resumed immediately after shock delivery
  - Student directs instructor to resume compressions *or*
  - Student resumes compressions

STOP TEST

Instructor Notes
- Place a ✓ in the box next to each step the student completes successfully.
- If the student does not complete all steps successfully (as indicated by at least 1 blank check box), the student must receive remediation. Make a note here of which skills require remediation (refer to Instructor Manual for information about remediation).

Test Results	Circle **PASS** or **NR** to indicate pass or needs remediation:	**PASS**	**NR**
Instructor Initials _____	Instructor Number _____	Date _____	

Child CPR and AED
Skills Testing Critical Skills Descriptors

1. **Assesses victim and activates emergency response system (this *must* precede starting compressions) within a maximum of 30 seconds. After determining that the scene is safe:**
   - Checks for responsiveness by tapping and shouting
   - Shouts for help/directs someone to call for help *and* get AED/defibrillator
   - Checks for no breathing or no normal breathing (only gasping)
     - Scans from the head to the chest for a minimum of 5 seconds and no more than 10 seconds
   - Checks carotid pulse
     - Can be done simultaneously with check for breathing
     - Checks for a minimum of 5 seconds and no more than 10 seconds

2. **Performs high-quality chest compressions (initiates compressions immediately after recognition of cardiac arrest)**
   - Correct hand placement
     - Lower half of sternum
     - 2-handed (second hand on top of the first or grasping the wrist of the first hand) or 1-handed
   - Compression rate of 100 to 120/min
     - Delivers 30 compressions in 15 to 18 seconds
   - Compression depth and recoil—compress at least one third the depth of the chest, about 2 inches (5 cm)
     - Use of a commercial feedback device or high-fidelity manikin is highly recommended
     - Complete chest recoil after each compression
   - Minimizes interruptions in compressions
     - Delivers 2 breaths so less than 10 seconds elapses between last compression of one cycle and first compression of next cycle
     - Compressions resumed immediately after shock/no shock indicated

3. **Provides 2 breaths by using a barrier device**
   - Opens airway adequately
     - Uses a head tilt–chin lift maneuver or jaw thrust
   - Delivers each breath over 1 second
   - Delivers breaths that produce visible chest rise
   - Avoids excessive ventilation
   - Resumes chest compressions in less than 10 seconds

4. **Performs same steps for compressions and breaths for Cycle 2**

5. **AED use**
   - Powers on AED
     - Turns AED on by pushing button or lifting lid as soon as it arrives
   - Correctly attaches pads
     - Places proper-sized pads for victim's age in correct location
   - Clears for analysis
     - Clears rescuers from victim for AED to analyze rhythm (pushes analyze button if required by device)
     - Communicates clearly to all other rescuers to stop touching victim
   - Clears to safely deliver shock
     - Communicates clearly to all other rescuers to stop touching victim
   - Delivers a shock
     - Resumes chest compressions immediately after shock delivery
     - Does *not* turn off AED during CPR

6. **Resumes compressions**
   - Ensures that high-quality chest compressions are resumed immediately after shock delivery
   - Performs same steps for compressions

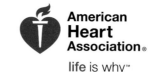

American Heart Association®

life is why™

American Academy of Pediatrics

DEDICATED TO THE HEALTH OF ALL CHILDREN™

Student Name _____   Date of Test _____

Hospital Scenario: "You are working in a hospital or clinic when a woman runs through the door, carrying an infant. She shouts, 'Help me! My baby's not breathing.' You have gloves and a pocket mask. You send your coworker to activate the emergency response system and to get the emergency equipment."

Prehospital Scenario: "You arrive on the scene for an infant who is not breathing. No bystander CPR has been provided. You approach the scene and ensure that it is safe. Demonstrate what you would do next."

Assessment and Activation

☐ Checks responsiveness   ☐ Shouts for help/Activates emergency response system   ☐ Checks breathing
☐ Checks pulse

Once student shouts for help, instructor says, "Here's the barrier device."

Cycle 1 of CPR (30:2)   *CPR feedback devices preferred for accuracy*

Infant Compressions

☐ Performs high-quality compressions*:

- Placement of 2 fingers in the center of the chest, just below the nipple line
- 30 compressions in no less than 15 and no more than 18 seconds
- Compresses at least one third the depth of the chest, about 1½ inches (4 cm)
- Complete recoil after each compression

Infant Breaths

☐ Gives 2 breaths with a barrier device:

- Each breath given over 1 second
- Visible chest rise with each breath
- Resumes compressions in less than 10 seconds

Cycle 2 of CPR (repeats steps in Cycle 1)   *Only check box if step is successfully performed*

☐ Compressions   ☐ Breaths   ☐ Resumes compressions in less than 10 seconds

Rescuer 2 arrives with bag-mask device and begins ventilation while Rescuer 1 continues compressions with 2 thumb–encircling hands technique.

Cycle 3 of CPR

Rescuer 1: Infant Compressions

☐ Performs high–quality compressions*:

- 15 compressions with 2 thumb–encircling hands technique
- 15 compressions in no less than 7 and no more than 9 seconds
- Compress at least one third the depth of the chest, about 1½ inches (4 cm)
- Complete recoil after each compression

Rescuer 2: Infant Breaths

This rescuer is not evaluated.

(continued)

Pediatric Advanced Life Support
Infant CPR
Skills Testing Checklist (2 of 2)

American Heart Association®

life is why™

American Academy of Pediatrics

DEDICATED TO THE HEALTH OF ALL CHILDREN™

Student Name _____   Date of Test _____

Cycle 4 of CPR

Rescuer 2: Infant Compressions
This rescuer is not evaluated.

Rescuer 1: Infant Breaths
☐ Gives 2 breaths with a bag-mask device:
- Each breath given over 1 second
- Visible chest rise with each breath
- Resumes compressions in less than 10 seconds

STOP TEST

Instructor Notes
- Place a ✓ in the box next to each step the student completes successfully.
- If the student does not complete all steps successfully (as indicated by at least 1 blank check box), the student must receive remediation. Make a note here of which skills require remediation (refer to Instructor Manual for information about remediation).

Test Results	Circle **PASS** or **NR** to indicate pass or needs remediation:	**PASS** **NR**

Instructor Initials _____   Instructor Number _____   Date _____

Infant CPR
Skills Testing Critical Skills Descriptors

1. **Assesses victim and activates emergency response system (this *must* precede starting compressions) within a maximum of 30 seconds. After determining that the scene is safe:**
   - Checks for responsiveness by tapping and shouting
   - Shouts for help/directs someone to call for help *and* get emergency equipment
   - Checks for no breathing or no normal breathing (only gasping)
     - Scans from the head to the chest for a minimum of 5 seconds and no more than 10 seconds
   - Checks brachial pulse
     - Can be done simultaneously with check for breathing
     - Checks for a minimum of 5 seconds and no more than 10 seconds

2. **Performs high-quality chest compressions during 1-rescuer CPR (initiates compressions within 10 seconds of identifying cardiac arrest)**
   - Correct placement of hands/fingers in center of chest
     - 1 rescuer: 2 fingers just below the nipple line
   - Compression rate of 100 to 120/min
     - Delivers 30 compressions in 15 to 18 seconds
   - Adequate depth for age
     - Infant: at least one third the depth of the chest (about 1½ inches [4 cm])
     - Use of a commercial feedback device or high-fidelity manikin is highly recommended
   - Complete chest recoil after each compression
   - Appropriate ratio for age and number of rescuers
     - 1 rescuer: 30 compressions to 2 breaths
   - Minimizes interruptions in compressions
     - Delivers 2 breaths so less than 10 seconds elapses between last compression of one cycle and first compression of next cycle

3. **Provides effective breaths with bag-mask device during 2-rescuer CPR**
   - Opens airway adequately
   - Delivers each breath over 1 second
   - Delivers breaths that produce visible chest rise
   - Avoids excessive ventilation
   - Resumes chest compressions in less than 10 seconds

4. **Switches compression technique at appropriate interval as prompted by the instructor (for purposes of this evaluation). Switch should take no more than 5 seconds.**

5. **Performs high-quality chest compressions during 2-rescuer CPR**
   - Correct placement of hands/fingers in center of chest
     - 2 rescuers: 2 thumb–encircling hands just below the nipple line
   - Compression rate of 100 to 120/min
     - Delivers 15 compressions in 7 to 9 seconds
   - Adequate depth for age
     - Infant: at least one third the depth of the chest (about 1½ inches [4 cm])
   - Complete chest recoil after each compression
   - Appropriate ratio for age and number of rescuers
     - 2 rescuers: 15 compressions to 2 breaths
   - Minimizes interruptions in compressions
     - Delivers 2 breaths so less than 10 seconds elapses between last compression of one cycle and first compression of next cycle

Initial Impression—Pediatric Assessment Triangle*

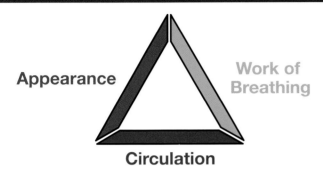

Appearance

From the doorway, your initial observation of the patient

Caregiver observes for

- Abnormal tone
- Decreased interaction
- Inconsolable
- Abnormal look/gaze
- Abnormal speech/cry

Work of Breathing

- Abnormal sounds
- Abnormal positioning
- Retractions
- Flaring
- Apnea/gasping

Circulation to the Skin

- Pallor
- Mottling
- Dusky
- Cyanosis

*If the patient is unresponsive, not breathing, or only gasping, initiate the BLS algorithm. Students can refer to Part 4 of the *PALS Provider Manual*.

Primary Assessment

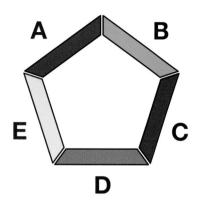

A | **Airway**

Assessment

- Is the airway maintainable?
- Is the airway clear?
- If no to any of these, below are the interventions*

Interventions

- Maintain airway patency by positioning, using OPA
- Suction as indicated
- Advanced airway (eg, supraglottic airway or endotracheal tube)
- If inserting an advanced airway, verify correct placement with waveform capnography

B | **Breathing**

Assessment

- Adequate depth and rate of respirations
- Chest rise
- Noisy breathing (eg, grunting, stridor, wheezing)
- Use of accessory muscles, nasal flaring
- Pulse oximetry*

Interventions

- Provide high-flow O_2
- Bag-mask device with or without OPA
- Advanced airway
- Avoid excessive ventilation

C | **Circulation**

Assessment

- Adequate peripheral and/or central pulse
- Heart rate
- Blood pressure*
- Capillary refill—peripheral and/or central
- Skin color and temperature
- Level of consciousness

Interventions

- Obtain IV/IO access
- Consider fluid resuscitation

(continued)

(continued)

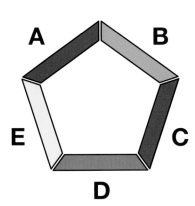

D	**Disability**
	Assessment
	• Quickly assess for responsiveness, level of consciousness, and pupillary response to light
	• AVPU: Alert, Voice, Pain, and Unresponsive
	• Check point-of-care glucose
	Interventions
	• Spinal motion restrictions
	• Correct hypoglycemia
	• Consider naloxone for acute opioid toxicity
E	**Exposure**
	Assessment
	• Remove clothing to perform a physical examination (anterior and posterior), looking for obvious signs of trauma, bleeding, burns, unusual markings, rashes, or medical alert bracelets
	• Temperature
	Interventions
	• Ensure normothermia
	• Control bleeding
	• Decontamination

*If at any part of this sequence you find that a patient has a life-threatening condition, correction of that condition takes precedence over establishing baseline vital sign measures, such as blood pressure or pulse oximetry. When the primary assessment is completed and after life-threatening problems have been addressed, the healthcare provider proceeds to the secondary assessment (Consensus Statement: Emergency Medical Services for Children—Definitions and Pediatric Assessment Approaches. April 2005. Updated July 2015).

Remediation

Any provider who does not pass both skills tests will practice and undergo remediation during the remediation lesson at the end of the course.

Providers who require remediation and retesting will be tested in the entire skill.

Skills Station Competency Checklists

Airway Management Skills Station Competency Checklist

Critical Performance Steps	For More Information, See
Verbalizes difference between high-flow and low-flow O_2 delivery systems • High flow: O_2 flow exceeds patient inspiratory flow, preventing entrainment of room air if system is tight-fitting; delivers nearly 1.00 FIO_2 (eg, nonrebreathing mask with reservoir high-flow nasal cannula) • Low flow (≤10 L/min): patient inspiratory flow exceeds O_2 flow, allowing entrainment of room air; delivers 0.23 to 0.80 FIO_2 (eg, nasal cannula, simple O_2 mask)	
Verbalizes maximum nasal cannula flow rate for standard nasal cannula (4 L/min)	
Opens airway by using head tilt–chin lift maneuver while keeping mouth open (jaw thrust for trauma victim)	Instructor demonstration
Verbalizes different indications for OPA and NPA • OPA only for unconscious victim without a gag reflex • NPA for conscious or semiconscious victim	
Selects correctly sized airway by measuring • OPA from corner of mouth to angle of mandible	
Inserts OPA correctly	
Verbalizes assessment for adequate breathing after insertion of OPA	
Suctions with OPA in place; states suctioning not to exceed 10 seconds	
Selects correct mask size for ventilation	"Bag-Mask Ventilation" in "Resources for Management of Respiratory Emergencies" at the end of Part 7
Assembles bag-mask device, opens airway, and creates seal by using E-C clamp technique	
With bag-mask device, gives 1 breath every 3 to 5 seconds for about 30 seconds. Gives each breath in approximately 1 second; each breath should cause chest rise	
Endotracheal Intubation • States equipment needed for endotracheal (ET) tube intubation procedure • Demonstrates technique to confirm proper ET tube placement by physical exam and by using an exhaled CO_2 device • Secures ET tube • Suctions with ET tube in place	"Pre-event Equipment Checklist for Endotracheal Intubation" in "Resources for Management of Respiratory Emergencies" at the end of Part 7
The following steps are optional. They are demonstrated and evaluated only when the student's scope of practice involves ET intubation.	
Endotracheal Intubation • Prepares equipment for ET intubation • Inserts ET tube correctly	

Rhythm Disturbances/Electrical Therapy Skills Station Competency Checklist

Critical Performance Steps	For More Information, See
Applies 2 ECG leads correctly (or local equipment if >3 leads are used) • Negative (white) lead: to right shoulder • Positive (red) lead: to left lower ribs • Ground (black, green, brown) lead: to left shoulder	Instructor demonstration
Demonstrates correct operation of monitor • Turns monitor on • Adjusts device to manual mode (not AED mode) to display rhythm in standard limb leads (I, II, III) or paddles/electrode pads	Instructor demonstration
Verbalizes correct electrical therapy for appropriate core rhythms • Synchronized cardioversion for unstable SVT, VT with pulses • Defibrillation for pulseless VT, VF	"Part 10: Recognition of Arrhythmias"; "Part 11: Management of Arrhythmias"
Selects correct paddle/electrode pad for infant or child; places paddles/electrode pads in correct position	"Part 11: Management of Arrhythmias"
Demonstrates correct and safe synchronized cardioversion • Places device in synchronized mode • Selects appropriate energy (0.5 to 1.0 J/kg for initial shock) • Charges, clears, and delivers current	"Part 11: Management of Arrhythmias"
Demonstrates correct and safe manual defibrillation • Places device in unsynchronized mode • Selects energy (2 to 4 J/kg for initial shock) • Charges, clears, and delivers current	"Part 11: Management of Arrhythmias"

Vascular Access Skills Station Competency Checklist

Critical Performance Steps	For More Information, See
Verbalizes indications for IO insertion	"Intraosseous Access" in "Resources for Management of Circulatory Emergencies" at the end of Part 9
Verbalizes sites for IO insertion (anterior tibia, distal femur, medial malleolus, anterior-superior iliac spine)	
Verbalizes contraindications for IO placement • Fracture in extremity • Previous insertion attempt in the same bone • Infection overlying bone	
Inserts IO catheter safely	
Verbalizes how to confirm IO catheter is in correct position; verbalizes how to secure IO catheter	
Attaches IV line to IO catheter; demonstrates giving IO fluid bolus by using 3-way stopcock and syringe	Instructor demonstration
Shows how to determine correct drug doses by using a color-coded length-based tape or other resource	"Color-Coded Length-Based Resuscitation Tape" in "Resources for Management of Circulatory Emergencies" at the end of Part 9
The following is optional:	
Verbalizes correct procedure for establishing IV access	

Rhythm Recognition Review

Rhythm Strip 1

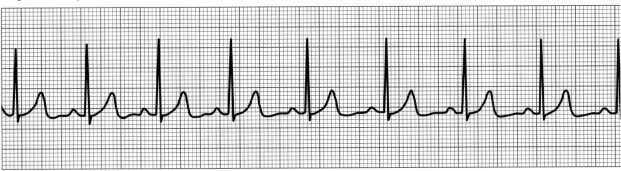

Figure 54. Normal sinus rhythm, rate 100/min.

Note that every P wave conducts to the ventricle, resulting in a QRS complex. Be aware that normal heart rates are age dependent in the pediatric population. For example, a heart rate of 75/min would be normal for a 10-year-old but brady-cardic for a neonate. Likewise, a rate of 140/min would be normal for an infant but tachycardic for an adolescent.

Rhythm Strip 2

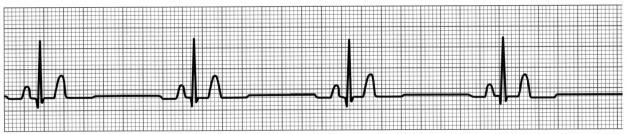

Figure 55. Sinus bradycardia.

Note that the P waves result in a QRS complex (conducted to the ventricle). The rate is very slow (approximately 45/min). Sinus bradycardia is often a manifestation of hypoxemia and acidosis. It may be seen in healthy children, particularly during sleep.

Rhythm Strip 3

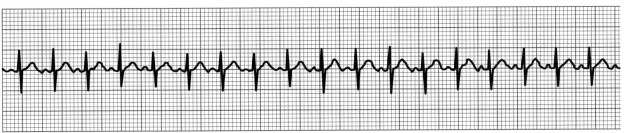

Figure 56. Sinus tachycardia, 180/min.

Note that P waves are visible preceding every QRS. The rate for sinus tachycardia may vary according to age. In an infant, sinus tachycardia could be as high as 220/min.

Rhythm Strip 4

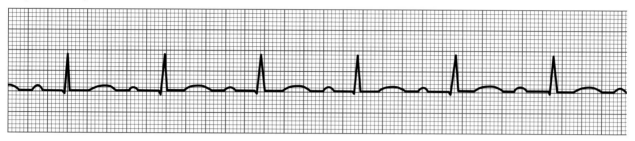

Figure 57. Sinus rhythm with first-degree heart block.

Note that the PR interval is prolonged (0.3 second). This is often a reflection of increased vagal tone and may be seen in healthy children. Less often, it can be a sign of intrinsic atrioventricular node disease, myocarditis, electrolyte disturbances (such as hyperkalemia), hypoxemia, drug toxicity (such as digoxin, ß-blocker, or calcium channel blocker), or acute rheumatic fever.

Rhythm Strip 5

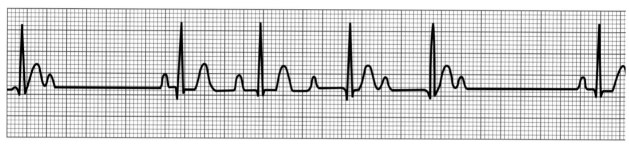

Figure 58. Second-degree heart block, Mobitz type I, or Wenckebach.

Note that the PR interval progressively prolongs until a P wave fails to conduct to the ventricle. Like first-degree heart block, this is often seen in healthy children, especially during sleep. It may also be a manifestation of drug toxicity, such as digoxin, ß-blocker, or calcium channel blocker.

Rhythm Strip 6

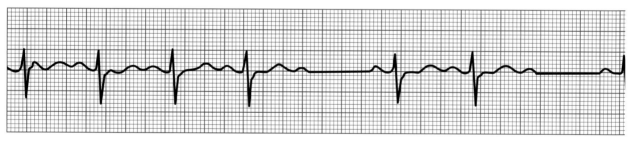

Figure 59. Second-degree heart block, Mobitz type II.

Note that some, but not all, of the P waves do not conduct to the ventricle. There is no progressive prolongation of the PR interval. This is a sign of intrinsic conduction system disease, typically related to cardiac surgery or myocardial inflammation or infarction.

Rhythm Strip 7

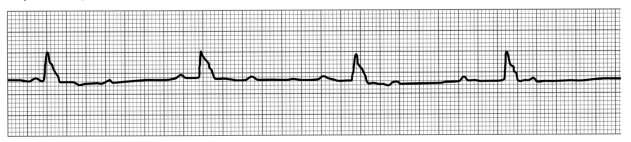

Figure 60. Third-degree (complete) heart block with ventricular escape rhythm.

Note that none of the P wave conducts to the ventricle. Often the QRS complex "marches" at a constant interval because of junctional or ventricular escape rhythm. There is no relation between P waves and QRS complexes. Occasionally this is a result of severe hypoxemia and acidosis. This may also be a manifestation of damage to the atrioventricular node or extensive conduction system disease, such as that seen after cardiac surgery, or myocarditis, or with congenital complete heart block.

Rhythm Strip 8

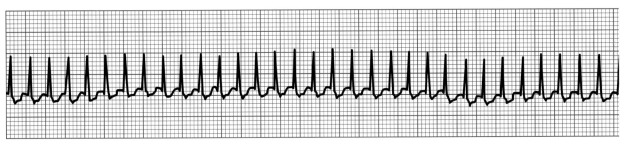

Figure 61. Supraventricular tachycardia, 230/min.

Note that the QRS complexes are narrow and regular, the rate is very fast (greater than 200/min), and P waves are not obvious.

Rhythm Strip 9

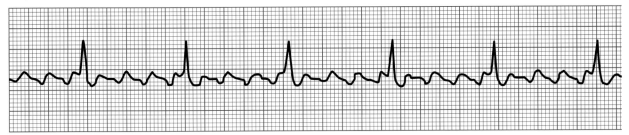

Figure 62. Atrial flutter.

Note that there is a "sawtooth" pattern to the P waves, reflecting an extremely rapid atrial rate. Conduction of the P waves to the ventricle may be variable, resulting in an irregular QRS rate.

Rhythm Strip 10

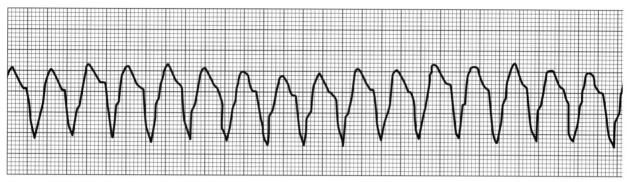

Figure 63. Ventricular tachycardia, 150/min.

Note that the QRS complexes are wide (greater than 0.09 second), regular, and fast. The QRS morphologies are all identical, characterizing it as monomorphic ventricular tachycardia. P waves are not identifiable.

Rhythm Strip 11

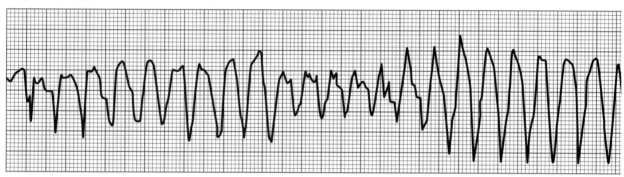

Figure 64. Polymorphic ventricular tachycardia.

Note that the QRS complexes are wide, irregular, and very fast (greater than 200/min). The QRS complexes vary in appearance, characterizing it as polymorphic. In fact, there is a phase change during this recording where the QRS complexes are initially positive and then become negative before returning to positive polarity. This is a torsades de pointes ("turning of points") type of polymorphic ventricular tachycardia, seen most often in states where the QT interval is prolonged during the baseline.

Rhythm Strip 12

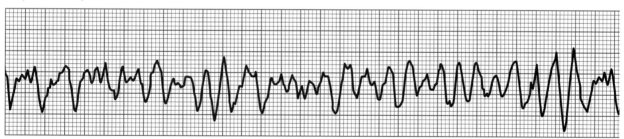

Figure 65. Ventricular fibrillation.

Note that there are no definable QRS complexes, just irregular disorganized electrical activity.

Rhythm Strip 13

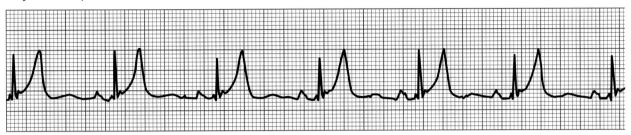

Figure 66. Sinus rhythm with peaked T waves.

Note how the T waves have increased amplitude and are even larger than the QRS complexes. This may be indicative of hyperkalemia.

Learning Station Competency Checklists

The learning station competency checklists provide detailed descriptions of the critical performance steps that you will perform at each learning/skills station.

Additionally, the case scenario testing checklists provide the steps you will perform during each case scenario test. Your instructor will evaluate your skills on the basis of these descriptions.

If you perform a specific skill exactly as described in the critical performance criteria details, the instructor will check that specific skill as "passing." If you do not perform a specific skill exactly as it is described, the skill will not be checked off and you will require remediation in that skill.

Study these checklists so that you will be able to perform each skill correctly.

Airway Management Skills Station Competency Checklist

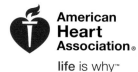

American Heart Association® life is why™

American Academy of Pediatrics
DEDICATED TO THE HEALTH OF ALL CHILDREN™

Student Name _____ Date of Test _____

Critical Performance Steps	✓ if done correctly
Verbalizes difference between high-flow and low-flow O$_2$ delivery systems • High flow: O$_2$ flow exceeds patient inspiratory flow, preventing entrainment of room air if system is tight-fitting; delivers nearly 1.00 FIO$_2$, eg, nonrebreathing mask with reservoir, high-flow nasal cannula • Low flow (≤10 L/min): patient inspiratory flow exceeds O$_2$ flow, allowing entrainment of room air; delivers 0.23 to 0.80 FIO$_2$, eg, standard nasal cannula, simple O$_2$ mask	
Verbalizes maximum nasal cannula flow rate for standard nasal cannula (4 L/min)	
Opens airway by using head tilt–chin lift maneuver while keeping mouth open (jaw thrust for trauma victim)	
Verbalizes different indications for OPA and NPA • OPA only for unconscious victim without a gag reflex • NPA for conscious or semiconscious victim	
Selects correctly sized airway by measuring • OPA from corner of mouth to angle of mandible	
Inserts OPA correctly	
Verbalizes assessment for adequate breathing after insertion of OPA	
Suctions with OPA in place; states suctioning not to exceed 10 seconds	
Selects correct mask size for ventilation	
Assembles bag-mask device, opens airway, and creates seal by using E-C clamp technique	
With bag-mask device, gives 1 breath every 3 to 5 seconds for about 30 seconds. Gives each breath in approximately 1 second; each breath should cause chest rise	
Endotracheal Intubation • States equipment needed for endotracheal (ET) tube intubation procedure • Demonstrates technique to confirm proper ET tube placement by physical exam and by using an exhaled CO$_2$ device • Secures ET tube • Suctions with ET tube in place	
The following steps are optional. They are demonstrated and evaluated only when the student's scope of practice involves ET intubation.	
Endotracheal Intubation • Prepares equipment for ET intubation • Inserts ET tube correctly	

STOP TEST

Instructor Notes
• Place a ✓ in the box next to each step the student completes successfully.
• If the student does not complete all steps successfully (as indicated by at least 1 blank check box), the student must receive remediation. Make a note here of which skills require remediation (refer to Instructor Manual for information about remediation).

Test Results	Circle **PASS** or **NR** to indicate pass or needs remediation:	**PASS**	**NR**

Instructor Initials _____ Instructor Number _____ Date _____

Rhythm Disturbances/ Electrical Therapy Skills Station Competency Checklist

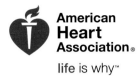 **American Heart Association®** life is why™

 American Academy of Pediatrics
DEDICATED TO THE HEALTH OF ALL CHILDREN™

Student Name _____   Date of Test _____

Critical Performance Steps	✓ if done correctly
Applies 3 ECG leads correctly (or local equipment if >3 leads are used) • Negative (white) lead: to right shoulder • Positive (red) lead: to left lower ribs • Ground (black, green, brown) lead: to left shoulder	
Demonstrates correct operation of monitor • Turns monitor on • Adjusts device to manual mode (not AED mode) to display rhythm in standard limb leads (I, II, III) or paddles/electrode pads	
Verbalizes correct electrical therapy for appropriate core rhythms • Synchronized cardioversion for unstable SVT, VT with pulses • Defibrillation for pulseless VT, VF	
Selects correct paddle/electrode pad for infant or child; places paddles/electrode pads in correct position	
Demonstrates correct and safe synchronized cardioversion • Places device in synchronized mode • Selects appropriate energy (0.5 to 1 J/kg for initial shock) • Charges, clears, delivers current	
Demonstrates correct and safe manual defibrillation • Places device in unsynchronized mode • Selects energy (2 to 4 J/kg for initial shock) • Charges, clears, delivers current	

STOP TEST

Instructor Notes
- Place a ✓ in the box next to each step the student completes successfully.
- If the student does not complete all steps successfully (as indicated by at least 1 blank check box), the student must receive remediation. Make a note here of which skills require remediation (refer to Instructor Manual for information about remediation).

Test Results Circle **PASS** or **NR** to indicate pass or needs remediation:	**PASS** **NR**
Instructor Initials _____ Instructor Number _____ Date _____	

Vascular Access
Skills Station
Competency Checklist

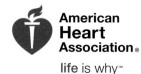

Student Name _____ Date of Test _____

Critical Performance Steps	✓ if done correctly
Verbalizes indications for IO insertion	
Verbalizes sites for IO insertion (anterior tibia, distal femur, medial malleolus, anterior-superior iliac spine)	
Verbalizes contraindications for IO placement • Fracture in extremity • Previous insertion attempt in the same bone • Infection overlying bone	
Inserts IO catheter safely	
Verbalizes how to confirm IO catheter is in correct position; verbalizes how to secure IO catheter	
Attaches IV line to IO catheter; demonstrates giving IO fluid bolus by using 3-way stopcock and syringe	
Shows how to determine correct drug doses by using a color-coded length-based tape or other resource	
The following is optional:	
Verbalizes correct procedure for establishing IV access	

STOP TEST

Instructor Notes
- Place a ✓ in the box next to each step the student completes successfully.
- If the student does not complete all steps successfully (as indicated by at least 1 blank check box), the student must receive remediation. Make a note here of which skills require remediation (refer to Instructor Manual for information about remediation).

Test Results	Circle **PASS** or **NR** to indicate pass or needs remediation:	**PASS**	**NR**

Instructor Initials _____ Instructor Number _____ Date _____

PALS Case Scenario
Testing Checklist
Respiratory Case Scenario
Upper Airway Obstruction

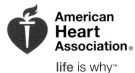

American **Heart** Association®

life is why™

American Academy of Pediatrics

DEDICATED TO THE HEALTH OF ALL CHILDREN™

Student Name _____ Date of Test _____

Critical Performance Steps	✓ if done correctly
Team Leader	
Assigns team member roles	
Uses effective communication throughout	
Patient Management	
Directs assessment of airway, breathing, circulation, disability, and exposure, including vital signs	
Directs administration of 100% oxygen or supplementary oxygen as needed to support oxygenation	
Directs application of cardiac monitor and pulse oximetry	
Identifies signs and symptoms of upper airway obstruction	
Categorizes as respiratory distress or failure	
Directs administration of nebulized epinephrine and corticosteroid (for croup), or IM epinephrine and IV corticosteroid (for anaphylaxis)	
States indications for bag-mask ventilation and/or other airway or ventilation support	
If the student does not verbalize the above, prompt the student with the following question: "What are the indications for bag-mask ventilation and/or other airway or ventilation support?"	
Directs establishment of IV or IO access, if indicated	
Directs reassessment of patient in response to treatment	
Case Conclusion/Debriefing	
The following step is evaluated only if the student's scope of practice applies	
Describes how to estimate correct endotracheal tube size for this patient	
If the student does not verbalize the above, prompt the student with the following question: "How would you estimate the endotracheal tube size for this infant with upper airway obstruction?"	

STOP TEST

Instructor Notes
- Place a ✓ in the box next to each step the student completes successfully.
- If the student does not complete all steps successfully (as indicated by at least 1 blank check box), the student must receive remediation. Make a note here of which skills require remediation (refer to Instructor Manual for information about remediation).

Test Results Circle **PASS** or **NR** to indicate pass or needs remediation:	**PASS** **NR**

Instructor Initials _____ Instructor Number _____ Date _____

PALS Case Scenario
Testing Checklist
Respiratory Case Scenario
Lower Airway Obstruction

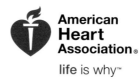

Student Name _____   Date of Test _____

Critical Performance Steps	✓ if done correctly
Team Leader	
Assigns team member roles	
Uses effective communication throughout	
Patient Management	
Directs assessment of airway, breathing, circulation, disability, and exposure, including vital signs	
Directs administration of 100% oxygen or supplementary oxygen as needed to support oxygenation	
Directs application of cardiac monitor and pulse oximetry	
Identifies signs and symptoms of lower airway obstruction	
Categorizes as respiratory distress or failure	
Directs administration of albuterol and corticosteroids (for asthma) or suctioning or possible additional laboratory studies (for bronchiolitis)	
States indications for bag-mask ventilation and/or other airway or ventilation support	
If the student does not verbalize the above, prompt the student with the following question: "What are the indications for bag-mask ventilation and/or other airway or ventilation support?"	
Directs establishment of IV or IO access, if appropriate	
Directs reassessment of patient in response to treatment	
Case Conclusion/Debriefing	
The following step is evaluated only if the student's scope of practice applies	
States indications for endotracheal intubation	
If the student does not verbalize the above, prompt the student with the following question: "What are the indications for endotracheal intubation?"	

STOP TEST

Instructor Notes

- Place a ✓ in the box next to each step the student completes successfully.
- If the student does not complete all steps successfully (as indicated by at least 1 blank check box), the student must receive remediation. Make a note here of which skills require remediation (refer to Instructor Manual for information about remediation).

Test Results Circle **PASS** or **NR** to indicate pass or needs remediation:	**PASS** **NR**

Instructor Initials _____   Instructor Number _____   Date _____

PALS Case Scenario
Testing Checklist
Respiratory Case Scenario
Lung Tissue Disease

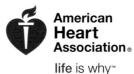

American **Heart** Association®

life is why™

American Academy of Pediatrics

DEDICATED TO THE HEALTH OF ALL CHILDREN™

Student Name _____ Date of Test _____

Critical Performance Steps	✓ if done correctly
Team Leader	
Assigns team member roles	
Uses effective communication throughout	
Patient Management	
Directs assessment of airway, breathing, circulation, disability, and exposure, including vital signs	
Directs administration of 100% oxygen (or supplementary oxygen as needed to support oxygenation) and evaluates response	
Identifies indications for bag-mask ventilation and/or additional airway or ventilation support	
Describes methods to verify that bag-mask ventilation is effective	
Directs application of cardiac monitor and pulse oximetry	
Identifies signs and symptoms of lung tissue disease	
Categorizes as respiratory distress or failure	
Directs establishment of IV or IO access	
Directs reassessment of patient in response to treatment	
Identifies need for involvement of advanced provider with expertise in pediatric intubation and mechanical ventilation	
Case Conclusion/Debriefing	
The following step is evaluated only if the student's scope of practice applies	
States indications for endotracheal intubation	
If the student does not verbalize the above, prompt the student with the following question: *"What are the indications for endotracheal intubation?"*	

STOP TEST

Instructor Notes
- Place a ✓ in the box next to each step the student completes successfully.
- If the student does not complete all steps successfully (as indicated by at least 1 blank check box), the student must receive remediation. Make a note here of which skills require remediation (refer to Instructor Manual for information about remediation).

Test Results Circle **PASS** or **NR** to indicate pass or needs remediation:	**PASS** **NR**
Instructor Initials _____ Instructor Number _____ Date _____	

PALS Case Scenario
Testing Checklist
Respiratory Case Scenario
Disordered Control of Breathing

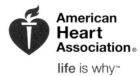

American Academy of Pediatrics

DEDICATED TO THE HEALTH OF ALL CHILDREN™

Student Name _____ Date of Test _____

Critical Performance Steps	✓ if done correctly
Team Leader	
Assigns team member roles	
Uses effective communication throughout	
Patient Management	
Directs assessment of airway, breathing, circulation, disability, and exposure, including vital signs	
Directs administration of 100% oxygen (or supplementary oxygen as needed to support oxygenation) and evaluates response	
Identifies indications for bag-mask ventilation and/or additional airway or ventilation support	
Describes methods to verify that bag-mask ventilation is effective	
Directs application of cardiac monitor and pulse oximetry	
Identifies signs of disordered control of breathing	
Categorizes as respiratory distress or failure	
Directs establishment of IV or IO access	
Directs reassessment of patient in response to treatment	
Identifies need for involvement of advanced provider with expertise in pediatric intubation and mechanical ventilation	
Case Conclusion/Debriefing	
The following step is evaluated only if the student's scope of practice applies	
States indications for endotracheal intubation	
If the student does not verbalize the above, prompt the student with the following question: "What are the indications for endotracheal intubation?"	

STOP TEST

Instructor Notes
- Place a ✓ in the box next to each step the student completes successfully.
- If the student does not complete all steps successfully (as indicated by at least 1 blank check box), the student must receive remediation. Make a note here of which skills require remediation (refer to Instructor Manual for information about remediation).

Test Results	Circle **PASS** or **NR** to indicate pass or needs remediation:	**PASS**	**NR**

Instructor Initials _____ Instructor Number _____ Date _____

PALS Case Scenario
Testing Checklist
Shock Case Scenario
Hypovolemic Shock

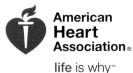

American Heart Association®

life is why™

American Academy of Pediatrics

DEDICATED TO THE HEALTH OF ALL CHILDREN™

Student Name _____ Date of Test _____

Critical Performance Steps	✓ if done correctly
Team Leader	
Assigns team member roles	
Uses effective communication throughout	
Patient Management	
Directs assessment of airway, breathing, circulation, disability, and exposure, including vital signs	
Directs administration of 100% oxygen	
Directs application of cardiac monitor and pulse oximetry	
Identifies signs and symptoms of hypovolemic shock	
Categorizes as compensated or hypotensive shock	
Directs establishment of IV or IO access	
Directs rapid administration of a 20 mL/kg fluid bolus of isotonic crystalloid; repeats as needed to treat signs of shock	
Reassesses patient during and after each fluid bolus. Stops fluid bolus if signs of heart failure (worsening respiratory distress, development of hepatomegaly or rales/crackles) develop	
Directs reassessment of patient in response to each treatment	
Case Conclusion/Debriefing	
States therapeutic end points during shock management	
If the student does not verbalize the above, prompt the student with the following question: "What are the therapeutic end points during shock management?"	

STOP TEST

Instructor Notes
- Place a ✓ in the box next to each step the student completes successfully.
- If the student does not complete all steps successfully (as indicated by at least 1 blank check box), the student must receive remediation. Make a note here of which skills require remediation (refer to Instructor Manual for information about remediation).

Test Results Circle **PASS** or **NR** to indicate pass or needs remediation:	**PASS** **NR**
Instructor Initials _____ Instructor Number _____ Date _____	

PALS Case Scenario
Testing Checklist
Shock Case Scenario
Obstructive Shock

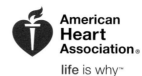

Student Name _____ Date of Test _____

Critical Performance Steps	✓ if done correctly
Team Leader	
Assigns team member roles	
Uses effective communication throughout	
Patient Management	
Directs assessment of airway, breathing, circulation, disability, and exposure, including vital signs	
Directs application of cardiac monitor and pulse oximetry	
Verbalizes DOPE mnemonic for intubated patient who deteriorates	
If the student does not verbalize the above, prompt the student with the following questions: *"What mnemonic is helpful to recall when the intubated patient deteriorates? What does this mnemonic mean?"*	
Identifies signs and symptoms of obstructive shock	
States at least 2 causes of obstructive shock	
If the student does not state the above, prompt the student with the following statement: *"Tell me at least 2 causes of obstructive shock."*	
Categorizes as compensated or hypotensive shock	
Directs establishment of IV or IO access, if needed	
Directs rapid administration of a fluid bolus of isotonic crystalloid, if needed (ie, for cardiac tamponade, massive pulmonary embolus)	
Directs appropriate treatment for obstructive shock (needle decompression for tension pneumothorax; fluid bolus, and pericardiocentesis for cardiac tamponade; oxygen, ventilatory support, fluid bolus, and expert consultation for massive pulmonary embolus; prostaglandin infusion and expert consultation for neonate with ductal-dependent congenital heart disease and constriction/closure of the ductus arteriosus)	
Directs reassessment of patient in response to treatment	
Case Conclusion/Debriefing	
States therapeutic end points during shock management	
If the student does not verbalize the above, prompt the student with the following question: *"What are the therapeutic end points during shock management?"*	

STOP TEST

Instructor Notes
- Place a ✓ in the box next to each step the student completes successfully.
- If the student does not complete all steps successfully (as indicated by at least 1 blank check box), the student must receive remediation. Make a note here of which skills require remediation (refer to Instructor Manual for information about remediation).

Test Results	Circle **PASS** or **NR** to indicate pass or needs remediation:	**PASS**	**NR**

Instructor Initials _____ Instructor Number _____ Date _____

PALS Case Scenario
Testing Checklist
Shock Case Scenario
Distributive Shock

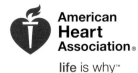

American Heart Association®

life is why™

American Academy of Pediatrics

DEDICATED TO THE HEALTH OF ALL CHILDREN™

Student Name _____ Date of Test _____

Critical Performance Steps	✓ if done correctly
Team Leader	
Assigns team member roles	
Uses effective communication throughout	
Patient Management	
Directs assessment of airway, breathing, circulation, disability, and exposure, including vital signs	
Directs administration of 100% oxygen	
Directs application of cardiac monitor and pulse oximetry	
Identifies signs and symptoms of distributive (septic) shock	
Categorizes as compensated or hypotensive shock	
Directs establishment of IV or IO access	
Directs rapid administration of a 20 mL/kg fluid bolus of isotonic crystalloid; repeats as needed (with careful reassessment) to treat shock	
Reassesses patient during and after each fluid bolus. Stops fluid bolus if signs of heart failure (worsening respiratory distress, development of hepatomegaly or rales/crackles) develop	
Directs initiation of vasoactive drug therapy within first hour of care for fluid-refractory shock	
Directs reassessment of patient in response to treatment	
Directs early administration of antibiotics (within first hour after shock is identified)	
Case Conclusion/Debriefing	
States therapeutic end points during shock management	
If the student does not verbalize the above, prompt the student with the following question: "What are the therapeutic end points during shock management?"	

STOP TEST

Instructor Notes
- Place a ✓ in the box next to each step the student completes successfully.
- If the student does not complete all steps successfully (as indicated by at least 1 blank check box), the student must receive remediation. Make a note here of which skills require remediation (refer to Instructor Manual for information about remediation).

Test Results Circle **PASS** or **NR** to indicate pass or needs remediation:	**PASS** **NR**

Instructor Initials _____ Instructor Number _____ Date _____

PALS Case Scenario
Testing Checklist
Shock Case Scenario
Cardiogenic Shock

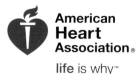

Student Name _____ Date of Test _____

Critical Performance Steps	✓ if done correctly
Team Leader	
Assigns team member roles	
Uses effective communication throughout	
Patient Management	
Directs assessment of airway, breathing, circulation, disability, and exposure, including vital signs	
Directs administration of 100% oxygen	
Directs application of cardiac monitor and pulse oximetry	
Identifies signs and symptoms of cardiogenic shock	
Categorizes as compensated or hypotensive shock	
Directs establishment of IV or IO access	
Directs slow administration of a 5 to 10 mL/kg fluid bolus of isotonic crystalloid over 10 to 20 minutes and reassesses patient during and after fluid bolus. Stops fluid bolus if signs of heart failure worsen	
Directs reassessment of patient in response to treatment	
Recognizes the need to obtain expert consultation from pediatric cardiologist	
Identifies need for inotropic/vasoactive drugs during treatment of cardiogenic shock	
If the student does not indicate the above, prompt the student with the following question: "What are the indications for inotropic/vasoactive drugs during cardiogenic shock?"	
Case Conclusion/Debriefing	
States therapeutic end points during shock management	
If the student does not verbalize the above, prompt the student with the following question: "What are the therapeutic end points during shock management?"	

STOP TEST

Instructor Notes
- Place a ✓ in the box next to each step the student completes successfully.
- If the student does not complete all steps successfully (as indicated by at least 1 blank check box), the student must receive remediation. Make a note here of which skills require remediation (refer to Instructor Manual for information about remediation).

Test Results Circle **PASS** or **NR** to indicate pass or needs remediation:	**PASS** **NR**

Instructor Initials _____ Instructor Number _____ Date _____

PALS Case Scenario Testing Checklist
Cardiac Case Scenario
Supraventricular Tachycardia

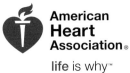

American Heart Association®

life is why™

American Academy of Pediatrics

DEDICATED TO THE HEALTH OF ALL CHILDREN™

Student Name _____ Date of Test _____

Critical Performance Steps	✓ if done correctly
Team Leader	
Assigns team member roles	
Uses effective communication throughout	
Patient Management	
Directs assessment of airway, breathing, circulation, disability, and exposure, including vital signs	
Directs application of cardiac monitor and pulse oximetry	
Directs administration of supplementary oxygen	
Identifies narrow-complex tachycardia (ie, SVT with adequate perfusion) and verbalizes how to distinguish between ST and SVT	
If the student does not verbalize the above, prompt the student with the following question: "How do you distinguish between ST and SVT?"	
Directs performance of appropriate vagal maneuvers	
Directs establishment of IV or IO access	
Directs preparation and administration of appropriate doses (first and, if needed, second) of adenosine	
States the rationale for the strong recommendation for expert consultation before providing synchronized cardioversion if the stable child with SVT fails to respond to vagal maneuvers and adenosine	
Directs or describes appropriate indications for and safe delivery of attempted cardioversion at 0.5 to 1 J/kg (subsequent doses increased by 0.5 to 1 J/kg, not to exceed 2 J/kg)	
Performs reassessment of patient in response to treatment	
Case Conclusion/Debriefing	
Discusses indications and appropriate energy doses for synchronized cardioversion	
If the student does not verbalize the above, prompt the student with the following question: "What are the indications and appropriate energy doses for synchronized cardioversion?"	

STOP TEST

Instructor Notes
- Place a ✓ in the box next to each step the student completes successfully.
- If the student does not complete all steps successfully (as indicated by at least 1 blank check box), the student must receive remediation. Make a note here of which skills require remediation (refer to Instructor Manual for information about remediation).

Test Results	Circle **PASS** or **NR** to indicate pass or needs remediation:	**PASS**	**NR**

Instructor Initials _____ Instructor Number _____ Date _____

PALS Case Scenario Testing Checklist
Cardiac Case Scenario
Bradycardia

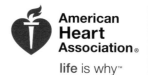

American Heart Association®
life is why™

American Academy of Pediatrics
DEDICATED TO THE HEALTH OF ALL CHILDREN™

Student Name _____ Date of Test _____

Critical Performance Steps	✓ if done correctly
Team Leader	
Assigns team member roles	
Uses effective communication throughout	
Patient Management	
Directs assessment of airway, breathing, circulation, disability, and exposure, including vital signs	
Identifies bradycardia associated with cardiopulmonary compromise/failure	
Directs initiation of bag-mask ventilation with 100% oxygen	
Directs application of cardiac monitor and pulse oximetry	
Reassesses heart rate and systemic perfusion after initiation of bag-mask ventilation	
Recognizes indications for high-quality CPR (chest compressions plus ventilation) in a bradycardic patient	
If the student does not indicate the above, prompt the student with the following question: "What are the indications for high-quality CPR in a bradycardic patient?"	
Directs establishment of IV or IO access	
Directs or discusses preparation for and appropriate administration and dose (0.01 mg/kg) of epinephrine	
Performs reassessment of patient in response to treatment	
Case Conclusion/Debriefing	
Verbalizes consideration of 3 potential causes of bradycardia in infants and children	
If the student does not verbalize the above, prompt the student with the following statement: "Tell me 3 potential causes of bradycardia in infants and children."	

STOP TEST

Instructor Notes
- Place a ✓ in the box next to each step the student completes successfully.
- If the student does not complete all steps successfully (as indicated by at least 1 blank check box), the student must receive remediation. Make a note here of which skills require remediation (refer to Instructor Manual for information about remediation).

Test Results Circle **PASS** or **NR** to indicate pass or needs remediation:	**PASS** **NR**

Instructor Initials _____ Instructor Number _____ Date _____

PALS Case Scenario
Testing Checklist
Cardiac Case Scenario
Asystole/PEA

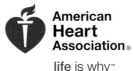

American Academy
of Pediatrics
DEDICATED TO THE HEALTH OF ALL CHILDREN™

Student Name _____ Date of Test _____

Critical Performance Steps	✓ if done correctly
Team Leader	
Assigns team member roles	
Uses effective communication throughout	
Patient Management	
Identifies cardiac arrest	
Directs immediate initiation of high-quality CPR, and ensures performance of high-quality CPR at all times	
Directs placement of pads/leads and activation of monitor/defibrillator	
Identifies asystole or PEA	
Directs establishment of IO or IV access	
Directs preparation and administration of appropriate dose of epinephrine at appropriate intervals	
Directs checking rhythm approximately every 2 minutes while minimizing interruptions in chest compressions	
Case Conclusion/Debriefing	
Verbalizes at least 3 reversible causes of PEA or asystole	

If the student does not verbalize the above, prompt the student with the following statement:
"Tell me at least 3 reversible causes of PEA or asystole."

STOP TEST

Instructor Notes
- Place a ✓ in the box next to each step the student completes successfully.
- If the student does not complete all steps successfully (as indicated by at least 1 blank check box), the student must receive remediation. Make a note here of which skills require remediation (refer to Instructor Manual for information about remediation).

Test Results Circle **PASS** or **NR** to indicate pass or needs remediation:	**PASS** **NR**

Instructor Initials _____ Instructor Number _____ Date _____

PALS Case Scenario
Testing Checklist
Cardiac Case Scenario
VF/Pulseless VT

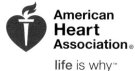

American Academy of Pediatrics
DEDICATED TO THE HEALTH OF ALL CHILDREN™

Student Name _____ Date of Test _____

Critical Performance Steps	✓ if done correctly
Team Leader	
Assigns team member roles	
Uses effective communication throughout	
Patient Management	
Identifies cardiac arrest	
Directs immediate initiation of high-quality CPR, and ensures performance of high-quality CPR at all times	
Directs placement of pads/leads and activation of monitor/defibrillator	
Identifies VF or pulseless VT cardiopulmonary arrest	
Directs safe performance of attempted defibrillation at 2 J/kg	
After delivery of every shock, directs immediate resumption of CPR, beginning with chest compressions	
Directs establishment of IO or IV access	
Directs preparation and administration of appropriate dose of epinephrine at appropriate intervals	
Directs safe delivery of second shock at 4 J/kg (subsequent doses 4 to 10 J/kg, not to exceed 10 J/kg or standard adult dose for that defibrillator)	
Directs preparation and administration of appropriate dose of antiarrhythmic (amiodarone or lidocaine) at appropriate time	
Case Conclusion/Debriefing	
Verbalizes possible need for additional doses of epinephrine and antiarrhythmic (amiodarone or lidocaine), and consideration of reversible causes of arrest (H's and T's)	

If the student does not verbalize the above, prompt the student with the following question:
"If VF persists despite the therapies provided, what else should you administer or consider?"

STOP TEST

Instructor Notes
- Place a ✓ in the box next to each step the student completes successfully.
- If the student does not complete all steps successfully (as indicated by at least 1 blank check box), the student must receive remediation. Make a note here of which skills require remediation (refer to Instructor Manual for information about remediation).

Test Results	Circle **PASS** or **NR** to indicate pass or needs remediation:	**PASS**	**NR**

Instructor Initials _____ Instructor Number _____ Date _____

Index